MEDICAL CARE
IN THE UNITED STATES

The Debate Before 1940

A documentary series, reproducing
in facsimile the most important
primary sources on medical care
in the United States to 1940

EDITED BY
Charles E. Rosenberg
UNIVERSITY OF PENNSYLVANIA

A GARLAND SERIES

Philanthropic Foundations and Resources for Health
An Anthology of Sources

EDITED WITH AN INTRODUCTION BY
Barbara G. Rosenkrantz and
Peter Buck

Garland Publishing, Inc.
NEW YORK & LONDON 1990

Library of Congress Cataloging-in-Publication Data

Philanthropic foundations and resources for health : an anthology of
sources / edited with an introduction by Barbara G. Rosenkrantz and
Peter Buck.
p. cm. — (Medical care in the United States)
Collection of articles reprinted from various sources.
ISBN 0-8240-8343-1 (alk. paper)
1. Public health—Research grants—United States—History.
2. Public health—Research—United States—Endowments—History.
I. Buck, Peter, 1943–   . II. Rosenkrantz, Barbara Gutmann. III.
Series.
[DNLM: 1. Charities—history—United States—collected works.
2. Foundations—history—United States—collected works. 3.
History of Medicine, 20th Cent.—United States—collected works.
WZ 70 AA1 P48]
RA440.87.U6P46 1990
361.7'632'0973—dc20
DNLM/DLC
for Library of Congress   89-25976

Printed on acid-free, 250-year-life paper.
Manufactured in the United States of America

CONTENTS

Introduction   ix

Hans Zinsser, "The Perils of Magnanimity:
A Problem in American Education,"
Atlantic Monthly, 139 (February, 1927), 246–50.   1

Editorial, "The Perils of Magnanimity,"
The Journal of the American Medical Association,
(March 5, 1927), 726.   7

Announcement, "Conference on Public Health,"
The Journal of the American Medical Association,
88 (April 2, 1927), 1083–84.   9

Participants, "Conference on Public Health,"
The Journal of the American Medical Association,
88 (February 25, 1927), 653.   11

Editorial, "The Health Conference," *The Journal
of the American Medical Association*, 88
(April 2, 1927), 1080.   13

Arthur T. Holbrook, "The Relations of the
Physician to Public Health," *The Journal of the
American Medical Association*, 89 (July 2, 1927),
1–4.   15

Harlow Brooks, M. D., "The Physician and the
Public Health," *The Journal of the American
Medical Association*, 89 (July 2, 1927), 8–11   19

Linsly R. Williams, M. D., "The Relation of
Voluntary Health Agency to Physicians and
Health Departments," *The Journal of the
American Medical Association*, 89 (July 9, 1927),
82–84.   23

Julius Rosenwald, "Principles of Public Giving,"
Atlantic Monthly, 143 (May, 1929), 599–606.   27

Julius Rosenwald, "The Trend Away from
Perpetuities," *Atlantic Monthly*, 146 (1930),
741–49.   35

Edwin R. Embree, "The Business of Giving
Away Money," *Harper's Magazine*, 161
(August, 1930), 320–29.   45

The Julius Rosenwald Fund

Edwin R. Embree, *Review of Two Decades,
1917–1936* (1936), selections.   55

Edwin R. Embree, "The New Philanthropy,"
from *A Review to June 30, 1929* (1929).   71

Michael M. Davis, *Eight Years' Work in
Medical Economics, 1929–1936* (1937).   75

The Commonwealth Fund

"Program for Child Health," from *Fifth
Annual Report* (1923).   103

"Division of Rural Hospitals," from *Eighth
Annual Report* (1926).   117

"Child Welfare, Health," from *Ninth
Annual Report* (1927).   125

Division of Rural Hospitals," from *Tenth Annual Report* (1928).   143

"Rural Health and Rural Medicines,"
"Division of Public Health and Health
Studies," "Division of Rural Hospitals,"
from *Fourteenth Annual Report* (1932).   149

The Milbank Memorial Fund

"Meeting of the Advisory Council," *Milbank
Memorial Fund Quarterly Bulletin*
(January, 1924).   175

*Milbank Memorial Fund Report for the Year
Ended December 31, 1923.*   213

John A. Kingsbury, "Two Years of Public Health
Demonstrations," *Milbank Memorial Fund
Quarterly Bulletin* (April, 1925).   359

Dorothy Gerard Wiehl, "Infant Mortality in
Cattaraugus County," *Milbank Memorial
Fund Quarterly Bulletin* (January, 1928).   365

Edgar Sydenstricker, "The Decline in the
Tuberculosis Death Rate in Cattaraugus
County," *Milbank Memorial Fund Quarterly
Bulletin* (January, 1928).   383

The Duke Endowment

William R. Perkins, "An Address on The Duke
Endowment. Its Origin, Nature and Purposes,"
(October 11, 1929).   395

*The Duke Endowment. Annual Report of the
Hospital Section, 1925* (selections).   427

*The Duke Endowment. Fourth Annual Report
of the Hospital Section, 1928* (selections).   483

*The Duke Endowment. Hospital Section.
A Six-Year Review of the Activities of Assisted
Tuberculosis Sanatoria in the Carolinas* (1930)
(selections).   495

The W. K. Kellogg Foundation

(Transcripts of microfilm in the Kellogg
Foundation Archive.)

William S. Sadler, Lena K. Sadler, "The
Foundation Plan and Purpose," from *Report of
a Survey of the W.K. Kellogg Foundation* (1937).   539

W. C. Smillie, "Confidential Report to the
Director of the Kellogg Foundation on
Community Health Centers, May 10, 1937."   544

W. C. Smillie, *A Report Upon the Organization
and Activities of the W. K. Kellogg Foundation*
(1937).   548

INTRODUCTION

Today, close to the end of the twentieth century, the name of
Rockefeller is almost a household word. If you ask a college
senior to say what the family name brings to mind, chances
are that the association will be to vast wealth; and then from
Rockefeller money to the Rockefeller Foundation. The choice
of that connection sharply contrasts with the more common
early twentieth-century linkage of the Rockefeller name with
monopoly control of industries that was seen to lead inexora-
bly to trusts and labor violence. A Congressional investigation
published in 1915 further stirred public antipathy to John D.
Rockefeller when it showed that his money and power were
used to arm strikebreakers and assault Colorado copper
miners and their families. In this context the "good works"
Rockefeller was known to support with his fortune were not
above suspicion, and Congress investigated the sinister
consequences of investing tainted money in philanthropy. At
the height of Rockefeller's first big venture in spreading the
gospel of scientific medicine to the ignorant and poor through
the crusade of his Sanitary Commission against hookworm in
the rural south, the organizers did their best to keep the
Rockefeller name out of the picture for fear that the association would undermine their efforts. Almost a century later the
connection of private wealth and institutionalized philanthropy is regarded as the necessary and natural evolution of a
tradition of charitable gifts to hospitals and schools that
began on a small scale and was swelled by gifts from John D.
Rockefeller, Andrew Carnegie, and other successful business-
men and captains of industry.[1]

    Private foundations today provide essential support to

individuals and institutions producing scientific research, humanistic studies, and the creative arts to name the most obvious beneficiaries of endowment income. Increasing corporate and personal wealth in the United States, particularly in the aftermath of two world wars, generated the resources for 22,000 foundations that award annual grants amounting to $4 billion. In the field of medicine alone, foundations have assisted or initiated programs that range from fundamental research on basic life processes to the evaluation of psychotherapy, from building hospitals in small towns to setting up county health departments, from professorships to training grants. The distribution of corporate wealth to encourage development of talent and practice is no longer denounced as potentially corrupting or intrusive even when the underlying rationale of a specific program is contested. The costly appetites of research and development have undoubtedly calmed recipients' fears of outside control, but more significantly, the American public now appears confident that there is no fundamental conflict between the interests of donors and recipients. On the contrary, social policy and social values are generally in agreement when it comes to the obligation to put private fortunes to work for the public good.

Despite the substantial contributions of voluntary organizations and foundations, the massive increase in government funding of individuals and institutions since World War II provides by far the largest resources devoted to the care and feeding of science, medicine, education, and the arts. Controversy over the impact of the government's involvement in support of specific projects in the sciences and arts has also raised troubling questions; do spokesmen in behalf of these projects thus gain access to power in high places? Are the criteria used in making awards biased to favor scientific and cultural elites? It has been difficult to find a consistent pattern of legislative or popular support for specific projects. The Golden Fleece "prizes" focus outrage on the obscurity of some research projects and get sympathetic news coverage, while at another moment the papers are eloquent in reporting arguments against restricting public funds for an esoteric museum exhibit of meager public interest. But on the whole, anxieties about the impropriety of spending taxpayers' money on pure science rather than practical applications has given way, particularly in the biomedical sciences, to confidence that generous support will pay off in the conquest of disease and the promotion of better health.

The National Institutes of Health annual budgets for training and research grew in the two decades after 1947 from $29 million to almost a billion and a half. Through the Hill-Burton Act Congress voted unprecedented aid for hospital construction, indirectly transforming the impact of medical services that had been the central concern of voluntary agencies and philanthropy in the health field. Foundations have continued to commit more money to support an increasingly varied menu of health-related programs, but since the end of World War II private funds are a small fraction of disbursements.[2] Despite this largesse, in the 1970s and 1980s competition for public and private support sharpened in the context of three distinct influences. First, advances in scientific knowledge and technologies that dramatize medical achievement much as the identification of specific disease carrying bacteria or the discovery of penicillin and broad-spectrum antibiotics caught earlier public enthusiasm. Second, dismay at the limits of medical science, most strikingly with respect to control and cure of a new disease menace—AIDS, but also in the face of age-old plagues represented in victims of addiction and famine. And third, inequities in health and comfort that persist despite the "conquest of disease" and assurances that health is both the business of government and the enduring concern of philanthropy. In these contexts, unease about the emphasis and efficacy of medical interventions have prompted questions about the

relation of costs and benefits to the public, all to the end that
the federal government is the largest investor in medical
research and services in a political and moral climate
charged, on many accounts, to return larger shares of this
responsibility to private funds and agencies.

Foundation watchers point to this sequence of events
as evidence of the unique contribution of American philanthropy to our political culture and draw conflicting conclusions. In one corner there are the advocates of public spending
for social and medical services who claim that history shows
how foundations provided the seed money to test provisional
claims in special "demonstrations," experiments that once
tested were adopted by government agencies and applied to
larger social problems. And in the other corner there are the
strategists of privatization for whom the key element in the
foundations' past success is their influence on the community
of citizens who were stimulated by money from outside to act
in their own interest. There is evidence for either conclusion,
but little to show that foundation executives were able to
predict that the need for additional support beyond the trial
period would turn out to be the most consistent outcome of
their initiatives.

Foundation boards and staff members are sometimes
credited with extraordinary foresight because of their prudent
investment in medical services at a time when faith in the
advice of good men and public servants was their guide to
action. The aggressive development of medical research and
its successful clinical applications over the past half century
in the context of public and private support of medical knowledge and institutions is cited as evidence of foundation
directors' wisdom at a critical moment in history. In the
aftermath of World War I the hope and confidence that
surrounded the incorporation of a second generation of
American foundations was indeed broad and inclusive,
although the repeated reference to advancing "the welfare of
mankind" reflected a shared vision that by later standards

seems more naive than prescient. Contrary to following any single-minded view of what lay ahead, the ambitious directors of new foundations at first favored proposals in education, law, industrial relations, and child welfare rather than in clinics, hospitals, and public health because they believed that the territory controlled by medicine was already well-occupied by the Rockefellers.

The five foundations represented in this collection of documents soon turned to support of medical and public health services and eventually became identified with the development of scientific research and social policy in these fields. Their initial involvements in projects for improving health were, however, relatively modest; each of them asserted their goals and established their programatic ambitions in distinctive assessments of social needs. Nonetheless, two characteristic objectives of contemporary social analysis were reflected in staff recommendations to their respective boards of trustees, and these objectives were in the end decisive to these foundations' support of medical and public health services. First, the expectation that the problems they chose to correct could in fact be remedied, and second, the intention that once corrected, that danger would be removed, the threat recognized and eliminated in some fundamental way. The latter ground led the officers of new foundations to break consciously with the tradition of charitable relief, and the former riveted their attention to information that a fourth of the deaths occurring annually in the United States were unnecessary and preventable. Foundation trustees heard from their executive officers and from consultants in other agencies about successful programs and new opportunities. Officers of the Metropolitan Life Insurance Company and the National Tuberculosis Association provided compelling data from a community health project they had first sponsored in Framingham, Massachusetts, a middle-class suburb located about 20 miles outside of Boston. In 1916 one third of the city's population had participated in a program of x-ray screening and regular physical examinations in order to diagnose undetected tuberculosis at an early stage, when prevention was considered more effective and treatment less expensive. Statistics collected for the sponsors showed that chances of increased longevity in Framingham improved at roughly twice the rate of neighboring towns, while the effect of health education and encouragement was to alert the whole community to the possibility of preventing many diseases. "Of primary importance is the development of an intimate, democratic, local interest and responsibility," noted the sponsors as they agreed to replicate their contribution of $100,000 for another three years. "Framingham's experiment . . . demonstrates that it is practical for a community, within reasonable expenditure limits, to 'sanitate' itself." Franz Schneider, a social scientist working for the Bureau of Surveys and Exhibits at the Russell Sage foundation produced a list of the contagious diseases responsible for 99 percent of preventable deaths in 1913 (*see table opposite*) and a menu of remedies to demonstrate how the proper choice of targets could transform certain common contagions into a novelty.[3] Recognizing that pinched public health budgets squeezed ambition dry, Schneider proposed criteria to differentiate among diseases that could be easily prevented, those that caused the most permanent "defects" and those that caused most fatalities. Evidence that attention directed to preventing tuberculosis and the common diseases of childhood was the key to a scientifically balanced program that could achieve multiple benefits was not lost on foundations. The documents published in this volume reflect the combination of grand hopes and trust with which foundation trustees and officers committed themselves to "the welfare of mankind" through priming opportunities for better health in America.

The first group of articles represents conflicts among contemporaries who layed some of the guidelines for relations between medicine and its multiple constituencies in the early twentieth century. Hans Zinsser was a leading figure in

TABLE 1.
PREVENTABLE DEATHS IN ALL REGISTRATION CITIES, 1913.

Cause of death.	Number of deaths.	Per cent. of preventable deaths.
Infectious Diseases	149,600	99.0
Tuberculosis—all forms:................	56,624	37.5
Lungs.......................	48,733	
Meningitis...................	3,861	
Other forms..................	4,030	
Diarrhea and enteritis (under 2).............	30,244	20.0
Bronchopneumonia..................	21,091	14.0
Common contagious diseases..............	19,058	12.6
Measles.......................	4,517	
Scarlet fever...................	3,854	
Whooping-cough..................	3,047	
Diphtheria and croup...............	7,640	
Typhoid fever....................	5,627	3.7
Syphilis—total...................	4,902	3.2
Syphilis.......................	3,422	
Locomotor ataxia................	1,020	
Softening of the brain.............	460	
Influenza.......................	3,000	2.0
Puerperal fever...................	2,825	1.9
Gonococcus infection................	191	0.1
Other infectious diseases..............	6,038	4.0
Erysipelas....................	1,599	
Dysentery....................	1,212	
Tetanus......................	876	
Cerebrospinal fever...............	834	
Malaria......................	644	
Infantile paralysis...............	392	
Cholera nostras.................	140	
"Other epidemic diseases".........	124	
Rabies.......................	67	
Smallpox.....................	44	
Intestinal parasites..............	30	
Mycoces.....................	24	
Hyatid tumor of liver.............	13	
Anthrax......................	12	
Ankylostomiasis................	10	
Glanders.....................	7	
Leprosy......................	4	
Typhus fever..................	3	
Relapsing fever................	2	
Plague.......................	1	
Nutritional Diseases..............	1,097	0.7
Pellagra.....................	702	
Rickets......................	335	
Scurvy.......................	53	
Beriberi......................	7	
Poisoning by Food.................	329	0.2
Industrial Poisonings..............	124	0.1
Lead poisoning.................	120	
Other chronic occupational poisonings.........	4	
Total—preventable deaths.............	151,150	100 00

Table 1 from Franz Schneider, "Relative Values in Public Health Work,"
American Journal of Public Health, 6:917 (1916)

academic medicine and scientific research whose work had important consequences for clinical medicine and public health. He also wrote and published for the well-read layman at a time of growing popular interest in science. Although this article does not speak for the university community in which Zinsser worked, his concerns were echoed in the ranks of the American Medical Association and this, combined with Zinsser's public visibility troubled foundation supporters. The AMA Conference on Public Health that took place almost simultaneously with publication of Zinsser's article reflects a more receptive climate with regard to cooperation between organized medicine, public health, and the voluntary organizations supported by philanthropy. In the last three articles of this section Julius Rosenwald, and Edwin R. Embree, the man Rosenwald brought from the Rockefeller Foundation to take over direction of the foundation he had established and managed for himself from 1917 to 1927, explain their opposition to permanence of any philanthropic endowment. This was not a view adopted by other foundations, and the Julius Rosenwald Foundation is the only philanthropy represented here that no longer exists.

Michael M. Davis's article in the section representing the Rosenwald Foundation reflects an important aspect of the pioneering work of other foundations as well in supporting the social and economic structure of medical services. Julius Rosenwald was a "self-made" man who combined his success in building the Sears Roebuck company with carefully planned contributions to Chicago charitable and cultural institutions, support of primary, college, and professional education for blacks, medical services, and institutions. In 1927 after Rosenwald retired, his successor continued to initiate independent projects that often were designed to provide better access for blacks to the benefits of medicine.

The Commonwealth Fund began its operations at the close of World War I with an initial endowment of $15,000,000 given by the widow of Stephen Harkness, a suc-

cessful financier whose wealth was connected to the fortunes
made in the development of oil and railroads at the end of the
nineteenth century. The Harkness family had long supported
worthy causes and Commonwealth's first board of directors
represented a close-knit group of friends and associates that
included Mrs. Harkness's youngest son Edward, men who
shared the expectation that the new projects endorsed by the
Fund would be carried out by "operating agencies" with
established reputations in social welfare rather than being
managed by a staff from the Fund itself. By the time the
annual reports reprinted here were published the Commonwealth Fund had staked out its own important territory
defined by the special health needs and opportunities of small
town and rural America. A tiny professional staff generated
important information about communities that could develop
"demonstrations" through child health programs and health
centers flowing from hospital services. As the Commonwealth
Fund grew in size and scope it continued to emphasize con-
nections between the trustees, staff, and local community
leaders, and to be committed to the exercise of national
influence through example.

The Milbank Fund also focused its activities in a
geographically circumscribed area. The Cattaraugus County
(NY) Health Demonstration represented in this collection was
the first of its three early "demonstration" programs in
preventive medicine and public health, this one in a rural
county, the others in the small city of Syracuse in upstate
New York and in a section of metropolitan New York City.
Each of these projects was influenced by an ongoing collabora-
tive relationship with the State Board of Health in New York.
The impact of the Milbank programs was extended well
beyond New York's state borders, in part through the distinguished scientists associated with Milbank. This contribution
of foundation work is represented by Edgar Sydenstricker, a
social investigator, statistician for the U. S. Public Health
Service, and epidemiologist who became Milbank's director of

research in 1928.

As documents in the last two sections show, the gifts establishing the Duke and Kellogg foundations were the product of fortunes made by men who grew up in the communities that were intended to be the major beneficiaries of their acquired wealth. In 1924 and 1930 when the Duke Endowment and the Kellogg Foundation began, their staffs saw their professional objectives as virtually indistinguishable from those of public institutions and agencies in the Carolinas and Michigan. The ambiguities that this somewhat parochial view involved are barely visible in the early days of work reflected here. The charters or indentures establishing the responsibility for managing these enormous endowments, among the largest of all private foundations, set geographic and social limits that became less constraining over time as medical and public health sciences and institutions developed programs that could easily be expanded.

The editors of this volume thank Kristin E. Peterson for assistance in selecting, transcribing, and reproducing these documents.

Barbara G. Rosenkrantz
Peter Buck

Notes

1. John Ettling, *The Germ of Laziness, Rockefeller Philanthropy and Public Health in the New South* (Cambridge, Mass., 1981) is the most recent study of the Sanitary Commission. Ellen Lagemann, *Private Power for the Public Good, A History of the Carnegie Foundation for the Advancement of Teaching* (Middletown, Conn., 1983). On Congressional and public reactions to the Rockefellers' social policies see Graham Adams Jr., *Age of Industrial Violence 1910–1915, The Activities and Findings of the United States Commission on Industrial Relations* (New York, 1966), especially chapters 3 and 9.

2. Victoria A. Harden, *Inventing the NIH, Federal Biomedical Research Policy, 1887–1937* (Baltimore, 1986). Waldemar A. Nielsen, *The Golden Doors, A New Anatomy of the Great Foundations* (New York, 1985).

3. *Framingham Monograph No. 1*, Framingham Community Health Station, April, 1918. Franz Schneider, "Relative Values in Public Health Work," *American Journal of Public Health*, 6:916–25 (1916). These data remained persuasive even though statisticians, physicians, and public health officers expressed doubts that mortality decline could so rapidly reflect the benefit of intervention, especially in the case of TB where rates had steadily diminished for decades.

THE PERILS OF MAGNANIMITY

A PROBLEM IN AMERICAN EDUCATION

BY HANS ZINSSER

It is easy to be clever at the expense of opulence and to jeer at the contrast of the barracks in which Pasteur achieved his wonders, or the rural milk route of Koch, with the palaces and equipment which have grown like mushrooms from the golden fertilizer scattered over our medical schools. Such triviality, however, obscures the accomplishments which have already resulted from this unexampled generosity, and which have placed American medicine upon a footing approaching equality with that of Europe.

Were it helpful, we could mention offhand a dozen important contributions and double that number of names which might have been to our credit without the Rockefeller donations (to mention only one of these agencies), but which probably would not have been — at least at this early stage. And even were this inaccurate, there is little risk in prophesying increased intellectual velocity from the potential energy now accumulating in young men and women who, for the first time in history, are being given that thorough medical education which furnishes the tools for high endeavor. And the nature of medicine, broadly conceived, is such that no school not highly endowed can furnish this.

These admissions are platitudes to the fair-minded. And it may well be that, such splendid accomplishments conceded, wisdom should remain blind

to the threatening centre of the cloud with such a golden lining. But in the minds of many who are in touch with medical institutions a feeling of apprehension is being aroused by the progressively increasing dependence of a great educational system upon one or more centrally controlled funds. And since, in our opinion, this apprehension is based on more than the unworthy caution of suspicious natures, we believe that it should be aired in frank discussion instead of being allowed to ferment in the dark corners of vague and irritated criticism. Our remarks of course do not apply to the Rockefeller organizations alone. The General Education Board idea has appealed to other philanthropists; and for this every sensible medical man should be grateful. But the best way to show gratitude, aside from cultivating one's own garden to the best of one's ability, is to contribute what one can to the reaping of the healthiest crop from the generous sowing.

It is true that the criticisms to which we refer are often based on differences of conception in which our own judgment inclines us to side with the foundations. And it may also be said that much of this criticism emanates from sources which have failed to obtain some of the money. On the other hand we believe that, if one searches below the surface, the basis for dissatisfaction, often not clearly understood by the

1

critics themselves, may be found in a foreboding that the guidance of medical education is to a considerable extent passing out of the hands of the universities themselves into the hands of a permanent or, at any rate, self-perpetuating body of gentlemen who, by the very force of the established relations, cannot help extending their influence over all the important centres of American education. Though the expressions of this feeling usually take the form of criticisms of the policies of the leaders of this movement, to whose labors American medicine owes a profound debt of gratitude, the heart of the problem lies not so much in a conflict of opinions as in the growth of a situation inevitably created by existing circumstances.

If, as we believe, there is amid the confusion of much trivial, irritated, and reactionary criticism an element that is objective and thoughtful, nothing can be lost and much may be gained by an attempt to formulate this element in order that it may be freely examined. For it would be unintelligent to bury our heads in the golden sand and, for lack of frank discussion, risk the slowing of a forward movement which owes most of its velocity to the group of public-spirited men who have already accomplished so much for our profession. They have devoted laborious and conscientious years to the development of sound medicine — thoughtfully, with study and contemplation. When they hastened the death of some of the obviously inferior schools and formulated policies of progress for the others, they liberated American medicine. They have ridden their lances into many dragons — but also into a number of windmills. The dragons expired and are gratefully forgotten. But the windmills keep on clattering and dulling the lances. We do not want these Saint Georges to become Don Quixotes

merely because, as in the classical case, altered conditions are calling for a change of methods.

We may grant — indeed, it seems to us quite self-evident, because of the nature of the relationship — that the purpose of the responsible governing bodies is solely to spend as much as possible of the available funds, as rapidly as is feasible, for the greatest good. It is inevitable that such boards must be besieged by requests for sums far greater than the endowments they administer, a considerable proportion of which could not be granted without unpardonable laxity in the spirit of trusteeship. Ergo, it has been necessary to have on hand one or more individuals who are constantly studying the problems involved in the development of medical institutions and who can give expert opinions in individual instances. Such experts, therefore, must form opinions and — naturally — must adhere to them after they have obtained all the information possible.

Immediately we have a situation. The expert and his board have opinions. They also have money. The universities, too, have opinions; but often no money; never enough. The trustee-experts with the money — in all honesty, we are convinced — disavow the desire to impose their own views upon the organization of the medical schools. But if they do not approve of such organizations, their methods, or intentions, how can they conscientiously give the money? The medical schools, on the other hand, need the money very badly. Often — we know of such cases — their existence may depend upon the control of a hospital, the possession of a laboratory building. They may have convictions of one kind or another, and they may — perhaps wrongly — believe that a certain procedure is peculiarly suited to their

2

traditions, locality, or what not. But the temptation is great to adjust in the direction that will lead to the needed assistance.

We are not leading up to a discussion of the 'full-time plan.' Specific differences of opinion do not properly enter our argument. The point is not who is right about this and who about that; but rather: Does the system which was necessary to achieve the indisputable good so far accomplished carry with it into the future an inevitable uniformity of educational methods; does it inevitably diminish local initiative in educational experiment; and does it, or does it not, by all these tokens, by its very uncontrollable evolution, lead to the establishment of a hierarchy of opinion on matters which, of all human endeavors, are the ones for which freedom of development is most necessary?

The question is not: Is the vast benefit accomplished worth the risk? It *has* been, so far, undoubtedly. But the question is rather, for the thoughtful: Is the great conception in danger of losing effectiveness? And the reply to this query depends upon the answers to a number of further questions. Is there a tendency among medical schools to adjust their organizations and the nature of some of their important appointments by a process of reasoning in which the influence of such adjustment upon prospective donations plays more than a secondary rôle? Have any of the leaders of individual schools put their pride into their pockets, reconsidered their own decisions, and wandered like Henry the Fourth to Canossa to say, 'Father, I have erred; give me the two millions'? In short, are there growing indications of an influence, well-intended and so far highly beneficial, which is formularizing our medical educational system by a uniform standard and subtly imposing the beliefs — however wise — of a single group?

None of this may be true. But we believe that there is enough truth in it to necessitate frank and friendly discussion; and we believe this discussion to be especially desirable because we are not among those — and there are such — who see in the situation the sinister tentacles of the octopus reaching for power. The situation is much simpler than that, and less dramatic. There is merely a group of conscientious and well-informed gentlemen who have taken over the arduous duties and responsibilities in connection with a fund which they are trusted to spend wisely and without too much delay. They are guided by a capable scholar who has made himself one of the foremost lay students of medical education. They are beset by a clamor of requests which it is their duty to gratify in so far as they properly can do so. Many of these requests are wise, some of them are less wise, others not wise at all. The trustees have wrought mightily by the only method possible when the field was rough, stony, and full of weeds. The situation that has arisen is not of their making — surely, we believe, not desired by them. But if it exists, why not face it before it has done the harm which may not easily be undone?

To all that we have said there are a number of obvious rejoinders. Indeed our discussion might be reasonably regarded as an entirely gratuitous attack upon an undertaking which is unmatched in the magnanimous application of financial resources. We should not care to risk lending support to reactionary obstinacy, inertia, or professional arrogance. But when these and other still smaller human motives for criticism are eliminated, there remain a number of factors in the situation which are causing misgivings in the minds of the thoughtful who hope for still greater results from these undertakings in the future. Foremost among these factors is this inevitable development of a power, superimposed upon the organized educational system of the country, which — however benevolent in its autocracy — must still retain the last word in any question in which its opinions differ from local judgments. If higher education is to develop in a wholesome manner it must be free to follow many paths, to experiment in many directions — if necessary, to make its own mistakes. The universities are the normal guardians of educational progress. Their organizations and their considerable resources in expert opinion and educational experience entitle them to autonomy of decision, both as to policy and as to details of method. Limit them in this regard and the future will inevitably pay for it. Left free, they may commit errors, fall behind, or even remain — for periods — unmindful of their obligations. But in the long run they will make progress, impelled by the varying problems they encounter, or by the enthusiasms of the particular brand of educational progressive who happens to gain local influence. At any rate they will remain individual and independent of guidance by a sort of superacademic general staff.

We know and repeat that none of these tendencies are deliberately intentional; but that they are bound to eventuate we must also endeavor to make clear. That they have begun to develop seems indicated to us by the considerable uniformity of organization already apparent in the clinical departments of almost all the schools that have received support, and by our impression that leaders in many of these schools — wisely, we admit, but none the less significantly — look to the foundations for advice and guidance at least as much as to their own university councils and colleagues.

It behooves us to ask ourselves whether these conditions are inevitable and inherent accompaniments of the foundation idea — in which case they may be accepted as minor evils overshadowed by a great good. But we note that similar developments have been completely avoided in the world-wide activities of the International Health Board, and it would appear to the observer a simple matter to eliminate them completely from the educational programme of the foundations by a relatively slight adjustment to recent changes in the management of medical schools. Largely owing to the activities of the trustees of the larger funds, these medical schools have matured and have become incorporated departments of universities. They are guided by educational wisdom and experience, and can be trusted to apply with studious conscientiousness any funds they may receive. Is it not reasonable to hope that future donations may be determined purely on the basis of demonstrated needs and bestowed for definite purposes, leaving the details of procedure and organization entirely to the governing bodies of the beneficiary institutions? Surely this would be safe in most cases, and would eliminate irritation and the apprehensions we have mentioned from a relationship which should be one purely of gratitude for great benefactions.

We feel neither called upon nor qualified to enlarge upon the remedy. We have endeavored to make a diagnosis. And we have thought it worth attempting because we believe the conception that underlies the return of great private fortunes to public service a very fine one that demands the coöperation of everyone interested in safeguarding its purposes.

There is, of course, still another way

of looking at the situation, but one that seems to us unworthy of the magnanimity which pervades the undertaking — to the effect that, after all, the great fund is a free donation, given under conditions which no one but the donors is entitled to determine; and that institutions which apply for assistance cannot expect to dictate the terms of acceptance. This we believe to be a complete misconception of the intentions of the givers, and far removed from the spirit of those who have administered expenditures; moreover, whatever misgivings we may have of the future, a point of view so crude is unjustified by the experience of the past.

THE JOURNAL OF THE AMERICAN MEDICAL ASSOCIATION

535 North Dearborn Street · · · Chicago, Ill.

Cable Address : · · · · "Medic, Chicago"

Subscription price · · · · · · Five dollars per annum in advance

Please send in promptly notice of change of address, giving both old and new; always state whether the change is temporary or permanent. Such notice should mention all journals received from this office. Important information regarding contributions will be found on second advertising page following reading matter.

SATURDAY, MARCH 5, 1927

"THE PERILS OF MAGNANIMITY"

Not only physicians but also sociologists, psychologists and economists have on frequent occasions in recent years devoted pages of anathema to the curse of philanthropy. Ever since it was realized that pauperization resulted from much of the practice of free medical clinics, committees of physicians and investigators have issued pronouncements against uncontrolled application of charitable funds to medical care. The great problem of the past quarter of a century has been to use for the public good the benefits to be derived from medical science. The possibilities for good logically have made medical research and medical education the beneficiaries of more philanthropy than has been accorded to art institutes, sculpture and general cultural and municipal improvements. They have also given rise to the new professions of social worker, public welfare counselor and the executive secretary, whose sinecure recently attracted the vitriol of Mr. Mencken's pen.

Prof. Hans Zinsser of the department of bacteriology in the Harvard Medical School, under the attractive title which heads this comment, cleverly tosses a series of shafted and veiled barbs into the control of medical education exerted by the General Education Board and similar endowments. In his contribution in the *Atlantic Monthly*, he asserts that the basis for such dissatisfaction as may exist with the work of such directorates is "a foreboding that the guidance of medical education is to a considerable extent passing out of the hands of the universities themselves into the hands of permanent or, at any rate, self-perpetuating bodies of gentlemen who, by the very force of the established relations, cannot help extending their influence over all the important centers of American education." Indeed, Dr. Zinsser seems to find most of his own disapproval of the situation in the fact that the leadership that has brought about the present high state of American medical education has largely fulfilled its purpose and is now without reason for perpetuation. The permanent existence of vast sums that must be applied to specific purposes creates a situation in which those who desire the use of such funds must conform to the requirements set up by the administrators in order to secure the advantages accruing through grants of money. Thus, medical education, according to Dr. Zinsser, is being compelled into fixed lines and systems in which initiative is destroyed and freedom of development made impossible. The situation is not unique in relation to medical education, which is the one point concerned in Dr. Zinsser's discussion. The existence of endowments for the perpetuation of the fight on animal experimentation has been a curse to medical progress in many communities, and has required the spending of equal sums to combat attempts at securing reactionary legislation. The existence of tremendous funds whose income must be devoted to certain types of public welfare work has resulted in bureaus which endeavor to promote such work without proper medical cooperation and indeed sometimes with antagonism to all the forces that make for individual freedom and that oppose paternalism and pauperization.

As a result of the dominance of fixed ideas in the field of education, Dr. Zinsser sees already a uniformity of organization in the clinical departments of all the medical schools that have received support. He sees universities deprived of autonomy of decision both as to policy and as to details of method. He notes that similar developments have been completely avoided in the activities of the International Health Board, but he does not reason from observation that this may be largely a matter of policy with the present directorate of the International Health Board, and that there is no guarantee as to future developments of that work. Dr. Zinsser's note of warning against standardization of medical education, through the economic pressures exerted by philanthropy, is timely. The medical professions in various communities have already protested against attempts by health demonstrations and similar movements to destroy initiative and individual relationships in medical practice.

Commonwealth Fund, Mr. Barry C. Smith, New York; Miss Barbara S. Quin, New York.

General Federation of Women's Clubs, Miss Mary E. Murphy, Chicago.

Gorgas Memorial Institute, Dr. Gilbert Fitzpatrick, Chicago.

International Health Board, Dr. John A. Ferrell, New York.

Life Extension Institute, Dr. Eugene L. Fisk, New York.

Milbank Memorial Fund, Mr. John A. Kingsbury, New York.

National Catholic Welfare Conference, Miss Raphael M. Foran, Washington, D. C.

National Committee for the Prevention of Blindness, Mr. Lewis H. Carris, New York; Dr. B. Franklin Royer, New York.

National Committee for Mental Hygiene, Dr. Edwin R. Eisley, Chicago.

National Congress of Parents and Teachers, Miss Mary E. Murphy, Chicago.

National Education Association, Miss Mary E. Murphy, Chicago.

National Health Council, Mr. T. C. Edwards, New York.

National League of Nursing Education, Miss Ada Belle McCleery, Evanston, Ill.

National Organization for Public Health Nursing, Miss Winnifred Rand, Detroit.

National Tuberculosis Association, Dr. Linsly R. Williams, New York.

Russell Sage Foundation, Mr. Evart G. Routzahn, New York.

State Charities Association, Mr. Homer Folks, New York.

Association News

THE WASHINGTON SESSION

Invitation to a Tournament to Be Held by the Washington Gun Club

The Washington Gun Club extends an invitation to the members of the American Medical Association to be guests of the club and to take part in a tournament to be held on May 16. Suitable prizes will be awarded.

The club is anxious to arrange its program, and would appreciate hearing from those members of the Association who intend to enter the tournament. The entries will be scratch.

CONFERENCE ON PUBLIC HEALTH

Held at the Headquarters of the American Medical Association, March 24 and 25

A complete report of the transactions of the conference on public health held at the headquarters of the Association will appear in future issues of THE JOURNAL. As an indication of its scope, THE JOURNAL presents herewith a list of the official representatives in attendance, of the guests, and of those taking part in the program.

The agencies represented included thirty-two volunteer health organizations, seventeen state boards or other official agencies, four welfare departments of insurance companies, the American Medical Association, and various medical schools and publications.

VOLUNTEER HEALTH AGENCIES

American Federation of Organizations for the Hard of Hearing, Dr. George Shambaugh, Chicago.

American Association of Hospital Social Workers, Miss Marie Lurie, Chicago.

American Association of Industrial Physicians and Surgeons, Dr. F. L. Rector, Chicago.

American Association for Medical Progress, Mr. Benjamin C. Gruenberg, New York.

American Child Health Association, Dr. S. J. Crumbine, New York; Dr. Clifford Grulee, Chicago.

American Conference on Hospital Service, Dr. John M. Dodson, Chicago.

American Heart Association, Dr. Linsly Williams, New York.

American Hospital Association, Dr. William H. Walsh, Chicago.

American National Red Cross, Dr. William R. Redden, Washington, D. C.; Mr. James L. Fieser, Washington, D. C.

American Nurses Association, Miss Evelyn Wood, Chicago; Miss Ada Belle McCleery, Evanston, Ill.

American Public Health Association, Dr. H. N. Bundesen, Chicago; Dr. H. F. Vaughan, Detroit; Mr. Homer N. Calver, New York; Mr. James A. Tobey, New York.

American Society for the Control of Cancer, Dr. Francis C. Wood, New York; Dr. George A. Soper, New York.

American Social Hygiene Association, Dr. W. M. Brunet, New York.

Carnegie Institution of Washington, Dr. Linsly R. Williams, New York.

Commission on Medical Education, Dr. W. C. Rappeleye, New Haven, Conn.

STATE BOARDS OF HEALTH AND NATIONAL OFFICIAL AGENCIES

Alabama, Dr. S. W. Welch, Montgomery; Mr. Charles M. Leach, Montgomery.

Florida, Dr. B. L. Arms, Jacksonville.

Georgia, Dr. M. E. Winchester, Atlanta.

Indiana, Dr. William F. King, Indianapolis; Dr. Ada Schweitzer, Indianapolis.

Iowa, Dr. James A. Wallace, Des Moines.

Kansas, Dr. J. C. Montgomery, Topeka.

Louisiana, Miss Agnes Morris, New Orleans.

Maryland, Dr. R. H. Riley, Baltimore.

Michigan, Miss Marjorie Delavan, Lansing.

Minnesota, Mr. H. A. Whittaker, St. Paul.

New York, Dr. Mathias Nicoll, Jr., Albany.

Pennsylvania, Dr. William G. Turnbull, Harrisburg.

Utah, Dr. P. W. Covington, Salt Lake City.

Wisconsin, Dr. C. A. Harper, Madison.

Children's Bureau, Department of Labor, Dr. Blanche Haines, Washington, D. C.

United States Department of the Interior, Office of Indian Affairs, Dr. M. C. Guthrie, Washington, D. C.

United States Public Health Service, Surg. Gen. H. S. Cumming, Washington, D. C.

WELFARE DEPARTMENTS OF LIFE INSURANCE COMPANIES

John Hancock Mutual Life Insurance Company, Prof. Ira V. Hiscock, New Haven, Conn.

Metropolitan Life Insurance Company, Dr. Donald B. Armstrong, New York.

Penn Mutual Life Insurance Company, Dr. J. C. Humphreys, Philadelphia.

Union Central Life Insurance Company, Dr. Emmett Fayen, Cincinnati

OFFICIAL PROGRAM

Dr. Harlow Brooks, New York.

Dr. Arthur T. Holbrook, Milwaukee.

Dr. John A. Ferrell, New York.

Mr. Evart Routzahn, New York.

Dr. Linsly R. Williams, New York.

Surg. Gen. H. S. Cumming, Washington, D. C.

Dr. Matthias Nicoll, Jr., Albany, N. Y.

Dr. Morris Fishbein, Chicago.

Mr. R. C. Smith, Chicago.

AMERICAN MEDICAL ASSOCIATION

Dr. A. J. Cramp, Bureau of Investigation.

Dr. D. Chester Brown, Board of Trustees, Danbury, Conn.

Dr. M. L. Harris, Judicial Council, Chicago.

Dr. Austin A. Hayden, Treasurer, Chicago.

Dr. E. B. Heckel, Board of Trustees, Pittsburgh.

Dr. J. H. Walsh, Board of Trustees, Chicago.

Dr. Wendell Phillips, President, New York.

Dr. A. R. Mitchell, Board of Trustees, Lincoln, Neb.

Dr. John M. Dodson, Bureau of Health and Public Instruction.

Dr. W. C. Woodward, Bureau of Legal Medicine.

Mr. J. W. Holloway, Bureau of Legal Medicine.

Dr. Morris Fishbein, Editor.

Mr. H. J. Holmquest, Council on Physical Therapy.

Dr. Paul N. Leech, Director of Chemical Laboratory.

Prof. W. A. Puckner, Secretary, Council on Pharmacy and Chemistry.

Dr. Olin West, Secretary and General Manager.

Mr. R. C. Smith, special investigator to report on public health literature.

Dr. R. G. Leland, Assistant Secretary, Bureau of Health and Public Instruction.

Dr. N. P. Colwell, Secretary, Council on Medical Education and Hospitals.

Dr. R. M. Hewitt, Assistant Editor.

OTHER VISITORS

Mrs. W. B. Meloney, Editor, New York Herald-Tribune Magazine, New York.

Dr. O. N. Auer, Michael Reese Dispensary, Chicago.

Dr. Everett S. Elwood, National Board of Medical Examiners, Philadelphia.

Dr. G. M. Fisher, president, Medical Society of the State of New York, Utica, N. Y.

Dr. W. S. Leathers, Vanderbilt Medical School, Nashville, Tenn.

Dr. Philip Marvel, Atlantic City, N. J.

Dr. Frank Overton, Medical Society, State of New York, New York.

Dr. William Allen Pusey, Chicago.

Dr. C. G. Smith, Iowa State Medical Society, Granger, Iowa.

Dr. H. G. Weiskotten, Syracuse University College of Medicine, Syracuse, N. Y.

THE CONFERENCE ON PUBLIC HEALTH

Elsewhere on this page appears the announcement of the conference on health agencies, arranged by the Board of Trustees of the American Medical Association with a view to aiding coordination of efforts in the field of public health work. During the last twenty-five years, agencies for applying to daily life the benefits of scientific progress in the field of medicine have multiplied exceedingly. Their ramifications extend into every phase of human existence. They are in some instances self-supporting; in others, the result of philanthropy; in others, the organizations of local, state or national governments, and in many instances, controlled by special bodies of persons employed in the field concerned. Obviously, such rapidity and fertility of growth must have been accompanied by much duplication of effort, much confusion of thought, much invasion of fields considered by their possessors as quite sacrosanct. Repeated efforts have been made in the past to secure understanding among these groups whereby the difficulties that have been mentioned might be obviated, but thus far a complete assembling of either data or representatives of the many agencies concerned has not been accomplished. Without accurate data, comprehension cannot be achieved or any workable plan developed for the clearing of the situation. The Board of Trustees of the Association hopes, no doubt, to secure through a conference of national organizations of good repute at least two major objects: better understanding among all concerned in public health work, and sufficient data to aid in producing team work in a campaign in which much of the energy has been diffuse.

practicing physician, to the workers in the field of public health and to the public itself. Since official organization is not contemplated, there will not be resolutions or voting. Invitations have not been extended to health organizations limiting their activities to local fields. Acceptances so far received indicate that the conference will be well attended.

Association News

CONFERENCE ON PUBLIC HEALTH

The Board of Trustees of the American Medical Association has issued an invitation to official and volunteer organizations engaged in public health work to attend a conference to be held at the headquarters of the Association in Chicago, March 24 and 25. The following program has been arranged:

1. *The Relations of the Physician to Public Health*

   HUGH S. CUMMING, M.D., Surgeon General, U. S. Public Health Service.

   LINSLY R. WILLIAMS, M.D., Director, National Tuberculosis Association.

   HARLOW BROOKS, M.D., New York.

   ARTHUR T. HOLBROOK, M.D., Milwaukee.

   FRANK W. CREGOR, M.D., Indianapolis.

2. *Public Health Education (with Especial Reference to the Use of the Printed Page)*

   MATTHIAS NICOLL, JR., M.D., Commissioner of Health of the State of New York.

   E. G. ROUTZAHN, Associate Director, Department of Surveys and Exhibits, Russell Sage Foundation.

   MORRIS FISHBEIN, M.D., Editor of THE JOURNAL OF THE AMERICAN MEDICAL ASSOCIATION.

3. *Some Phases of the Economics of Public Health*

   J. A. FERRELL, M.D., Director for the United Stated States of the International Health Board.

Dr. Wendell C. Phillips, President of the American Medical Association, will preside over the conference.

An exhibit of printed material of an educational nature, being used by official and volunteer health agencies, will a feature.

This conference has been called with the view of securing open discussion of subjects of vast importance to the

THE JOURNAL OF THE AMERICAN MEDICAL ASSOCIATION

535 North Dearborn Street · · · Chicago, Ill.

Cable Address · · · · "Medic, Chicago"

Subscription price · · · · · · Five dollars per annum in advance

Please send in promptly notice of change of address, giving both old and new; always state whether the change is temporary or permanent. Such notice should mention all journals received from this office. Important information regarding contributions will be found on second advertising page following reading matter.

SATURDAY, APRIL 2, 1927

THE HEALTH CONFERENCE

Representatives of almost one hundred voluntary, official and professional organizations interested in preventive medicine and in public health education met last week at the headquarters of the American Medical Association at the call of the Board of Trustees. The primary purposes of this meeting were coordination of effort with avoidance of duplication in public health work and the reaching of a better understanding as to the specific opportunities and duties in this field for each of the organizations concerned. That clashes have occurred in the past among representatives of these groups is not a secret. In some instances, physicians have felt that the efforts of volunteer agencies and of official agencies were leading to forms of medical practice that could only be detrimental to the public. In other instances, public health officials have felt that volunteer agencies had infringed on their prerogatives or that physicians had not properly cooperated for the good of the community. Finally, representatives of volunteer health agencies have thought at times that the actions of the other groups concerned were guided, or perhaps misguided, by selfish motives and that it was their special function to protect the public interest.

Apparently the time was ripe for open discussion which would lead to more efficient cooperation in the future, since the motives of all the groups concerned were, beyond question, in the interest of the public welfare. The results of the conference, including the original manuscripts that were read and the discussions on them, will be made available through The Journal. Especially significant was the recognition of all those present of the necessity for medical leadership and guidance in any effort in this field. Such leadership would not necessarily involve origination of the procedure in the medical mind, but would concern the planning of the effort so as to preserve the personal relationship of physician to patient and the scientific factors necessary for ultimate good.

Among the interesting side-lights of the conference was the impression of leaders in volunteer health activities that physicians could not be educated or constrained to act as a group, that many did not have a social consciousness, and that organized medicine was not sufficiently organized to fulfil satisfactorily its obligation in this respect. The discussion opened up many other problems for consideration in medical societies or medical groups. Today medicine—and particularly preventive medicine—is the property of all mankind. A progressive physician must be aware of his relationships to the civic and economic problems of the community and the nation.

The Journal of the
American Medical Association

Published Under the Auspices of the Board of Trustees

| Vol. 89, No. 1 | Chicago, Illinois | July 2, 1927 |

THE RELATIONS OF THE PHYSICIAN TO PUBLIC HEALTH

FROM THE STANDPOINT OF THE PHYSICIAN IN THE SMALL CITY *

ARTHUR T. HOLBROOK, M.D.

MILWAUKEE

The cardinal sin in medical discussion is to wander from the topic. My topic is traversed by so many trails and crossroads that it becomes quite necessary at the outset to determine those conditions of public health control and medical practice in the small city which are essentially different from those of larger or smaller organized communities.

It is perfectly clear that all physicians should take an interest in public health—that would be ideal; but the conditions before us are real and not ideal. It also seems clear that the real attitude of the profession is that the interest of the practicing physician in the administration of public health is of far less importance in the large cities than it is in the rural communities. In the large cities the matter is in the hands of full-time, well paid, presumably competent health officers with an ample staff of assistants, while the unofficial public health agencies are well organized, well financed, and directed for the most part by expert officers and workers. In the rural community too often the part-time, underpaid, inexperienced health officer has no resources, personal or acquired, with which to meet his problem and usually does not receive any assistance from unofficial organizations. The interest and aid of the physicians in this community are imperatively demanded, whereas in the large city the practicing physician realizes that the public health affairs are in competent hands and does not feel any particular urge to interest himself or to assist, outside of a conformity with the laws and rules.

The interest of the average physician, therefore, may be stated as varying inversely as the number of people in his community; and somewhere in this scale comes the district, town or city that concerns each individual physician. What, then, are the conditions peculiar to the smaller city designated as my topic?

Such a city has gone past the stage where the personal attention of the public health officials to individual cases and minor problems is demanded, and yet is in the stage where the officials have a personal knowledge of the city's physical condition, housing conditions, the various factors entering into individual health problems; not a knowledge by report or by hearsay but by personal

* Read before the Conference on Public Health, Chicago, March 24, 1927.

contacts. Furthermore, the health officer of such a city has a personal acquaintance with perhaps a majority of its physicians and knows by reputation most of those he has not met. He is expected by the profession to do more than mere executive directing. Although it is not demanded of him, it is no unusual experience for the health officer to take up directly with physicians or families specific problems of quarantine, garbage disposal, odor nuisances and the like. Because of the personal relation he prefers not to delegate the duty. He knows the family concerned either personally or by reputation; he knows where it lives and the conditions of the neighborhood; he probably knows the physician in the case and calls him by his first name.

A comparable condition exists between the physicians of the smaller city and the unofficial public health organizations.

The average physician of such a city knows personally and perhaps intimately some of the officers, workers and members of the Red Cross, family welfare, antituberculosis and practically every such local organization. He is consulted by the members concerning their problems; he feels at liberty to make suggestions to his friend, who is a director of the society. He attends some of the annual dinners, contributes a moderate sum, and may be on one or two committees.

Without doubt there are many medical conditions affecting our topic peculiar to these communities, but in my opinion the outstanding, distinguishing characteristic is in the *personal contact*. In the larger city the health department and allied organizations are probably maintained at a higher development, but the personal touch is lost. In the smaller community the personal relation is even closer, but the health department and the organizations are missing. The small city combines the two.

Granting this personal contact to be an important element, what advantage can be taken of it in developing the most satisfactory relationship between the small city practitioner and the agencies for public health?

In the first place, if a hundred private practitioners in my community were to pick up a journal containing an article with the title of this paper, at least eighty-five of them would pass it by. Of the other fifteen there would be eight who consistently read journals from cover to cover, and the other seven would include the specially trained public health physicians, the men who have a grievance against public health agencies and are looking for more arguments, and the man who has been asked to write a paper on the subject. This fairly expresses the interest of the profession in a small city, and the general lack of a feeling of personal responsibility to problems of public health.

I wish to make clear my belief that practically every ethical practitioner in every department of medicine

15

recognizes the importance of public health control through agencies both official and unofficial. No body of professional or nonprofessional men of which I have knowledge has shown the unselfish, altruistic support of any program for public welfare that has characterized the efforts of our profession to safeguard the public health. Nevertheless, I am certain that under our present conditions the vast majority of private practitioners feel that the actual responsibility for the carrying out of this program rests with those who have chosen to specialize in this branch, those who volunteer for such service, and particularly those who are selected as officials and are paid to do the job. Each of the eighty-five would argue earnestly in favor of the program. He signs birth and death certificates punctiliously; he reports communicable diseases scrupulously; he favors milk inspection, increased taxes to insure better sewage disposal, and all the rest of that long list of needs so familiar to those who read health reports. Over the cigars after dinner he enthusiastically explains how the health department has cut down typhoid so that he has not seen a case in two years, whereas twenty years ago he thought his practice was falling off if he had less than a half-dozen cases on hand. He believes in it heart and soul; but he doesn't study it; he doesn't attend public hearings on questions affecting the city's health; he joins some of the allied societies, but he doesn't attend the meetings; he favors public clinics, but he couldn't tell where they are located. He is something like the Christian who never goes to church.

He certainly furnishes a tempting morsel of food for the thought of public health workers. How is this man to be sold the idea that every practitioner of medicine who is granted a license has a definite obligation to the state and that it is nothing short of duty for him actively to assist in the work of the health department? If he chances to live in New York State, the law and the sanitary code of his state specifically point out to him this duty and the penalties for evading the duty.

He perhaps is one of those who believe in a definite line between preventive and curative medicine. Possibly without giving it much analytic thought he takes the attitude that his job is to take care of people after they are sick, and that it is the concern of the health department and volunteer organizations to formulate regulations and enforce measures for the prevention of disease. He certainly is on thin ice. If he were a surgeon where would he draw the line between the prevention and cure of tetanus, anthrax, erysipelas, or of many other types of infection that have surgical aspects? If he were a laryngologist, what about diphtheria, toxin-antitoxin, control of carriers? If a pediatrician, how about the milk supply, prenatal management, the handling of a poliomyelitis outbreak, the Dick procedures? Each specialty would readily present its proof that no department of practice can definitely separate preventive from curative medicine. With the importance of quarantine, of surveys in limiting infections, the use of laboratory methods in diagnosis and control of therapeutic measures, the use of vaccines and serums, the resources presented by the public health department and allied organizations for the intelligent use and aid of practicing physicians, it is quite difficult to see how any thinking man would attempt to segregate preventive and curative medicine and lose the benefits of the cooperation of the two branches.

Among these eighty-five men there will be surely found a definite type of successful practitioner. He

does consistently good work and he is well paid. His days are filled from early to late. He works in a little time for studying cases and for journals and meetings. He squeezes in an occasional nine holes of golf and a few rubbers of bridge. He has not had a vacation in three years. How in heaven's name, he demands, can he be expected to attend public health meetings, join the Infant's Welfare Club, read *Hygeia*, and let his assistant put in two hours at the county dispensary every Tuesday and Friday—a couple of his busiest days. He is perfectly willing to pay his taxes and help hire the best specialists possible for the job, but he certainly has not the time for any such "outside" work as public health.

Now, this sort of man is the very one needed in public health work. He is very sure to be well prepared, he is a so-called live wire, he can do things and understand people. He has to be convinced that if all the men like him should refuse an active participation, the health program of our smaller city would fail.

Also in this eighty-five will be another distinct type. He is the man who is an ultraspecialist, puts in all his spare time on an arbeit, and harbors the impression that on the upper rounds of the medical ladder are poised those who are doing research work, while down below in an indefinite somewhere are the physicians who are taking care of sick people or trying by practical means to prevent sickness. He would feel that public health matters should be entirely in the hands of those who have made an exclusive study of the subject and that it is not a matter for his concern. Honor to the microbe hunters, the laboratory problem workers. Grateful are the acknowledgments to them for the weapons and ammunition they place in the armamentarium of the health workers. But equal honor, at least, to the earnest, studious, ethical men who are working to prevent and cure sickness. A good salesman is needed to tell a thing or two to this hyperdeveloped man.

The unsuccessful man may be in the eighty-five or in the fifteen. Usually he does not matter so much, for he lacks preparation, or force, or common sense or industry. Possibly—and probably—he has a grievance against the health department and the volunteer organization. They vaccinate his patients free; they take his baby to the welfare meeting and have its food prescribed; the clinics and dispensaries get many of the people in his neighborhood and he just plainly has no show. Well, this man in many communities probably has a right to complain. In the zeal to build up dispensaries and clinics; to better conditions of motherhood, infant care and feeding; to stamp out tuberculosis, and other laudable enterprises, the case of this struggling doctor in a poor neighborhood may be overlooked. It is an old, old controversy and no matter how long or how loud it is argued it will always come back to the one common sense conclusion of recognizing on the one hand the absolute need of free clinics and dispensaries, and on the other hand the absolute requirements that they be carefully regulated and supervised so as not to work an injustice to the physician who could not survive if the government or volunteer organizations indiscriminately offered free treatment to those who should pay. Fairness, tact, a mutual understanding and common sense are the remedies.

There are probably a few men who snapped back the page on public health matters with some show of feeling. They are the ones who rarely lose an opportunity to warn of the perils of state paternalism and the regulation of one's private affairs by commissions and societies, by long haired men and short haired women and other cranks, who feel that they have a mission to save the world. One of these physicians tells of the nurse who came from the welfare society to show one of his patients how to make her bed and wash her baby. He deplores the circumstance that he was not there to throw the nurse out the window. Another knows of two women in the motherhood association who are not fit to be in the same theater with his scrub woman, and he has heard that the treasurer of the Red Cross chapter beats his wife. It is an easy thing to let personalities influence one's estimation of a movement or an organization with which these personalities are associated. Let a popular, highly esteemed and trusted man head an organization, and success and achievement are fairly certain to follow. On the contrary, a weak president or an uninterested, carelessly chosen board may ruin for a time any organization. It becomes important, therefore, for these groups not to organize loosely or carelessly and stand vulnerable to opponents who are only too ready to wreck what may be a splendidly conceived movement for great public good.

In my opinion the medical profession leaves the work of the allied organizations too much in the hands of the laity. Some one has said that "medicine has a poor vision when it comes to seeing socially," and the indictment is more or less true. There would be far less criticism to offer these organizations if physicians were a bit more far-seeing, if they sought membership and activity in these agencies, gave freely of expert medical advice, interpreted and explained technical aspects to lay members, gave talks before clubs and other groups to help educate the public in the objects and activities of antituberculosis, Red Cross, family and infant welfare and like activities. On their side these organizations should realize that their greatest usefulness is attained when they supplement the work of the public health authorities and work in close cooperation with them. Kipling's oft-quoted lines might well be made familiar to their membership · "It ain't the individual nor the army as a whole, but the everlasting team-work of every bloomin' soul."

So far I have been considering chiefly what the public health agencies should expect of the physician. Let us shift the point of view and ask what the physician of a small city has a right to expect of his public health department.

First of all, the head of the health department in a small city must be a scientifically trained man, adequately prepared for his job. Too often these requirements are subordinated to the political qualifications that influence his appointment. I quote the statement of a recent report that "the greatest handicap to municipal health work in Illinois arises from the harmful influence of local partisan politics;" and if department heads are politicians instead of single-purposed, scientific workers the health of the public is going to suffer. In the selection of this trained official, for a smaller city at least, I feel strongly that he would be a far more efficient public servant if he were a local man rather than an imported stranger. I can conceive of local situations which would demand the seeking of an outsider for the health officer, but this would be a distinct disadvantage in losing the personal contact and acquaintanceship which I have urged as an important asset.

The physicians have a right to know definitely the attitude of the health officer toward medical practice in the community. Is he going to insist on protection of the rights of physicians in the dispensaries and clinics, on the courteous cooperation in the public city hospitals, on the proper reference of cases back to the original attending physician? I myself have never met a public health officer who, if approached in a reasonable spirit, was not perfectly willing to cooperate with me in all fairness in the consideration of my patient. Probably the other sort of health officer exists, but he is not an avis vulgaris and he would be very short-sighted not to realize that without cordial relations with the medical profession he is doomed to absolute failure, no matter how highly trained he may be.

In the smaller city the fact of a severe or unusual illness is general news or gossip and is given daily newspaper notice. It becomes a matter of no small importance to the physician to keep his conducting of the case free of criticism. If he has a clash with health officers about quarantine, removal to hospital, attendance in school of exposed children, or similar situations, and is openly and tactlessly opposed by the health department, he is very liable to unfair criticism and to being discredited by a large number of people. Consideration, tolerance and tact on both sides are all that is needed.

The advent of quacks and irregular practitioners in a small city presents its special problem. Contrary to conditions in a larger city, through hearsay and the newspaper practically the whole population of the smaller city knows of the presence of the impostors and prompt dealing with them and deportation become necessary to the medical morale of the community. This is a task the ethical physicians have a right to demand of the health department.

It would be tiresome to continue the list of the many situations affecting the relations of small city public health workers and practicing physicians. Enough has been said to indicate some of the more important problems, and I should like to recapitulate and emphasize three of them.

1. *The personal element in the relationship.* This means the selection of a properly qualified, local man at the head of the health department; the stimulation of interest in official and unofficial public health work on the part of practitioners and laymen; the cooperation of these men; the taking advantage of personal acquaintanceship with conditions and people in establishing a mutual, cordial and efficient relationship.

2. *The groundless fear that the public health administration will deprive deserving physicians of a competent livelihood.* This is a matter which simple fair-mindedness and common sense will settle among men who have a disinterested desire to cooperate.

3. *The fallacy of trying to define the exact and separate responsibilities of preventive and curative medicine.* There is no line of cleavage between these two. Of necessity they overlap, and where they run together each department must cooperate with the other. When the field of each becomes distinct, there the individual responsibility of each begins.

CONCLUSION

What measure or measures can be offered to secure most satisfactorily a proper handling of these three important considerations? I believe that Dr. John P. Koehler, health officer of my city of Milwaukee, has devised an effective means to the end we are seeking in the appointment of his advisory board. I am aware that the appointment of advisory boards and committees is not new, and have no doubt that other health officers have appointed boards along similar lines; but I do know that Dr. Koehler's plan has been particularly carefully studied and carried out and that there are small cities where such an advisory board is not being used although it would form a valuable adjunct.

The advisory board of the Milwaukee health department is composed of fourteen members. It includes six physicians and eight laymen. The physicians are appointed as representatives of the leading local medical societies, include the head of the milk commission, and are well distributed among the staffs of different hospitals, forming a group that is comprehensive of the various medical specialties and interests. The laymen include representatives from the allied volunteer health and social organizations, chairmen of the federated trades council, building trades union, etc., and the chairmen of the health committees of the county and city councils.

The health officer presides over and directs the activities of the board. When a question of general interest is before the health department, the entire board is asked to attend meetings for its consideration. It is definitely understood by the health officer and the members of the board that any member or group of members is subject to call and to consultation by the department on problems of which such members may have particular knowledge.

The results of such an arrangement are manifold. The health officer is able to avail himself of the advice of experts. The various interests represented by the board have a ready means of intelligent, practical appeal to the health authorities. Mooted questions after discussion at the general meeting may be carried by individual members to the organizations they represent, and the sense of these groups be carried back to help the satisfactory decision of the board.

When some important measure is before the common council, the county supervisors, the state legislature, the mayor or the governor, a great deal of influence will be carried with the expression of opinion of the fourteen men who have been chosen because of recognized qualifications and who represent the opinions of hundreds of other citizens composing the organizations from which they are delegated. In the small city where these men are personally and presumably favorably known, such influence is very potent, and the effect of the newspaper published personnel of such a board with their expressed opinions is of much importance in stimulating that active public interest on which the health of every city must largely depend. The cooperation of the medical profession and the volunteer health agencies with the health department, and the mutual confidence inspired by this intimate contact of lay interests and medical interests have earned for this board of advisers the title it has been given of the "Unofficial Guardian of the City's Health."

711 Goldsmith Building.

THE PHYSICIAN AND THE PUBLIC HEALTH *

HARLOW BROOKS, M.D.

NEW YORK

I speak today from the point of view of a medical man engaged in active practice in one of the great urban centers. I shall consider particularly those various points on which the medical practitioner in these centers is likely to be, or may be, out of complete sympathy with the activities of lay organizations that have largely interested themselves in questions pertaining to public health matters.

At the outset I wish to state that I, and I believe all my fellow practitioners, honor, respect and crave the assistance of every lay person and organization that is devoted to altruistic service to the public, to the alleviation of suffering, and to the betterment of mankind. Whatever I may say in the way of criticism is meant to be in the nature of a constructive one. Our purpose is, and should be, identical. As to the methods by which this may be best accomplished, I believe that there is often room for argument and full consideration.

If we may grant, at least for the sake of argument, that my point of view is to be that of the professional in regard to matters of health as contrasted to that of the amateur in health matters, I do not think that I am asking too much. I will consider also as professional health workers equal with ourselves all those who in their training in hygiene, bacteriology, pathology, anatomy, physiology and therapeutics have equaled the requirements in these subjects of a Class A medical college. In this assumption I feel that whether or not such persons have a medical degree and a license to practice, they are equipped to be grouped with us as professionals and not as mere amateurs.

Sanitation, epidemiology and the executive features of public health work must be considered only as specialties in medicine, just as we practitioners group ourselves as neurologists, surgeons, internists, and so on. Without a basic training in the elemental medical sciences there cannot be true specialization in such work any more than the surgeon can be permitted to practice his craft without a careful training in physiology, in bacteriology and in the other essential fundamentals.

I wish also to advance as my ideal of the specialist in public health that splendid group of officers comprising the U. S. Public Health Service, and those in the medical departments of the army and navy, whose everyday function it is to apply the problems of public health in a practical way. To such men the medical profession as a whole gives its sincere confidence and full cooperation. I do not know of any exceptions. We have every confidence in all those specialists in

* Read before the Conference on Public Health, Chicago, March 24, 1927.

public health who are legitimately specialists. We have a quite natural suspicion of those lawyers, politicians, business men, preachers, and otherwise unoccupied ladies, grouped so loosely and so thoughtlessly as "social workers," who do not have basic training or understanding of those subjects to which we have so seriously and with single hearted zeal devoted our whole preparation and life.

I was astonished the other day to read the statement of a worker in public health that the practicing medical profession was often found in conflict with public health activities. I cannot understand such a position unless the public health service in that instance was interested, as are some of the lay organizations, in activities basically contrary to the teachings of medical science and to the welfare of the public and its infirmities, just as some lay organizations advocate antivivisection, antivaccination, and various quack institutions and projects.

The statement has also been made that because the medical man is chiefly concerned with the sick person he cannot, therefore, be interested in the problems of the community, which, if I understand it properly, is made up merely of collections of individuals. The absurd accusation has also been laid against the medical practitioner that he is not interested in the prevention of sickness but only in its alleviation. I am sure that the individual who made such a silly and entirely unfounded statement never had a family doctor. The family doctor is and always has been the very bone and sinew of all successful methods for the prevention of disease. Little has ever been produced in the prevention of disease which has not been based on the preliminary work of a physician, or on that of the trained scientist who has the identical preliminary schooling which the physician must secure before he is permitted to graduate or to take out his license to practice. The doctor has never opposed true medical progress, but bitter experience has taught him to view with great caution the emanations of untrained, unthinking, irresponsible and often unscrupulous dabblers in health and medical practice. The practitioner is slow to accept unreasonable theories, to jump at cure-alls or to contract the hysteria which in every epidemic is likely to develop in the largely unoccupied masses.

The accusation has also been made that the medical practitioner is not public spirited, not a nationalist—this, mind you, of a profession that recently voluntarily gave 20 per cent of its personnel, old and young, in a great national calamity; of a profession the members of which are acting generously, anxiously and efficiently on the boards of every educational advance, every church and charitable venture; a profession that has always identified itself personally and as a united front in every good project of humanity. I know that there are those who feel that hospitals would be beautifully efficient institutions if only there were no doctors to demand that business step aside for the welfare of the sick, and that organized charity reach the unfortunate instead of spending its efforts and funds on a perfect business institution. That the doctor is not a business man, I confess. The recent revelations of the income tax proves that definitely.

We are that single profession which statistics show devotes voluntarily from 25 to 45 per cent of its time to unremunerated personal charities, mostly to that large and generally inarticulate mass of the unfortunate which are the secret wards of every honest medical man. Do any of you know a single practitioner who does not devote to the very best of his ability a large percentage of his time, without remuneration, to the care of the unfortunate sick?

But enough of this foolishness. Criticisms of this ganglion cell-less type simply indicate the motivation of its authors. As General Harbord, a great soldier and a greater citizen, has recently said, most of this propaganda originates from the activity of a pathogenic bacillus known as the paid executive secretary. He has never flourished in the culture medium supplied by the medical profession.

Misunderstandings have arisen, it is true, honest misunderstandings between the profession and some worthy public health activities. Was there ever progress without argument and criticism? There is little or none in those activities controlled by the United States Public Health Service or in those of the state or city health departments when they have been controlled and directed by trained medical men. The commissioner of health of our great, generous and progressive city has in a recent bulletin thanked the state and county medical societies and the Academy of Medicine of New York, all of which he terms his allies, for the full cooperation and assistance we have given him. I have never known it to be otherwise when we have had, as we now have, as our commissioner a physician who still remembers his training and his origin, and who still believes in medical ethics, which, I take it, is only a concrete application in our profession of the Golden Rule.

Misunderstandings between the profession and social activities along the line of public health have almost without exception originated when we have been asked to abrogate, to forget, our scientific training, or when our code of ethics has been ruthlessly ignored. Are we ready to scrap our code of ethics? If so I wish to leave medicine and become an arctic explorer or a field archeologist and be no longer a doctor. There is no more reason why medical ethics may not be applied in public health than in any other specialty in our profession. No efforts at progress will succeed until lay organizations are brought to realize that we shall first uphold the principles that have made modern medicine and the true physician of all times.

I believe that I may rightfully claim an intimate acquaintance with the members of my profession in the large community in which I live. I know few rascals in the profession; I know very few men who do not value their professional standard as high as life itself. I do not know of any practitioners who do not gladly give up a very considerable portion of their time to unremunerative and largely secret charities. I know but a few men who do not read the current journals and who do not buy, even at the prevailing high prices, standard text and other professional books. I know very few doctors who do not try to keep abreast of the times. I know few doctors who die rich; I know many who might do so if they were willing to conduct their profession as a business. I am sorry to say that I also know a few doctors of very exceptional ability who never attend medical meetings and who give none of their time to the necessary routine of society work. They are unknown outside their personal practice and perhaps to a few specialists and consultants, yet they are also an honor to their calling. I know many doctors who devote their time as employees of business

institutions. Some of them are men of considerable capabilities, but they have been dwarfed and curtailed by business control. Few of them frequent the libraries or medical societies. Eventually they become worth no more than the salary they receive. They are the result of the vaunted "business control of medicine." Many of them devote their time as secretaries and agents for organized charities. They are despised by their employers, who would never trust to them their lives; they are useless to the profession, and they eventually become so "organized" that they might as well be classed merely as lay secretaries.

What does the physician in family practice resent in the activities of public health? He resents nurses doing the work of physicians, making diagnoses and dictating treatment which the family physician shall carry out. Do you blame him? He resents the underpaid, time-serving employee of the department who from the wealth of his inexperience minimizes to school children the work and ridicules the respect of their family doctor. He resents, too, wholesale septic vaccinations and other evidences of legal but bad practice. He resents the snap diagnosis of an employee of the department on a case to which he has perhaps given serious and experienced study. He resents being directed the institution of treatments which he knows from his journals and from his societies to be still in the experimental stage. He has often just cause for his complaints, for he knows himself to be the better man.

This is all easily correctable. Nurses are nurses until they have studied medicine and legally qualified themselves as practitioners of medicine. They should not be allowed to do as an agent of public medicine work which the law does not permit them to do as private individuals.

Physicians working under the direction of public health institutions must be sufficiently remunerated so that competent men may be retained. Such men will always meet courtesy, compliance and cooperation; the cheap man will not.

In a recent publication, attention has been drawn to the great economic waste which results in the duplication of work prosecuted by the many lay directed organizations. This could be avoided were these activities directed by professional, and not jealous lay, skill. Concentration under professional control would result in such economy that the money of the public would not be so wasted, and at the same time adequate salaries could be paid so that professional workers in this special field of medicine might properly compare their lot with that of the successful teacher or practitioner of medicine.

Employment of young physicians at meager salaries robs the profession of the material from which it should recruit its general practitioners, now the greatest need of the profession. I often tell my interns as they graduate that the worst thing that could happen to them would be to receive a salary on which they could live from some lay institution in which the professional experience does not reward the service; for many of them later in life would not dare to give up their salaries and start out for themselves. Some of the brightest youngsters I have ever known have been ruined by such activities. They typify the business and non-professional controlled society.

Another matter in the control of professional institutions by the layman lies in the demands made on the

young men for service inadequately repaid either by
the experience gained or by the pay received. Many
of our private lay controlled hospitals are sinners in
this matter. Some of them are notorious for their
ruthless but entirely businesslike exploitation of the
young physician.

Wealth, under the guise of charity and public health
progress, more than seldom dominates even medical
education. High endowments without professional control have dwarfed medical teaching in more than one
institution. This is a matter for your attention.

Public medicine cannot be divorced from private
medicine, except at a loss by both. The most potent
and influential teacher of public medicine and of practice is the physician in contact with his patient. No
public medicine can succeed professionally that has not
the endorsement of the average physician.

The value and the influence of the average practitioner is beyond the comprehension of the executive
who is himself not conversant with the details of medical practice or who has through lack of experience so
estranged himself from his profession and its practitioners that he fails to comprehend even its purposes.
He is likely to develop from his ignorance of real
medicine and its problems a superiority complex of
particularly inexcusable type. This is the disease from
which many public health workers suffer; they are the
ones who criticize the average physician. The public
health worker must keep in touch with the general
science of medicine and not criticize his brother who
perhaps in the stress of his work has neglected to
remain fully conversant with the special methods of
public health. There are few surgeons who appreciate
the labor of the psychiatrist; each considers the other
something of a medical invert.

We of the medical profession believe that a license
to practice should be granted only after four or more
years of study in an accredited school, superimposed
on a preliminary education of no mean extent or small
cost. That this idea is not held by the public at large
is only too vividly shown in each state each year by all
manner of cults, often backed by the clergy, well intentioned philanthropists, financiers and people of all sorts,
intelligent and otherwise.

If we are correct and well founded as to our requirements as regards the private practitioner, why is it that
the practitioner of public health may be self anointed,
as it were? Is the public to be less protected than the
individual? May we not apply here also the invidious
comparison dictated by the Egyptians of old, who
admitted that Saul had slain his thousands, but David
his tens of thousands? And there are many Davids
engaged in their favorite avocation of public health,
how many only the properly prepared medical practitioner is able to judge.

Surely there are few of you who have not read in
a recent number of the *Atlantic Monthly* the exceedingly covert but telling and just arraignment of the
control of medical education by self perpetuating bodies
such as the General Education Board and other similar
endowments. Is it not apparent to most of you that
we are allowing precisely the same condition of affairs
to dominate the field of public medicine? An exceedingly thoughtful and just editorial [1] appeared in The
Journal, March 5, on this very subject.

I have also noted in The Journal an editorial
entitled "The Physician's Responsibility in Preventive
Medicine." [2] There are few, if any, practitioners
among my colleagues in New York who are not willing,
more than willing, to accept these implied responsibilities, few who do not subscribe whole heartedly to every
word expressed in this timely editorial.

I recall a time not so long ago when the medical
profession of my city did all in its power to increase
the authority and powers of the United States Public
Health Service, even to the extent of turning over to
them the sanitary control of our port. Those of you
who know the enormity of this agency in our city life
can appreciate what this meant. The project was
defeated. Can any of you surmise why, when the great
body of our practitioners wished it? Again the subtle
workings of Bacillus harbordensei.

I should like to ask General Cumming whether his
wonderful organization has felt a lack of cooperation
on the part of the practitioners of my city toward the
activities of his workers. I do not believe it possible,
and as I said at the outset of my paper, I think that I
know my practicing colleagues of New York.

It seems to me that it is a very simple matter to
readjust our differences and to bring to us the whole
hearted support of the public. We need them, they
need us. We particularly need their money, for we
are a poor people financially—we give already, perhaps,
too much of ourselves and of our funds to the unfortunate. Let us do all in our power to unite the public
to us, let us acquaint them with our purposes, with our
needs, let us invite them into our confidence. Let us
frankly give our ideas to the public press, let us warrant in every way the full confidence of those whom
we serve. Please remember, however, that every one
of our public has his doctor, and that he has not and
cannot have a higher opinion of the profession than
he has of his own doctor. We and our reputation in
every respect are absolutely in the hands of the
practicing physician. May it never be otherwise!

With all this, with the breaking down of our no
longer necessary brahministic seclusion, let us not for
one moment give up our professional ideals, our traditions and our ethics. If we do we become no more
than business men. In the eyes of the public we still
constitute a priesthood. This reputation has been built
up on the example of the family practitioner. If we
lose this we lose all, and most of all the confidence of
the public whom we still seek to serve, yes, even more
than the God of science.

I take it that this meeting is called for something
constructive. To an astonishing degree the American
Medical Association possesses the confidence of the
physicians of this land. It is our professional repub-
lic, a rule of ourselves by ourselves. What can
the American Medical Association do to solve this
problem?

It seems to me that the answer is a simple one,
though the trail is rough and the desired objective far
ahead. There are many wire entanglements, difficult
trenches to take, machine gun nests to dislodge, and
in many instances a well organized resistance against
the "Medical Trust"—that is, against us, serious
minded, progressive and ethical men who make up this
organization. There are many Elijahs, mostly of the
Bryanesque type, commanding against us. Old "Gen-

---

1. "The Perils of Magnanimity," editorial, J. A. M. A. 88: 726
(March 5) 1927.

2. The Physician's Responsibility in Preventive Medicine, editorial,
J. A. M. A. 88: 484 (Feb. 12) 1927.

eral Reformer" has already laid down his barrage against us; heaven knows what he is going to do without the doctor when he has so hemmed us in by restrictions and decimated us by levies that we have as a profession become entirely secularized. But that does not concern him. It does concern us and our future usefulness.

Let us win the enemy over to us by concerted action by the same devoted and disinterested zeal which has always typified the profession, and to which alone is progress in medical science due.

Let this great body insist on the control of its own members. Let it demand that it, and not the zealous amateur, shall control our education, our position in this nation, and even our discussion of medical matters.

Let us through our state and county societies, under the direction of the great parent body, enlist every member in the work of public health. Let us invite the cooperation of every honest lay body; but we must dominate and insist that the professional standards which have made medicine shall still prevail, and that medical science shall still control medicine, in all its applications.

Through our medical organizations let us detail lecturers for public occasions. Through our own authorized members let us give out to the public press of the land authoritative statements of such an enlightening character that the public will listen and take heed.

Let us take over the city, the county and the state public health organizations; too many of them are now taking us over. Let us teach our students and young practitioners the essentials of public health as we now teach them an outline of medicine, of therapeutics and of surgery. Let us in general so prepare ourselves that we are qualified to act as public health officers. Then, and then only, shall we be able to take over and to control public health in its every aspect. But we must demand at all times that the traditions and ethics of medicine shall be respected, that only the competent shall rule.

I believe that the intelligent public is really with us. I believe that they are more than willing to meet us half way, and to devote under scientific professional control the enormous sums which are now dissipated at a tremendous economic waste, mostly under the debauched name of "charity." Encourage in public health such leaders and creators as we have developed in bacteriology, in chemistry, in physics, in surgery, in physiology and in all other essential components of medicine. Insist that they shall also enjoy a commensurate reward financially, and the dignity of a professional, and not of a social or political, position. This cannot be achieved except through professional control.

Finally, may I say for the practitioners of New York that we are back of every sensible measure of accredited preventive medicine. We are more than willing to play our essential part in the program of public medicine. We are not, however, a class prone to accept without due consideration the vaporings of every volunteer amateur Moses. We are prepared and waiting for the leadership of qualified, scientific medicine in this great undertaking. We shall as a body welcome the control of this great project by accredited representatives of American medicine, whether it be by the American Medical Association or by any other similar body of equal ability and proved authority, if such other there be.

RELATION OF VOLUNTARY HEALTH
AGENCY TO PHYSICIANS AND
HEALTH DEPARTMENTS *

LINSLY R. WILLIAMS, M.D.

NEW YORK

The term "public health" has been somewhat loosely applied to everything which has to do with keeping people well, preventing disease and caring for the sick. Although care of the sick is not considered as a health activity, activities organized for the prevention of disease grow out of the movement for the care of the sick.

The care of the sick was carried on by religious orders during the middle ages and later by private organizations, particularly in England. The colonies and the United States followed the English tradition in organizing private hospitals and later dispensaries for the care of the sick. There were relatively few efforts made by governmental authority in this country for the care of the sick until the middle of the last century. Health departments were organized primarily for the suppression of epidemics; and as the knowledge of disease became more definite, their efforts were also directed to the prevention of other diseases which were known to be noncommunicable.

Hospitals and dispensaries, having begun as institutions for administering medical relief, that is, in caring for the sick, started to expand their work at the end of the last century to the prevention of disease, primarily in the field of tuberculosis. The antituberculosis movement took on more active work at the beginning of this century and has continuously expanded, so that an association exists in every state for the prevention of tuberculosis.

Although there were several voluntary agencies interested in health work, these antituberculosis societies were the first that formulated a definite policy which has been adopted with various modifications by voluntary health agencies interested in the prevention of other diseases. The voluntary health agencies have not formulated a definite policy that is the same throughout the country, yet there are certain similarities which may be expressed as follows: In general, they conceive of their function as being one of investigation, the inauguration of a new activity, the demonstration of its usefulness, transferring the activity to the official agency or discontinuing it. In certain places where the governmental authorities have not made any provision for the care of the sick, the voluntary agencies have carried on a continued activity for the care and relief of the sick poor.

These principles immediately bring up the age-long conflict in regard to the government—whether there should be a great deal of government and the state should do everything or whether the individual should be left to help himself or whether a voluntary group should undertake to secure funds which are contributed in addition to taxation for the carrying on of a special activity.

As tuberculosis work is perhaps the best known, this will be taken as an example. A voluntary health agency organized for the purpose of assisting in the prevention of tuberculosis desires aid in the situation, and its first problem is to determine how many cases of tuberculosis

* Read before the Conference on Public Health, Chicago, March 24, 1927.

there are in the community. This is the period of investigation. This study is known as a tuberculosis survey and should be made with the knowledge and assent of the health authorities. The survey is usually made by a nurse or social worker consulting hospital and dispensary records and visiting the poor farm and the physicians practicing in the community; the individual data giving names and addresses of patients with tuberculosis is not divulged. It is usually found as a result of such surveys that there is a far larger amount of tuberculosis in the community than is suspected by the physicians or health authorities.

It is then suggested, perhaps by the voluntary health agency, that the official health authority should create a local dispensary for tuberculosis or a special class for tuberculosis in the existing outpatient department of a hospital, or that a special hospital should be created in the county for tuberculosis or a special pavilion for tuberculosis should be established in connection with the municipal hospital. Whichever of these activities is agreed on is recommended to the local board of health, community council or county board with the usual reply that funds are not available and it is not necessary, that the people won't stand for it, etc. The voluntary agency then determines perhaps to establish a dispensary in the community, and its organization is worked out with the knowledge and advice of the health officer and is maintained for several years.

During this period, it is found that a number of cases need institutional care and no place is available for them. An effort is then made to transfer the maintenance of the dispensary to the local health department and very commonly with success; and as it has been shown that hospital beds are needed, another effort is made to bring about the creation of a special tuberculosis sanatorium or pavilion at the general hospital. This work may be called the period of inaugurating an activity and a demonstration of need.

During this period, the relationships between the health department, the voluntary agency and the medical profession have pushed themselves into the foreground because the health department has insisted on certain regulations for the administration of the dispensary, a private agency, and the local medical society has demanded certain privileges in regard to work in the dispensary or exacted certain conditions in regard to the payment of the dispensary physician and his method of appointment. Let us assume for the moment that the tuberculosis dispensary has been taken over by the health department and the local tuberculosis hospital established, and the voluntary agency has made a study of the relation of tuberculosis to children and has finally concluded that it may with profit to the community direct its efforts to keeping well babies well, this being determined on the theory that if children do not become ill they are less liable to develop tuberculosis. Consequently, the voluntary association organizes a child welfare station for children under school age.

Here again, a number of new questions are brought up in regard to the management of the child health station. There are certain differences between the problems arising in regard to the maintenance of the tuberculosis dispensary and the child welfare station. Tuberculosis is a communicable disease, and any patient believing that he has the disease should have the right to go to a dispensary for an examination and diagnosis, irrespective of his financial status. There is no valid objection to this procedure, although it has been contested by county medical societies. The child health station, however, is primarily an institution for education and not for treatment. It is supposed to examine children, weigh them, and advise the mother how to keep them well.

What parents should be permitted to bring their children to such a center? It is my own belief that parents should be permitted to bring their children for examination and diagnosis, irrespective of financial status, in the same manner as in the tuberculosis dispensary; but this point of view is highly contested by many members of the medical societies on the ground that this will pauperize the family and that such parents should go direct to their physician. The appointment of the physician also creates a difficulty in both instances. The institution or organization that has created the tuberculosis dispensary or the child health station has the responsibility of maintaining the medical efficiency of its work; and as it employs the physician in charge and presumably pays him for his services, it is incumbent on the organization to have the final authority in nominating the physician. On the other hand, many jealousies arise on the part of certain members of the local medical society who criticize the physician in charge on the ground that he is not a specialist, that he is not competent, that he is using the dispensary or child welfare station for advertising, that he is building up his practice by asking patients to come to his office instead of to the dispensary, and so on. The local society may endeavor to secure either the direct appointment of the physician in charge, the rotation in office of the physicians in charge, the appointment of a full-time physician who shall not engage in practice, and the rigid examination of all patients as to their capacity to pay, or that no patients shall be admitted to the dispensary or station except on the recommendation of their physician.

There are two essential difficulties which must be met in the future:

1. The health department and the voluntary agency desire to see diagnostic facilities and adequate medical care provided for every individual in the community. Theoretically, the private practitioner has a similar desire, but feels that every one in the community should have his own private physician. The health department and the voluntary agency advertise their clinics and health stations and do everything in their power to increase their trade. The private physician, on the other hand, may do nothing but wait until the patient calls.

2. The health department and the voluntary agency desire to show in their annual reports the largest number of new applicants and total visits possible, irrespective of financial status of their clients. On the other hand, the private practitioner feels very strongly that neither the governmental authority nor the voluntary agency should give diagnostic service or medical care to those who can afford to pay a private physician, and with certain modifications this is evidently a just point of view. However, there are many people who could afford to pay a modest fee but who cannot be persuaded to go to see a private physician when they or their children seem to be perfectly well, but who might be persuaded to go to a clinic for examination and diagnosis if they knew that no fee would be exacted.

Jour. A. M. A
July 9, 1927

There are also differences between the point of view of the voluntary agency and that of the health department. The health officials are embarrassed at times by the activities of the voluntary agency, and there are two chief reasons:

1. The voluntary agency frequently employs a publicity agent and is able to secure more notices in the press than does the health department, and it not uncommonly gives the impression that it is doing more work than the health department. The voluntary agency has been known at times to be confused in the minds of the public with the health department. There are also times when the policy of the health department is not agreed to by the voluntary agency, or the activity of the voluntary agency may not be approved of by the health department. How. can these difficulties be adjusted? They must be settled for the better promotion of public health and for the avoidance of disagreement and for the improvement of the health and medical care of the public and the practice of medicine.

In the autumn of 1925, a physician in New York invited representatives of the voluntary health agency, the state health department, and the state medical society for dinner and an informal conference. At this conference a number of these problems were discussed in considerable detail. This meeting was followed by a series of conferences which brought about a definite realization of the difficulties and finally resulted in the appointment of a committee on public health relations of the state medical society, which has been holding meetings regularly during the present winter with representatives of the voluntary health agency. Although no definite agreement has as yet been reached, both groups are in definite agreement that the health department and ·oluntary agency must both carry on their activities and that the advice and counsel of the county or local medical society must be sought before a new activity is inaugurated, in particular in regard to matters relating to the appointment and remuneration of physicians. This seems to be the most profitable method of securing progress—conference and agreement, and if not complete agreement, compromise.

2. In the relations between the voluntary health agency and the health department there is a greater difficulty, for the voluntary agency must primarily work in harmony with the health department in order to secure the best results; but occasions do arise when a large number of prominent physicians and health workers and others are in agreement that a definite step in advance should be taken by the health department or a marked change in method of administration of a particular health department activity. In instances of this kind there are health officials who believe that no matter what the health officer desires to do he should be supported.

On the other hand, the voluntary health agency believes that it has the right as a group of citizens definitely to criticize and oppose a policy, plan or method of a governmental official. The latter question can never be solved completely, but many disagreements could be avoided by more frequent conference between the interested parties, by the health department seeking the cooperation and support of the voluntary health agency, and by the latter taking counsel with the health officer and advising him of its plans.

25

PRINCIPLES OF PUBLIC GIVING

BY JULIUS ROSENWALD

I

THERE are few colleges in the land to-day which are not striving for 'adequate endowment.' Museums, orchestras, operas, homes for the aged, hospitals, orphanages, and countless other charitable and remedial organizations, are aiming at the same goal. It was recently estimated that more than two and a half billion dollars were given to various endowments in this country in the last fifteen years. The sum is vast, equal to the total national wealth a hundred years ago, but institutions continue to solicit more and greater endowments, and men of wealth are encouraging them with ever-increasing gifts.

All of this giving and receiving is proceeding without much, if any, attention to the underlying question whether perpetual endowments are desirable. Perhaps the time has come to examine, or rather reëxamine, this question, for it is not a new one in the long history of philanthropy.

I approach this discussion neither as an economist nor as a sociologist, but simply as an American citizen whose experience as a contributor to charitable causes and as a trustee of endowed institutions has given him some insight into the practical side of the problem. My only purpose is to raise the question of how best we may aid in the advancement of public welfare.

We can learn much from British experience, which has been more varied as well as longer than our own.

Monasteries, in the earlier centuries, received such enormous grants that Edward I and his successors undertook to limit their possessions. Despite these efforts, it is estimated that shortly before Henry VIII secularized the monasteries between one third and one half of the public wealth of England was held for philanthropic use. This first great struggle between the living State and the dead hand indicated, as Sir Arthur Hobhouse has pointed out, that the 'nation cannot endure for long the spectacle of large masses of property settled to unalterable uses.'

This experience was reflected in laws intended to restrict charitable bequests in perpetuity, but the endowment of charities of all kinds continued until there was hardly a community in all England without its local fund. So obvious had abuses become that a Parliamentary Commission was created to inquire into the situation. Its preliminary report, published in 1837, filled thirty-eight folio volumes and listed nearly thirty thousand endowments with a combined annual income of more than £1,200,000.

Those who view endowments uncritically might think the condition of English charities fifty years ago happy in the extreme, for less than 5 per cent of the population lived in parishes without endowed charities, all sorts of human needs had been provided for by generous donors, and funds were increasing rapidly. But Mr. Gladstone, who certainly was a humanitarian, rose in the House of

Commons to say that the three commissions which had investigated the endowed charities 'all condemned them, and spoke of them as doing a greater amount of evil than of good in the forms in which they have been established and now exist.'

The history of charities abounds in illustrations of the paradoxical axiom that, while charity tends to do good, perpetual charities tend to do evil. James C. Young, in a recent article, 'The Dead Hand in Philanthropy,' reports that some twenty thousand English foundations have ceased to operate because changing conditions have nullified the good intentions of the donors; and a large number of American funds, many of them of comparatively recent origin, have likewise become useless.

II

When I was a boy in Springfield, Illinois, the covered wagons, westward bound, rolled past our door. The road ahead was long and full of hardships for the pioneers. They were hardy and self-reliant men and women, but many of them were so inadequately equipped that if misfortune overtook them, as it frequently did, they were almost certainly doomed to suffering, and perhaps death.

The worst hardships and dangers of the Western trail had passed in my boyhood, but there was still use, then, for the Bryan Mullanphy fund, established in 1851 for 'worthy and distressed travelers and emigrants passing through St. Louis to settle for a home in the West.' A few years later the trustees could with difficulty find anyone to whom the proceeds of the fund might be given. Some years ago, for lack of beneficiaries, the income had piled up until the fund totaled a million dollars. I have not followed its later

fortunes, but, unless the courts have authorized a change in the will, that money is still accumulating, and will accumulate indefinitely. The Mullanphy gift was a godsend in its brief day. The man who gave it found one of the most urgent needs of his time and filled that need precisely. He made only one mistake: he focused his gift too sharply. He forgot that time passes and nothing — not even the crying needs of an era — endures. He deserves to be remembered as a generous-hearted man who realized, perhaps better than anyone else in his generation, that a wealth of pioneer blood and energy was being dissipated in the creation of our American empire. If he is remembered at all, it is more likely as the creator of a perpetuity which lost its usefulness almost as soon as it was established.

Mullanphy's mistake has been made not once but countless scores of times. It has been made by some of the wisest of men. Benjamin Franklin in drawing his will assumed that there would always be apprentices and that they would always have difficulty when starting in business for themselves in borrowing money at a rate as low as 5 per cent. In addition, he assumed that a loan of three hundred dollars was enough to enable a young mechanic to establish himself independently. With these assumptions in mind, Franklin set up two loan funds of a thousand pounds each. One was for the benefit of 'young married artificers not over the age of twenty-five' who had served their apprenticeships in Boston, and the other for young men of similar situation in Philadelphia. The accumulated interest as well as the principal was to be lent out for a hundred years. By that time, Franklin's calculations showed, each thousand pounds would have amounted to £135,000. One hundred thousand pounds of each fund was then to be spent. The Boston fund was to be used in constructing 'fortifications, bridges, aqueducts, public buildings, baths, pavements or whatever may make living in the town more convenient for its people and render it more agreeable to strangers.' In Philadelphia, he foresaw that the wells which in his day supplied the city with water would become polluted; accordingly, he proposed that Philadelphia's fund should be used for piping the waters of Wissihicken Creek into the city. Fortunately, Boston provided herself with pavements, and Philadelphia herself with a water supply, without waiting for Franklin's money. Great as his intellectual powers were, he had miscalculated at every point. The class he proposed to benefit gradually became nonexistent; therefore the funds failed to accumulate as rapidly as he had anticipated. At the end of a hundred years, instead of the $675,000 he had expected in each fund, there were only $391,000 in Boston and $90,000 in Philadelphia, and meanwhile the good works which he had chosen as the grand climax of a career devoted to good works had long been provided.

Benjamin Franklin was a wise man, and so was Alexander Hamilton; yet it was Hamilton who drafted the will of Robert Richard Randall, who in the first years of the last century left a farm to be used as a haven for superannuated sailors. A good many years ago the courts were called upon to construe the word 'sailor' to include men employed on steamships. Even so, the fund for Snug Harbor, I am assured, vastly exceeds any reasonable requirement for the care of retired seafarers. The farm happened to be situated on Fifth Avenue, New York. To-day it is valued at thirty or forty million dollars.

I have heard of a fund which provides a baked potato at each meal for each young woman at Bryn Mawr, and of another, dating from one of the great famines, which pays for half a loaf of bread deposited each day at the door of each student in one of the colleges at Oxford. Gifts to educational institutions often contain provisions which are made absurd by the advance of learning. An American university has an endowed lectureship on coal gas as the cause of malarial fever. In 1727, Dr. Woodward, in endowing a chair at Cambridge, England, directed that the incumbent should lecture for all time on his *Natural History of the Earth* and his defense of it against Dr. Camerarius. It did not occur to the good doctor that his scientific theories might eventually become obsolete; yet, with the passing of years and the progress of scientific knowledge, the holder of the chair had to admit his inability to comply with the founder's instructions and at the same time execute Dr. Woodward's plain intent — namely, to teach science. The list of these precisely focused gifts which have lost their usefulness could be extended into volumes, but I am willing to rest the case on Franklin and Hamilton. With all their sagacity, they could not foresee what the future would bring. The world does not stand still. Anyone old enough to vote has seen revolutionary changes in the mechanics of living, and these changes have been accompanied and abetted by changing points of view toward the needs and desires of our fellow men.

I do not know how many millions of dollars have been given in perpetuity for the support of orphan asylums. The Hershey endowment alone is said to total $40,000,000 and more. Orphan asylums began to disappear about the time the old-fashioned wall telephone went out. We know now that it is far better for penniless orphans, as for other children, to be brought up under home influence. The cost of home care for orphans is no greater than the cost of maintaining them in an orphanage. But the question is not one of cost, but of the better interest of the children. Institutional life exposes them needlessly to contagion, and is likely to breed a sense of inferiority that twists the mind. The money which the dead hand holds out to orphan asylums cannot be used for any other purposes than maintaining orphan asylums; it therefore serves to perpetuate a type of institution that most men of good will and good sense no longer approve.

To protest twenty-five years ago that orphans were not best cared for in asylums would have been considered visionary; fifty years ago it would have been considered crack-brained. There is no endowed institution to-day which is more firmly approved by public opinion than orphanages were within the lifetime of any man of middle age. Let that fact serve as a symbol and a warning to those who are tempted to pile up endowments in perpetuity.

III

There is another and to my mind no less grievous error into which many givers still are likely to fall. They conceive that money given for philanthropic purposes must be given, if not for a limited object, then at least in perpetuity: the principal must remain intact and only the income may be spent. The result has been, as many a trustee knows, that institutions have become 'endowment poor.' Though they have many millions of dollars in their treasuries, the trustees can touch only the 4 or 5 per cent a year that the money earns. There is no means of meeting an extraordinary demand upon the institution, an extraordinary oppor-

tunity for increasing its usefulness. Research suffers; museums are unable to purchase objects that never again will be available; experiments of all sorts are frowned upon, not because they do not promise well, but because money to undertake anything out of the ordinary cannot be found, while huge sums are regularly budgeted to carry on traditional and routine activities. And nothing serves more successfully to discourage additional gifts than the knowledge that an institution already possesses great endowments.

As a trustee of the University of Chicago, I know how difficult the problem is. Opportunities for purchasing libraries or for extending the work of some department into new fields are continually coming before us, and though we have endowments of $43,000,000, we have frequently been unable to authorize the use of even a few thousands for some object which would add much to the University's resources and usefulness, to say nothing of its prestige. We may not even convert the principal of our endowments into books or men, which are the real endowment of any university.

A number of years ago the University started collecting more endowment. I did not contribute to the fund, but instead turned over a sum of which the principal may be exhausted. That fund, I am assured, has been of considerable service. It has been used for such diverse purposes as the purchase of the library of a Cambridge professor; for paying part of the cost of Professor Michelson's ether-drift experiments; for reconstructing the twelve-inch telescope at Yerkes Observatory; for a continuation of research in glacial erosion in the State of Washington, and for research in phonetics. If the fund had been given as permanent endowment, it is obvious that some of the objects could not have been achieved. The men who desired to undertake experiments and research might have been forced to postpone their investigations; the books purchased might have been scattered among a dozen libraries, never to be reassembled. It is true that money disbursed now will not yield income to the University fifty years hence, but it is also true that fifty years hence other contributors can be found to supply the current needs of that generation.

I am convinced that the timidity of trustees themselves is often responsible for their inability to spend principal. Donors would in many cases be willing to give greater discretion to trustees in such matters if they were asked to do so. A notable example in point is the consent by Mr. Carnegie, more than ten years ago, to the current use of funds which he had given originally for endowment to Tuskegee Institute. At a time when this school was in desperate need of money, I proposed at a meeting of the board of which Honorable Seth Low was chairman and Theodore Roosevelt was a member that we request Mr. Carnegie to permit us to spend not only the interest but also a small portion of the principal of his gift. My suggestion was at first frowned upon. Finally the board agreed, and a letter, dated January 24, 1916, was sent to Mr. Carnegie by Mr. Low which read in part as follows: —

I am writing to submit to you a suggestion which has been made to me by one or two of my fellow trustees of the board of the Tuskegee Institute. Mr. Rosenwald, in particular, who is a generous supporter of the Institute, feels very strongly that a permanent endowment fund is less useful than a fund the principal of which can be used up in fifty years, his idea being that every institution like a school ought to commend itself so strongly to the living as to command their interest and support. ... In accordance with this suggestion, I am writing to ask whether you would be willing to permit the trustees to use, each year, at their discretion, not more than 2 per cent of the principal of the fund which you so generously gave some years ago toward the endowment of the Institute. It is always possible that within the lifetime of the next generation industrial training for the negro race will be assumed by the state or national government. Should any such change or any unforeseen change in conditions take place, a fund so firmly tied up in perpetuity that the principal cannot be touched, except possibly through an act of the legislature, might be a disadvantage rather than an advantage.

To this Mr. Carnegie's secretary, Mr. John A. Poynton, replied on February 23, 1916, giving Mr. Carnegie's approval to the suggestion in the following terms: —

Mr. Carnegie has given careful thought to the proposal that your trustees be permitted to use each year a portion of the principal of the fund which he contributed toward endowment.

In establishing his foundation Mr. Carnegie has favored the plan of giving the trustees and their successors the right to change the policy governing the disposition of the principal as well as interest when to them it might seem expedient, believing it impossible for those now living to anticipate the needs of future generations. Mr. Carnegie would be happy to have the trustees of Tuskegee assume a similar responsibility in connection with the fund which he contributed toward the endowment of that institute, and asks me to say that he is willing to have a small percentage of the principal used annually for current expenses if three fourths of the members of your board should decide in favor of such a plan.

Here is evidence that Mr. Carnegie might have relaxed the terms of his other gifts had he been asked to do so. It was not the donor but the trustees who were timid. (I have seen trustees act in much the same way in matters of financial administration. Men accustomed to investing a large part of their private fortunes in sound common stocks have felt that as trustees they must invest only in first mortgages or bonds. Of late a good many boards of trustees have enjoyed a change of heart, to the vast benefit of the institutions they serve. But that is a digression.) In some of the institutions with which I am best acquainted, funds given with no strings attached have been added to the perpetual endowment as a matter of course. It is a noteworthy fact, though not as widely known as it should be, that the Rockefeller foundations are not perpetuities. If any of them to-day are wealthier than at their establishment, it is not because the trustees are not free to spend principal when the occasion rises. As a matter of fact, I am told these boards have expended about seventy-five million dollars of their capital or special funds, and it is probable that at least two of them will disburse all of their principal funds within another decade or two.

IV

I am opposed to gifts in perpetuity for any purpose. I do not advocate profligate spending of principal. That is not the true alternative to perpetuities. I advocate the gift which provides that the trustees *may* spend a small portion of the capital — say, not to exceed 5 or 10 per cent — in any one year in addition to the income if in their judgment there is good use at hand for the additional sums. Men who argue that permission to spend principal will lead to profligate spending do not know the temper of trustees and the sense of responsibility they feel toward funds entrusted to them;

nor do they appreciate the real difficulties which face donors and trustees of foundations in finding objects worthy of support. I am prepared to say that some of the keenest minds in this country are employed by foundations and universities in seeking such objects; yet, when a real need is discovered, it often cannot be met adequately, simply because of restrictions placed on funds in hand.

The point has been raised that great institutions must have perpetual endowments to tide them through hard times when new money may not be forthcoming. Those are precisely the times when it is most important to have unrestricted funds which will permit our institutions to continue their work until conditions improve, as they always do. A great institution like Harvard ought not to have to restrict its activities merely because its income for one reason or another has been temporarily curtailed. The spending of a million or two of principal at such a time is not imprudent. Sound business sense, indeed, would commend it.

I am thinking not only of university endowments, but also of the great foundations established to increase the sum of knowledge and happiness among men. Too many of these are in perpetuity. It is an astonishing fact that the men who gave them — for the most part, hard-headed business men who abhorred bureaucracy — have not guarded, in their giving, against this blight. I think it is almost inevitable that as trustees and officers of perpetuities grow old they become more concerned to conserve the funds in their care than to wring from those funds the greatest possible usefulness. That tendency is evident already in some of the foundations, and as time goes on it will not lessen but increase. The cure for this disease is a radical operation. If the funds must exhaust themselves within a generation, no bureaucracy is likely to develop around them.

What would happen, it might be asked, if the billions tied up in perpetuities in this country should be released over a period of fifty or one hundred years? What would become of education and of scientific research? How could society care for the sick, the helpless, and the impoverished? The answer is that all these needs would be as well provided for as the demands of the day justified. Wisdom, kindness of heart, and good will are not going to die with this generation.

Instead of welcoming perpetuities, trustees, it seems to me, would be justified in resenting them. Perpetuities are, in a measure at least, an avowal of lack of confidence in the trustees by the donor. And it is a strange avowal. The trustees are told that they are wise enough and honest enough to invest the money and spend the income amounting to 4 or 5 per cent each year; but they are told in the same breath that they are not capable of spending 6 or 10 or 15 per cent wisely.

If trustees are not resentful, it is because they know that donors of perpetuities are not thinking in those terms. Sometimes perpetuities are created only because lawyers who draft deeds of gifts and wills have not learned that money can be given in any other way. More often, probably, perpetuities are set up because of the donor's altogether human desire to establish an enduring memorial on earth — an end which becomes increasingly attractive to many men with advancing years.

I am certain that those who seek by perpetuities to create for themselves a kind of immortality on earth will fail, if only because no institution and no foundation can live forever. If some men are remembered years and centuries after the death of the last of their contemporaries, it is not because of endowments they created. The names of Harvard, Yale, Bodley, and Smithson, to be sure, are still on men's lips, but the names are now not those of men but of institutions. If any of these men strove for everlasting remembrance, they must feel kinship with Nesselrode, who lived a diplomat, but is immortal as a pudding.

V

There has been evolution in the art of giving, as in other activities. The gift intended to meet a particular need or support a particular institution in perpetuity was once generally approved, but is now outmoded. There are evidences that all perpetuities are becoming less popular, and I look forward with confidence to the day when they will become a rarity. They have not stood the test of time.

To prove that I practise what I preach, it may not be out of place to say that every donation that I have made may be expended at the discretion of the directors of the institution to which it is given. The charter of the foundation which I created some years ago provides that principal as well as income may be spent as the trustees think best. This year, as the management of this fund was being reorganized, I was anxious to make sure that the trustees and officers would meet present needs instead of hoarding the funds for possible future uses. I have stipulated, therefore, that not only the income but also all of the principal of this fund *must* be expended within twenty-five years of my death. This I did in the following letter to the board of trustees, approved and accepted by the board at its meeting in Chicago on April 29, 1928: —

I am happy to present herewith to the Trustees of the Julius Rosenwald Fund certificate for twenty thousand shares of the stock of Sears, Roebuck and Company.

When the Julius Rosenwald Fund was created and sums of money turned over, it was provided that the principal as well as the income might be spent from time to time at the discretion of the Trustees, and it was my expectation from the beginning that the entire principal should be spent within a reasonable period of time. My experience is that trustees controlling large funds are not only desirous of conserving principal, but often favor adding to it from surplus income.

I am not in sympathy with this policy of perpetuating endowment, and believe that more good can be accomplished by expending funds as trustees find opportunities for constructive work than by storing up large sums of money for long periods of time. By adopting a policy of using the fund within this generation we may avoid those tendencies toward bureaucracy and a formal or perfunctory attitude toward the work which almost inevitably develop in organizations which prolong their existence indefinitely. Coming generations can be relied upon to provide for their own needs as they arise.

In accepting the shares of stock now offered, I ask that the Trustees do so with the understanding that the entire fund in the hands of the Board, both income and principal, be expended within twenty-five years of the time of my death.

I submitted this letter, in advance, to a wide circle of men and women experienced in philanthropy and education, anticipating a good deal of dissent. There was almost none. Twenty years ago when I, among others, spoke in this vein, our ideas were considered visionary; to-day they are receiving an ever wider approval.

I believe that large gifts should not be restricted to narrowly specified objects, and that under no circumstances should funds be held in perpetuity. I am not opposed to endowments for colleges or other institutions which require some continuity of support, provided permission is given to use part of the principal from time to time as needs arise. This does not mean profligate spending. It is simply placing confidence in living trustees; it prevents control by the dead hand; it discourages the building up of bureaucratic groups of men, who tend to become overconservative and timid in investment and disbursement of trust funds. I have confidence in future generations and in their ability to meet their own needs wisely and generously.

THE TREND AWAY FROM PERPETUITIES

BY JULIUS ROSENWALD

I

FOR many years I have been convinced that it is wasteful to tie up money in perpetual trusts and that these trusts are often actually harmful in their influence. In May 1929, the *Atlantic Monthly* published an article by me on this subject. Since that time the movement away from perpetuities has made great progress. Several new trusts have been created with the stipulation that principal as well as income must be spent within a generation, trustees of existing endowments have begun to free themselves from legal restrictions as to the use of capital, and hundreds of people have written that they fully share my views as to the desirability of leaving trust funds free for use as from time to time they may be needed.

Some present readers may recall the previous article in the *Atlantic*. I sought first to show that perpetuities for specific objects are a mistake because times change and with them needs and circumstances change. I did not anticipate any serious opposition on that point because the evidence is too overwhelming to admit of doubt. The dead hand has been proved, time after time, to be a hindrance, if not indeed a menace, to the progress of mankind. A dozen or so instances were cited by way of proof. Hundreds might have been mentioned. I went further and criticized not only perpetual trusts for special causes but also perpetuities of any sort, however general their

purposes. I made a plea for conferring upon trustees the right, if not the duty, to use a part of the principal as well as the income of funds in their care, should occasions arise which, in their judgment, warranted the additional expenditure. This is a somewhat advanced position, and I expected that it would meet opposition in many quarters.

I was pleasantly surprised by the chorus of Amens. I cannot quote them all, but a few of the letters will suggest the others.

Dr. George E. Vincent, for many years President of the Rockefeller Foundation, has probably had as much experience in the handling of large philanthropic funds as any man now living. He writes: —

THE ROCKEFELLER FOUNDATION
61 BROADWAY, NEW YORK
June 19, 1929

MY DEAR MR. ROSENWALD:

Mr. Embree has told me that you would like to have me comment upon your article in the May 'Atlantic.' I have just reread this and here are my comments in succinct form:

1. As to specific permanent endowments, there can be no question. The case against them has been proved over and over again.

2. You are unquestionably right about permanent endowments even for philanthropic purposes with the widest discretion granted to the trustees. Power to spend not only interest but principal should be given to those who hold and administer such funds. This ought to apply also to the community trusts which are being organized in a number of our cities.

741

3. As to educational institutions, I have in the past been a little in doubt. It has seemed to me that the maintenance of colleges and universities ought to be ensured by having a large part of their activities cared for by permanent endowment. I have thought that such a central core of endowment might be usefully supplemented by such gifts as you have been making which give the trustees greater opportunities to deal with special emergencies and unforeseen needs. I have thought that both kinds of gifts would together make a very useful combination.

On further reflection I think I realize that this conservative feeling is traceable to my long experience in university work. It is very hard to escape the bias of any particular kind of activity. More recently I have come to the conclusion that your philosophy is essentially sound. After all, if trustees make unwise investments in funds there is no way of avoiding loss. A trust in perpetuity cannot ensure perpetuity unless there is sound and conservative business management available.

One sees in the same way that if trustees are wise they can use their wisdom in administering funds which are not legally restricted. If an institution can secure sound leadership and the right sort of trustees, it is safe under the plan you propose. Lacking these conditions, nothing can protect it against decay and disaster.

So a little belatedly, but none the less heartily, I find myself in complete accord with your views on the subject of endowments in perpetuity.

Yours sincerely,
GEORGE E. VINCENT

Many others wrote briefer comments in the same general vein. The following excerpts are selected almost at random from files of hundreds of letters from persons who are in positions of great responsibility in connection with endowments. Here, for example, is a note from Dr. John Grier Hibben, President of Princeton University: 'I might add that it [the article] has been a help to me in bringing to the attention of our Finance Committee several items of our budget which should be provided for from our endowed funds, rather than from the annual income of the same.'

And this is from Thomas Cochran, of J. P. Morgan and Company, New York: 'It [the article] has changed my conception of how I ought to handle a substantial gift that I am planning to make in the near future. Thus, I am indebted to you.'

Albert Britt, President of Knox College, says: 'There is something extremely stimulating in your belief that each generation will and must care for its own problems. And this is more an opportunity than a burden. Conditions change so fast in our American life that we must plan broadly rather than particularly for the long future, and the more we confer upon our children the right of responsibility in solving their own problems, the more we shall benefit.'

And here speaks Mr. Lewis E. Pierson, chairman of the board of the Irving Trust Company, New York: 'Ordinarily when we hear of a public benefaction we visualize something perfect or nearly so. You have made it clear that excellent intention is only part of a perfect gift and that it is possible for the best-intended public giving to result in harm instead of benefit.'

This comes from a fellow townsman, Mr. E. J. Buffington, the president of the Illinois Steel Company: 'I heartily agree with your thought that the wisdom and goodness of men in the future may be relied upon for correct administration of endowment funds, and that it is wise and safe of donors to rely upon the judgment and character of trustees rather than the stipulation of fixed rules to govern in perpetuity.'

A letter from Mr. S. Stanwood Menken is especially gratifying, since it reports not only conviction but aggressive action. This distinguished member of the New York Bar writes: 'From my experience in drawing wills, I heartily concur in all your conclusions — so thoroughly, in fact, that I am writing to a client of mine who has just made a trust of five million dollars, sending him your pamphlet and urging him to take a lesson from your wide experience.'

It would be possible to go on quoting from these letters for pages, but space forbids. These few must stand for the rest.

II

Even more impressive than opinions are a number of recent actions which show the trend away from perpetuities. In my previous paper in the *Atlantic Monthly*, it will be remembered that I called attention to the fact that in the case of the foundation which I had established I had stipulated that the entire fund must be expended, both capital and income, within a period of twenty-five years of the time of my death.

A number of the older foundations permit trustees to spend capital as well as income. This is true of all of the foundations established by Mr. Rockefeller. As a matter of fact, in addition to expending all of the income year by year, more than $100,000,000 of principal has been expended by the several Rockefeller boards. The reports of these foundations indicate that in recent years greater and greater amounts of the capital funds are being expended. Evidently the Rockefeller trustees are convinced that funds need not be preserved for possible future generations, but may best be used when promising opportunities are found for social betterment and while ideas and enthusiasm are fresh. The Commonwealth Fund, established by the late Mrs. Stephen V. Harkness, is also using principal as well

as income, and the hope has been expressed that the entire fund will be expended within a generation.

Equally significant are the tendencies of boards of trustees of university endowments and other trust funds to free themselves from limitations, not only as to specific objects to which funds may be given, but also from the necessity of holding their funds in perpetuity even under the most general conditions.

The Association of Near East Colleges has set an example in raising funds for working capital rather than permanent endowment. In the recent campaign for a total of $15,000,000 of endowment for the five Near East Colleges in this association, I offered to make a contribution to Beirut University if my gift could be made a part of a temporary endowment rather than a perpetuity. The trustees of this university were attracted by the idea and immediately designated the larger part of their endowment as a temporary fund. The trustees of Robert College and Constantinople College for Women, after considering the matter, were convinced that it was wise to follow the same course of action, and use a part of the endowment each year for the present pressing needs of these colleges.

The provision in all these cases is not only that the trustees shall have the privilege of spending a part of the capital of this temporary endowment each year, but that they must set aside at least a small part of the capital either for current uses or for a reserve for future needs. The formal votes of the Board of Trustees of the American University of Beirut which embody these principles were adopted April 2, 1929, as follows: —

That every possible effort be made by the Trustees to bring up the endowment fund of the American University of Beirut to $4,500,000 by July 1st, 1929, and that $3,000,000 of this amount be placed in a temporary endowment and $1,500,000 into a permanent endowment.

That the Trustees of the University have the privilege not only of spending the income on the temporary endowment from year to year, but also may and will set aside from the principal not less than 2 per cent and not more than 5 per cent each year. These sums taken annually from the principal are to be used at the discretion of the Trustees either for the current expenses of the University for that year or placed in a reserve fund to be drawn upon from time to time for buildings, increase in salaries, pensions, development of new departments, or some unforeseen need.

It will be noticed that a part of the capital is still held as a permanent trust. This was necessary because certain bequests and donations had already been accepted as perpetuities. The larger part, however, of the funds has been placed in the temporary endowment.

The argument for not tying up funds in perpetuity is particularly strong in the case of these American-controlled institutions in foreign countries. Who can tell what the situation in the Near East will be in another hundred years, or even in twenty-five years? Political conditions may be such that it will be undesirable or even impossible for foreign institutions to continue in these countries. In such a case how unfortunate it would be to have $15,000,000 tied up in perpetual endowments which could not serve their designated objects and in consequence might be debarred from serving any useful purpose.

Somewhat similar considerations bear upon Negro colleges and universities which have been established in a number of Southern states, largely from private gifts. The changes in the condition of the Negro have been so rapid since the Civil War that it is almost impossible to follow them, let alone forecast them. Migration has removed two millions of the Negroes to the North. Meanwhile the Southern states are making increasingly liberal appropriations for the support of Negro education in the form of both public schools and Negro state colleges. In view of the swift changes in Negro conditions, it seems foolhardy to tie up in perpetuity funds for any particular Negro institution, however valuable its work may be at the moment. In fact, the crying demands of Negro schools and colleges are reasons for throwing all available resources into these present needs and leaving to coming generations the meeting of future requirements, which are certain to be different from those of to-day.

With such considerations in mind a number of Negro institutions, including Morehouse and Spelman Colleges in Atlanta and Lincoln University in Pennsylvania, have recently accepted endowment funds not as perpetuities but as working capital under essentially the same provisions as those adopted by the Near East Colleges. At the same time increasing support is being given to all Negro education on the basis of current gifts and public appropriations, as in the case of Howard University, Washington, D. C., the several state agricultural and normal colleges for Negroes, and an increasing number of private institutions.

It is also hazardous to endow in perpetuity agencies for social welfare. However fully an organization may be meeting current social needs, conditions change so rapidly that there is no guarantee that exactly the same requirements will hold for future generations. In fact, it is a certainty that these conditions will not persist. In my earlier paper I called attention to a number of examples of charities which met the needs of their time but have now ceased to have any meaning whatever. I cited the Bryan Mullanphy Fund, established in 1851 for 'worthy and distressed travelers and emigrants passing through St. Louis to settle for a home in the West'; the endowments set up by Benjamin Franklin for the training of apprentices in Boston and for a water supply in Philadelphia; endowments for orphan asylums — an outworn form of child care. I might have mentioned the trust funds established for education in Liberia, where one hundred years ago it was expected that American Negroes would colonize in large numbers, and innumerable other examples familiar to anyone who turns the pages of social records.

Yet all of these causes seemed as enduring in their time as public-health nursing or settlement houses do in ours. As unusually fine examples of institutions which are serving current needs might be mentioned Hull House in Chicago and the Henry Street Visiting Nurse Service in New York. These agencies have been built up in response to pressing demands through the vision and resourcefulness of two remarkable women, Miss Jane Addams and Miss Lillian Wald. There can be no question about the value of their service to-day. Yet we may be certain that conditions are changing and that the acute social need of to-morrow will be different from that of to-day and will doubtless call for a new kind of agency to meet it. The splendid service that Hull House and Henry Street are giving under their present leaders is the strongest argument for putting all the resources they can obtain into their present activities.

An example of an important private agency which has agreed to use its funds currently rather than as a perpetual trust is the National Institute of Public Administration, an organization with headquarters in New York City which is helping to analyze and improve various functions of government. In replying to a suggestion in this connection, Raymond B. Fosdick, a trustee of the several Rockefeller boards and an active director of the National Institute, wrote as follows: —

I am delighted, too, with your idea of setting up at least $900,000 of the $1,500,000 to be raised on the basis of a temporary endowment rather than in perpetuity. This is a forward-looking step which I hope will be widely followed in connection with other gifts and other institutions. Your continued emphasis on this matter is bound to liberalize the whole character of American philanthropy, and so far as the National Institute of Public Administration is concerned, we shall gladly adopt your condition.

For a number of years the University of Chicago has been urged not to tie up in perpetual endowments those funds which are given without restrictions, but rather to hold as large a part as possible of such resources for use at any time when needs arise. The University has recently decided to follow this course and the trustees have adopted the following vote: —

Conditions and restrictions specifically imposed by donors or testators will always be scrupulously observed by the University, but where no limitations of any character either expressed or implied have been placed upon the use of the gift, we believe that it is not only permissible but that it may be considered the definite duty of the Trustees to devote such unrestricted funds, both principal and income, to such purposes as in their judgment shall best serve the needs of the institution.

In view of the fact that the giving by the Rockefeller family and the Rockefeller boards has been conspicuous not only for its magnitude but no less for the wisdom with which the causes and institutions have been selected, it is gratifying to see that the influence of these givers is being thrown toward current use of funds and away from perpetual trusts. The elder Mr. Rockefeller continues to be a model in keeping his donations free from petty restrictions. Mr. John D. Rockefeller, Jr., has made many of his recent gifts with the formal understanding that after twenty-five years the trustees of the given institution may use the funds, both capital and income, for whatever purpose may then seem most desirable.

Two of the newest foundations have gone further than any of their predecessors in insisting upon current use of funds.

One of these is the Falk Foundation. The donor, Mr. Maurice Falk of Pittsburgh, has authorized the board to spend any or all of the fund of $10,000,000, principal as well as interest, within thirty-five years.

Another example was provided by Senator James Couzens of Michigan, who established in 1929 a fund of $10,000,000 'to promote the health, welfare, happiness and development of the children of Michigan primarily and elsewhere in the world.' He has stipulated that the entire fund, capital and income, be spent within twenty-five years.

When I congratulated Senator Couzens on this act he smiled and said, 'You see, I have gone you one better. You said that your fund must be expended within twenty-five years of some remote day when you die; I require my fund to be used up within twenty-five years of to-day.'

To make sure beyond any doubt that the instructions of Senator Couzens will be carried out, actuaries have been employed to determine just how much must be distributed each year to exhaust the funds in a quarter of a century. As a result of these computations

the trustees of this fund now know that they must spend $700,000 a year to achieve this object, and newspapers report their decision to proceed to disburse the funds at not less than this rate.

In all, $17,500,000 will be expended. The total may seem unduly high to those inexperienced in such computations. The explanation lies, of course, in the comparatively small demands on the capital in the first years. At 5 per cent, for example, the fund in its first year will yield $500,000 in interest, requiring only an additional $200,000 of the capital to meet the budget. The next year the income from interest will be only slightly less, $490,000, requiring only $210,000 reduction in the capital. The reduction of capital, of course, will be gradually speeded up until, in the last years, the expenditure will be almost entirely from capital, and interest will become the negligible factor.

We need not become unduly alarmed at the thought that the whole fund will be exhausted. Long before that day, other donors no doubt will have provided ample sums for future work. And meanwhile a vigorous administration can be expected to accomplish more for humanity with the increased sums at its disposal than could be expected in generations of spending in smaller amounts by men unacquainted with the donor. Such trustees who have not caught the donor's enthusiasm and his will to achieve decisive results are more than likely to take as much interest in conserving the capital as in finding the best uses for it.

III

These instances (practically all of them occurring within the past year or two) are remarkable evidence of the growing conviction that it is unwise to try to set up endowments in perpetuity. The fact that donors and trustees are coming to recognize the objections to perpetual trusts is encouraging evidence that the human race can learn from past experience.

As a matter of fact, it is not only unwise to create a perpetuity — it is impossible. There is evidence that the Egyptians attempted to set up perpetual trusts. In Greece and Rome endowments were apparently as common as they are to-day. All these carefully laid plans for perpetuities, needless to say, have crumbled to dust. They have succumbed to conquest, confiscation, expropriation, and the decline in the purchasing power of money, to mention only the more conspicuous causes of decay.

One of the earliest historical records of foundations, I am told, was a perpetuity set up in Greece in support of the Delphic Oracle. This endowment was established during the fifth century B.C. and entrusted to the administration of eight trustees whose successors were to be chosen under careful legal provision for all the rest of time. Does anyone to-day think that the Delphic Oracle would be worth supporting? Yet probably no one now believes in university education or public health more ardently than the Greeks only twenty-five hundred years ago believed in this Oracle. It is as impossible for us to judge the needs and wants of the future as it was for the Greeks to do so.

Perpetuity means not a thousand years or a million years, but eternity. No one in the history of the world has been able to establish a trust which has endured even for a thousand years. The word, in the sense in which it is employed by donors in making gifts or by lawyers in drafting wills, is simply the expression of a fond hope.

The very idea of a perpetual trust is strange and abnormal. It may have originated from the desire of men to gain favor in the world to come. 'Lay up for yourselves treasures in heaven' is a command that has been taken literally by many people, who wished to have their good deeds made a matter of perpetual record on earth and thus a source of eternal credit in Heaven. In a somewhat similar spirit the old Chaldean and Egyptian kings left wealth to colleges of priests who were to tend their tombs for all time and provide food for the departed spirits. In many countries trusts have been left to ensure perpetual prayers for the donor. There is also doubtless the desire to be remembered endlessly on earth as well as to gain favor in Heaven. Surely no one to-day would condone perpetuities established because of such purely selfish motives.

The obstructions to social progress that may come from perpetual trusts, at least as they apply to individual beneficiaries, have been recognized in law. The old common-law rule, which applies in most states of this country, prohibits the establishment of beneficiary trusts set up for more than twenty-one years beyond the life or lives of persons in being at the time the trust is created. The New York State law is even more rigid and prohibits the setting up of a personal fund to continue beyond the lives of any two designated persons living at the time of the creation of the trust.

Other legal devices have grown up to protect society from the ill-advised stipulations of donors. The principle known to lawyers as the cy-pres doctrine provides that, when an endowment can no longer be used for the specific cause designated in the will or deed of gift, the courts under certain conditions may transfer its use to other objects as nearly as possible in line with the original purpose. This principle serves as a safety valve in flagrant cases of out-moded charities. The difficulty is that very seldom is any group interested enough to take the time and trouble necessary for court action to revise the terms of the gift. In fact often the only parties directly interested are trust companies or salaried officers who are benefiting from the existing terms of the trust, however obsolete they may be. Under these conditions untold millions are tied up in the support of perfunctory services some of which actually retard progress. Instances in point are endowments of religious bodies no longer active, of orphan asylums which obstruct modern ideas of child care, and charity hospitals which, however beneficial in times past, now tend to retard the development of self-supporting organizations for medical care which offer proper compensation to the physician and self-respect to the patient.

A striking example of the inflexibility of perpetual trusts was the refusal of the courts a few years ago to allow the McKay bequest to Harvard to be used in a proposed consolidation of resources and activities of the Lawrence Scientific School and the Massachusetts Institute of Technology. Although this union was desired by the trustees of both institutions and seemed clearly to be in the public interest, the courts ruled that since funds had been given to Harvard they must forever be held and administered solely by the trustees of that specific corporation, rather than in a great coöperative effort in the Boston area. Following is an excerpt from the decision of the Massachusetts Supreme Judicial Court: —

It may be assumed also that a coöperative plan like that proposed would be advantageous to both of these great institutions by creating one school of applied science of the highest efficiency, with economy in expenditure and effort, to take the place of two competitive schools. But so far as the agreement attempts to dispose of the income of the McKay gift, the controlling question is whether it is authorized by the terms and conditions of the trust upon which the gift was made and accepted. The income of the McKay endowment must be administered according to the intention of the founder, Gordon McKay, even though it be at variance with our views of policy or expediency.

This case brought vividly before the educational world the power of the dead hand, expressed in a perpetual trust, to block change and reorganization even when these are recognized to be desirable.

The real contributions of philanthropy are not so much in money alone as in the support of new ideas or agencies which may prove to have great social value. Hospitals were built and in part endowed during the Middle Ages. The Hôtel-Dieu in Paris was founded more than a thousand years ago. St. Bartholomew's Hospital in London recently celebrated its eight-hundredth anniversary. These institutions have been continued not because of their initial endowments, for these were insignificant. They were recognized to be meeting a human need, and this recognition has been expressed in financial support generation after generation.

The ancient seats of learning abroad and in this country similarly have been kept alive, not because of their initial endowments, but because of their continued usefulness. In 1638 John Harvard left £750 and a library of 300 volumes to the college which now bears his name. The college in New Haven was named for Governor Elihu Yale in gratitude for an endowment of a few hundred books and about £600 in cash. Can anyone pretend that these original endowments of Harvard and Yale are responsible for the continuation of these universities throughout the centuries? The funds originally contributed simply made possible the experiments. The work has continued and expanded because of its support in every generation.

It is often said that the great contribution made by Mr. and Mrs. Leland Stanford was not so much to the institution which bears the name of their son as to the University of California, which, under the stimulus of the founding of Stanford University, has received greatly increased support from the State. To-day the appropriations of the State of California to its own institutions of higher learning are each year larger than the entire initial gift for the endowment of Stanford.

Similarly Mr. Rockefeller's gifts to the University of Chicago were valuable not only in themselves and to that university, but even more for the funds which were indirectly released for universities in neighboring states because of the high standards and leadership maintained in the Mid-West area by the University of Chicago.

Real endowments are not money, but ideas. Desirable and feasible ideas are of much more value than money, and when their usefulness has once been established they may be expected to receive ready support as long as they justify themselves. We may be confident that if a public need is clearly demonstrated, and a practicable way of meeting that need is shown, society will take care of it in the future.

THE BUSINESS OF GIVING AWAY MONEY

THE PROBLEM FACING THE AMERICAN FOUNDATIONS

BY EDWIN R. EMBREE

A NEW class, the multi-millionaire, is a small but growing one into which any of us by the accidents of commerce may be flung to-morrow. While romantic imagination has hovered over the rich man from time immemorial, little attention has been given to the real situation of a person possessed of funds immeasurably beyond his capacity to spend and enjoy.

George Bernard Shaw in a Fabian tract entitled "Socialism for Millionaires" is the first of the moderns to discuss this plight. "The unfortunate millionaire," he points out, "has the responsibilities of prodigious wealth without the possibility of enjoying himself any more than any ordinary rich man." "Indeed," he adds, "in many things he cannot enjoy himself more than many poor men do, nor even so much; for a drum-major is better dressed; a trainer's stable-lad often rides a better horse; the first-class carriage is shared by office boys taking their young ladies out for the evening; and of what use is it to be able to pay for a peacock's-brain sandwich when there is nothing to be had but ham or beef?"

The condition of the English man of wealth is exaggerated a hundredfold in the case of Americans, who during the past half-century have been heaping up fortunes hitherto undreamed of. And often the American millionaire has even less desire or capacity to use money for his own pleasure. In Europe habits of lavish spending have been built up over generations. Louis XIV poured a na-tion's riches into a great playhouse at Versailles. Huge estates, retinues of hundreds of servants and thousands of retainers, gaming at Monte Carlo, decorative and expensive mistresses—in such simple pastimes Europeans have sunk entire fortunes.

American men of great wealth have small tendency to such lavish expenditures. Their wives help a little; but after a few Paris gowns, a couple of town houses or country estates and the grand tour of the world even a wife gives up the unequal struggle of keeping pace with a husband's constantly swelling income. As American fortunes have grown by geometrical progression there has been literally nothing that could be done but either supinely to let them grow and so pass on the problem to the next generation or else to give them away. And the giving could not be done personally and piecemeal; huge sums had to be turned over *en bloc*.

Now the giving away of large amounts of money is no easy matter. The average person who contemplates longingly a large fortune thinks only of the joys of spending and the delights of giving to friends and pet charities. It seems pleasant and simple enough, but it isn't. Appeals pour in; insistent and ingenious beggars persistently hound any man suspected of charitable inclinations. It is difficult after the first flush of generosity for a rich man to take any joy in giving. Where gratitude is expected there appears only bitterness because the gifts were not larger.

45

Secretaries and assistants have to be employed simply to read mail and answer calls, to say nothing of looking into the merits of the thousands and tens of thousands of supplications.

One of the commonest criticisms of philanthropy is that it does not give freely to poor and unfortunate individuals. But the futility of alms is quickly recognized by any who try it. To give to a man to-day is simply to have that same man back to-morrow asking for twice as much. The answer at once is, "Do not give to the shiftless and unworthy; give only to the deserving." This is sound reasoning, but it implies some system of selection between the worthy and the unworthy. It is this process of investigating individual appeals that is most frequently objected to by many critics of organized charity. And it is the shiftless man who really needs the money—and who is most certain to keep on needing it. Beggars are real people. They are not simply industrious persons temporarily out of funds. They are usually life members of a large and very ancient profession which exists by living off others. These people can always make out cases for themselves, and as new sources of supply appear sycophants multiply egregiously.

If, on the other hand, a philanthropist tries to help only the deserving, he will find that he has to take infinite pains to sort them out from the thousands of clever beggars who beset him. Except for education or for some other very special purpose, giving even to worthy persons is dangerous. It is sinful to do for any individual what that individual can do for himself. This deprives a man of one of his greatest privileges, that of making his own place in the world in his own way.

Almost every rich man who is charitably inclined starts out with the idea of helping the poor and needy. Without exception he finds that he cannot do it directly. He can help to prevent the causes of misfortune such as disease and commercial exploitation. He can offer opportunities for education, for medical treatment, for self-respecting employment. He can better the general conditions of sanitation and social environment. But protection and opportunity having been provided, the individual must be left to take advantage of these for himself. That is the individual's obligation not only; it is one of his most precious prerogatives.

It is not easy to act wisely even in providing better general conditions. It is possible to do actual harm by indiscriminate giving. It takes brains as well as money to do any kind of good in the world.

For centuries the care of the sick poor was thought to be one of the highest forms of charity. Now we have found that it is possible to prevent a great many diseases as well as to cure them. The significant reduction of sickness and death came not from the centuries of charity but from the statesmanship that has wiped out smallpox and typhoid fever, that has greatly reduced malaria and diphtheria and tuberculosis, that has saved mothers at childbirth and nourished infants into robust health.

Even to-day the endowment of free hospitals is a favorite form of charity. Yet modern experience tends to prove that if medical services were organized half as effectively as the merchandising of other necessities the average man could pay for his medical care as well as for his food and shoes. And the average man would prefer to pay as he goes for what he gets in medicine as in other things. Wise philanthropists, therefore, are now giving attention to pay clinics, hourly nursing service, and health insurance.

Examples of generous but unwise giving are all about us. A few years ago a Pennsylvania millionaire made a sensation by leaving forty million dollars to build and support orphan asylums. His was a charitable aim at aiding innocent and unfortunate children, but there is doubt as to its wisdom. Orphan asylums do not offer the best environment. Modern thought and experience favor the placement of dependent children in foster homes. There is little difference of opinion on this matter among people who have devoted themselves to child care. Yet the very magnificence of this Pennsylvania gift will probably retard for decades the growth of home placement of children in that section of the country. By an irony which does not respect mere good intentions, this millionaire's generous impulse will very likely mean that the children of his State will be cared for under worse conditions than those in other parts of America.

A temptation to public-spirited men of wealth is to set up private agencies to perform public services. It is true that both stimulus and high standards often result from private efforts in such matters as schools, colleges, visiting-nurse agencies, and child-welfare clinics. But all these in a well-organized society are proper obligations of the State. If the private institutions are maintained only as a means of demonstrating to public authorities the value of these services or of keeping standards at a high level they are well justified. But too often the managers and patrons of private organizations become vain and desire to prolong their pet societies long after their usefulness is ended. Sometimes private groups actually enter into rivalry with public agencies and obstruct or postpone the proper development of important State services.

It requires painstaking thought and study to make sure that money is used not merely to perpetuate outworn forms of service. It takes courage to choose the slow road of prevention rather than the sentimentally pleasant path of present relief. Tact and imagination are necessary if one is to give in such a way as to strengthen rather than weaken the individual or group that receives help.

II

It was the sudden acquisition of huge fortunes in this country, together with the recognition that large-scale giving requires careful planning, which led to the creation of a great new force in society—the American foundations. At the turn of the century Mr. Carnegie and Mr. Rockefeller almost simultaneously hit upon this instrument for divesting themselves of huge blocks of their fortunes and of putting these funds to work constructively.

A few smaller foundations had been set up before the close of the nineteenth century. Mr. George Peabody had established a fund for Southern education and teacher training; Mr. John F. Slater had set up a trust for the aid of negro schools; and of course hospital and college endowments had received gifts for many centuries in both America and Europe. But the large general foundations of Rockefeller and Carnegie established new precedents, and started on a magnificent scale the American foundations as we know them to-day.

There are now some two hundred general foundations in America; their capital assets run to well over two billion dollars. And the newspapers report every few weeks the creation of another new fund by another new millionaire who either despairs of disposing of his money himself or desires to see it accomplish most for the benefit of society.

The distinctive features of these foundations are that large endowments are turned over with practically no restrictions to boards of trustees, and the administration and expenditure of the funds are in the hands of officers who devote their whole time to this work and are paid for their services. These officers often act also as advisers to the donor in his personal giving.

Since the giver himself is termed a philanthropist, and the recipient a philanthropee, some wag has suggested that these professional intermediaries between the donor and the recipient be called philanthropoids. The success of the given foundation is often found in the capacity of the philanthropoid—in the wisdom and resourcefulness of the directing head.

Foundations have usually chosen some special, limited field of activity and have cultivated that field intensively. A characteristic of the successful funds is that they are not charitable organizations in the regularly accepted sense; they are constructive forces, initiating or stimulating activity in a definite province. Some confusion has arisen in the public mind on this point. Many people, knowing of the large resources and broad powers of these trusts, have supposed they were ready and, in fact, morally obligated to give to any worthy cause which was properly presented. Disappointment and even resentment follow when foundations decline to consider projects which are of unquestioned merit in themselves. Yet a moment's reflection will convince anyone that only by aiming at definite goals can results be attained worthy of the potential power of these funds. To run deep it is necessary to keep the channel narrow; to exert power there must be concentration. To scatter attention and resources is simply to dissipate the great power for social good which is in the hands of modern foundations.

Hundreds of letters and personal calls come to each of the larger foundations every week. There are great numbers of appeals from individuals in distress. These must be referred to local relief agencies. Other calls come for the most bizarre causes. One man wants to establish a negro navy; another, who has operated for the correction of cross-eyes, suggests in all seriousness the establishment of a Cross-Eyed Foundation; another suggests the vast potentialities for social welfare in the manufacture of "gum garages"—small squares of paper provided in public places for the convenient parking of chewing gum. Endless varieties of quack medicines and sure cures for all diseases abound. One does not realize until he has been with a foundation how many ingenious devices there are for the salvation of the world.

Many requests of course are for significant enterprises. But even among these it is impossible to weigh the relative merits of each. Who can say whether the Shady Hill School in Cambridge is more meritorious than a tuberculosis sanitorium in Arizona; a concert singer more valuable to society than an anthropological explorer? Should one support educational broadcasting by radio and decline the appeal of the local relief society? Is chemistry at Harvard or history at Stanford the better subject for subsidy?

Confronted by diverse appeals pouring in by the scores and hundreds, and often sponsored by competent and influential persons, the individual rich man might answer according to his special interest, his changing whim, or his friendship for the particular applicant. But the president of a foundation, who must make out a case for each proposal he recommends to his trustees, must establish some basis of selection, some close limitation upon the kinds of appeals he will consider. And he must do so promptly if he is not to be submerged by appeals or torn asunder by enthusiastic and fanatical applicants.

Most of the foundations, therefore, however general their chartered purposes, have elected to pursue one or at most a very few types of work. Several of the funds already have made notable records in their special fields. Instances in point are the Rockefeller activities in medicine and health, the support of the social sciences by the Laura Spelman Rockefeller Memorial, the researches in natural science by the Carnegie Institution of Washington, and the negro school program of the Julius Rosenwald Fund.

III

The story of foundation achievements may properly start with the Rockefeller activities in medicine and health. There are a number of Rockefeller boards; their relationships are as difficult to untangle as those of the British Empire or

48

A total of more than two hundred million dollars has been spent by the Rockefeller boards in medicine and health. This is magnificent spending and it has produced magnificent results. When one includes the fundamental studies in medical science, the promotion of medical education and the world-wide stimulus to public health, it is safe to say that no influence in world history has been greater in advancing medicine and in reducing preventable sickness than that of the boards set up by Mr. Rockefeller.

IV

The foundations established by Mr. Carnegie have been more diffused in their activities. No one of them has made so distinctive a contribution as that of the Rockefeller group in medical science or public health. Probably the most significant of the activities of this group is the least generally known, the research in the natural sciences of the Carnegie Institution of Washington.

One of the ways of creating social energy that has been recognized by modern philanthropy is to produce new knowledge through research. The scientists who found a way to prevent typhoid and yellow fever furnished the means and created an urge in society to rid itself of these scourges. The researches of Faraday and the inventions of Edison aroused new demands in a thousand directions for the application of electricity to the service of men. Pure research of the most recondite sort must precede any progress in the application of science. Acting upon this principle, the Carnegie Institution for a quarter of a century has been supporting basic studies in many fields.

At Cold Spring Harbor on Long Island biologists have watched the fascinating vagaries of growth and evolution in such primitive forms of life as the jimson weed and the fruit fly, and have built up huge files of records of human families with a view to their possible bearing on eugenics—the purposeful control of human evolution. Stations in Carmel, California, in the Island of Tortugas, and in Baltimore and Boston are investigating plant and ocean life, the development of the human embryo, and the influence of various types of nutrition. In Guatemala and Yucatan spectacularly beautiful temples of the ancient Mayas have been unearthed. The researches of the Institution have been significant in themselves and have exerted throughout the country wide influence upon scientific standards and methods.

Another fundamental contribution to scientific research in a different group of subjects—the social sciences—has been made by the Laura Spelman Rockefeller Memorial under the leadership of Beardsley Ruml, one of the youngest of the philanthropoids and one who compares in his imagination and daring with Frederick T. Gates, the elder statesman. When Doctor Ruml began the direction of this newest of the Rockefeller boards he insisted that the same kind of sincere and realistic study which had brought striking results in medicine and machinery might if applied to economics, psychology, social problems, and political science bring findings of even greater benefit to mankind. This stand required courage, not alone because medicine at that time engaged the loyalty of the influential Rockefeller officers, but also because it was thought impolitic for any of the great foundations to take active part in social and economic questions.

Those whose memories go back to 1910 will recall that when the Rockefeller Foundation was attempting to obtain a federal charter from Congress the gravest fears were expressed as to the possible subversive influence upon the nation of these great agglutinations of wealth. Critics reported themselves as fearful that a private corporation with one hundred millions dollars at its disposal might become even more powerful than the Government itself and might use this great influence to destroy or pervert democratic institutions and the free play of liberal forces.

In view of the actual work of foundations and of the insignificance of their funds as compared with the expenditures which arose during the war period, these fears ceased to trouble and even began to appear absurd; nevertheless, there was natural hesitation on the part of responsible officers to see any organization bearing the Rockefeller name undertake activities in economics and politics. Ruml's reply to this was that his board would follow the usual foundation custom of not carrying on work directly but by supporting studies and demonstrations by other responsible bodies—universities, research institutes, and social agencies—and that the aim would be not to propagate any special theories but to bring about objective study of fundamental problems.

The program was started eight years ago. Contributions have been made to the social-science departments of a dozen leading American universities and to a number of institutions abroad. A national board of strategy has been set up—the Social Science Research Council —largely with support from this Fund. Opportunities have been provided at a number of University centers for realistic study of local problems. Stimulus has been given to efforts to apply the objective findings of research to improvement of government services and other types of social organization. In all, over twenty-five million dollars has been put into the social sciences and their application.

The Julius Rosenwald Fund, the largest of the foundations west of New York, has made its distinctive contribution in the building of negro schools. It is now beginning to promote pay clinics and organized medical services for the average man and is giving some consideration to the mental sciences and child development. But it will doubtless always retain a major interest in the negro, and its historic record is in the rural school program.

Mr. Rosenwald's interest in negro schools began fifteen or twenty years ago, when, as a trustee of Tuskegee Institute, he saw the great benefits that came to that race from the instruction which was being given under Booker Washington's direction in elementary subjects and farming and simple trades. He wanted to enlarge the influence of Tuskegee and to multiply these practical training courses throughout the South. He could have done this by building a number of private institutes. But Mr. Rosenwald knew something about the difficulties of making money really useful. He realized that the provision of schools for all groups of the population was a duty of the State. He saw that real progress could be made only as the local communities recognized this responsibility and acted upon it. Therefore, he offered not to build schools himself, but to co-operate with counties and states which wished to build their own public schools for negroes. The result has been five thousand new schools, trade shops, and teachers' homes in eight hundred and twenty-five counties of fifteen Southern States built with help from Mr. Rosenwald and from the Fund that he created. Of even greater significance than the schools themselves is the fact that the South has recognized its obligation for public schools for all groups. Momentum has been given to negro education and good race relations. The method of the giving has been worth many times the amount of money contributed.

The cost of the five thousand "Rosenwald Schools" is well above twenty-four million dollars, in addition to millions each year for maintenance and teachers' salaries. Of these sums the Fund and Mr. Rosenwald personally have given in all less than four million dollars. More than that has been contributed by the negroes themselves in collections of dimes and quarters and dollars from thousands of villages and farms—a striking evidence of the negro's eagerness for schooling for his children.

White citizens have provided by personal gifts more than another million. The great bulk of the money has come from the regular taxes. The task of the Julius Rosenwald Fund has been simply to prime the pump, to start a stream which has continued to flow in an ever-increasing volume. Yet the influence and stimulus of this Fund has transformed school conditions in the rural South for one great group of the population.

Other foundations have made distinctive contributions in their chosen fields. The activities that have been discussed are simply illustrative of the general principles and procedures common to many of these new trusts.

V

The subjects most popular with foundations are education, health, and scientific research. Two fields seem to have received less attention than they deserve: the mental sciences and the fine arts.

In mental hygiene, it is true, the Commonwealth Fund has made important contributions, and other foundations have flirted with the subject. But when one realizes that as many patients are in mental hospitals in this country as in hospitals for all other diseases put together, that in so progressive a country as Canada more persons in 1926 entered insane institutions than were graduated from all the colleges of the Dominion; when the individual suffering and the social havoc that follow mental disease and deficiency are kept in mind, one would suppose that the great forces of the foundations would turn to these problems however difficult and complex they may be.

The omission of the fine arts is more in keeping with the times and the American spirit. We worship just now social betterment as represented in public health, literacy, and prosperity; we revel in active combat whether in commercial business or in a struggle to search out the secrets of nature.

The arts still seem a bit ladylike to the robust American. The Juilliard Foundation in music is the only large fund devoted exclusively to any of the arts. The General Education Board has made one or two studies in industrial art, and the Carnegie Corporation is fingering somewhat gingerly a program in the fine arts; but no board has actually dirtied its hands with paint or clay or fabrics, or risked its morals with the drama or with the popular embodiment of the fine arts to-day—the talking movies.

This aloofness to art is not the historic attitude of wealth. Of old the monarchs and nobles and rich men of Europe and the East lavished their patronage upon religious temples and creations of art. Pericles is remembered not so much for his wealth or his civil administration as for the public buildings and statues and frescoes which flowered in Athens under his nourishing care. The Medicis have been exonerated for much of their cruelty because of their sympathetic support of artistic expression. Elizabeth's reign is memorable for its writers and dramatists. The pride of former European men of wealth was their patronage of arts and of artists.

As America absorbs her frontiers, and as wealth mellows in the possession of the third and fourth generations, doubtless there will be a revival of interest in creative expression. Meanwhile philanthropy probably does well to concentrate upon those things which are in accordance with America's present peculiar genius: intensive accumulation of knowledge (as well as of wealth) and the active application of scientific findings to organized social welfare.

If one were making general criticisms he might say that aside from a few notable instances, foundations have not found sufficiently capable men for their directors and that there is still some tendency on the part of founders to dictate or exert pressure as to the expenditure of funds which legally they have turned over completely to trustees and their elected officers.

The potential power of these concentrations of wealth can be realized only if there is freedom of action, coupled with imagination and resourcefulness in their direction.

If millionaires in their own giving are often actuated by whim and vanity, it is equally true that foundation officers and trustees may be a prey to timidity and lack of vision. To suppose that any social worker or former college professor will work miracles simply because he is in the presence of wealth is nonsense. Mediocrity, which is the curse of democracies, cannot be transformed merely by millions.

The fear that foundations will subvert democracy is pretty well answered. They have neither money enough nor brains enough to do it if they wished. The real danger is that they will have no influence of any consequence in any direction; that they will fritter away their potential power in small and insignificant enterprises.

There is danger also that as time goes on the officers and trustees of foundations will become perfunctory and routinized; that they will grow fat in posts which may easily become sinecures; that the whole organization will sink into commonplace bureaucracy. There is already some evidence of this in certain of the foundations. To guard against it several recent founders have stipulated that their funds, both capital and income, must be expended within a generation. There is much to be said for using resources while enthusiasm is fresh and while the group is fired by almost religious fervor for some cause. Succeeding generations may be counted upon to provide new resources, through new foundations or otherwise, for the recurring needs and the fresh opportunities.

VI

Underlying the various activities of practically all of the foundations is a common philosophy which is the essence of modern philanthropy and the antithesis of traditional almsgiving. The aim is to give as little as possible for as short a time as possible. Should any of their projects become permanently dependent upon their help, foundations would feel that they had failed. To anyone imbued with the ancient ideal this will seem strange philanthropy. But a moment's reflection will reveal the soundness of the principle.

It is a safe rule never to do anything for the public, any more than for an individual, that the public will do for itself. Private funds should be used not to satisfy existing "social appetites" but to stimulate new appetites. Thus benefactors can create energy in the only fundamentally possible way—by creating fresh needs and by getting these new needs recognized by the public.

Inertia and human contentment with things as they are often prevent or postpone new movements, though these movements may promise much for the welfare and happiness of men. The chief contributions of foundations are in the creation of new knowledge through scientific research and in getting new enterprises started and proving to society that these proposals are desirable and feasible.

The new philanthropy does not want or need endowments in perpetuity. If a cause is good it can count upon current support, once its usefulness is made evident. We may be confident that if a public need is clearly demonstrated and a practicable way of meeting that need is shown society will take care of it in the future. Thus one of the purposes of foundations is to make themselves unnecessary.

The Julius Rosenwald Fund

JULIUS ROSENWALD FUND

REVIEW OF
TWO DECADES
1917-1936

BY
EDWIN R. EMBREE
PRESIDENT OF THE FUND

CHICAGO
1936

JULIUS ROSENWALD FUND

CLASSIFICATION OF EXPENDITURES
DURING THE TWO DECADES OF ITS LIFE
1917-1936

I.	Negro School Building Program	$5,165,281
II.	Negro University Centers	1,276,508
III.	Negro Colleges and High Schools	822,083
IV.	Negro Fellowships	437,615
V.	Negro Health	857,507
VI.	Other Negro Activities	257,860
	Total Negro Activities	$ 8,816,854
VII.	Medical Services	994,794
VIII.	Library Service	653,118
IX.	General Education	902,317
X.	Social Studies	279,883
XI.	Race Relations	331,289
XII.	Rural Education	60,453
XIII.	Miscellaneous Gifts	620,496
	Total General Activities	$ 3,842,350
XIV.	Administration	576,879
	Grand Total	$13,236,083

Of this total, $4,039,051 was expended during the early period, 1917-1927, almost exclusively on the Negro school building program, and $9,197,032 was expended during the second period, 1928-1936, on the enlarged activities.

TWO DECADES

OF THE

JULIUS ROSENWALD FUND

THE life of the Fund has covered two distinct periods of approximately a decade each. During the first period, from its creation in 1917 through the year 1927, the Fund was devoted to a special program of helping to build schoolhouses for Negroes in the southern states and was administered directly by its founder, Julius Rosenwald. During the second period, the Fund was enlarged into a general foundation under the control of an active and responsible Board of Trustees and under the direction of a group of officers who gave their full time to the work. In this period the activities of the Fund were expanded to include various aspects of Negro education and welfare and also programs in medical economics, library service, general education, social studies, race relations, and, more recently, a special effort in rural education.

In order that our activities over the entire period might be reviewed, the officers prepared and presented to a recent meeting of the trustees of the Fund detailed reports of expenditures and services since the establishment of the trust on October 30, 1917. It seems appropriate to take advantage of the material assembled for the trustees to give also a public accounting of our stewardship.

The table on the opposite page gives a list of the expenditures by the Fund for all of its philanthropic activities from its incorporation to the close of the past fiscal year, June 30, 1936. Of the total payments of

[1]

approximately thirteen and a quarter million dollars ($13,236,083) slightly less than one third ($4,039,051) was expended during the first period (1917 to 1927), almost exclusively on the school building program, while more than two thirds ($9,197,032) was expended during the eight years of the second period (July 1, 1928, to June 30, 1936) on its enlarged activities. On pages 22 to 49 are given detailed reports, consisting of financial tables and verbal statements, of the expenditures and services under the various programs which the Fund has undertaken.

The Julius Rosenwald Fund was incorporated on October 30, 1917, under the laws of the State of Illinois as a corporation not for profit. It was authorized to receive and disburse funds for philanthropic causes, the purpose as stated in the charter being, "for the well-being of mankind." The corporation was established at the initiative of Julius Rosenwald, Chicago merchant and philanthropist, who furnished the original endowment and from time to time contributed additional large sums. While Mr. Rosenwald was the founder and chief patron, gifts have from time to time been received from other donors, for example, from the estate of Theodore Max Troy of Jacksonville, Florida, $20,195; from the Rosenwald Family Association, $69,119; and from the Carnegie Corporation for support of the program of library extension, $200,000. Small gifts have also been received from individuals who were interested in one or another of the activities of the Fund.

The gifts from Mr. Rosenwald were chiefly in the form of shares of the capital stock of Sears, Roebuck and Co. These gifts of stock, together with stock

[2]

dividends upon them, reached a total of 227,874 shares, which at one time in the autumn of 1928 had a market value of slightly more than forty million dollars.

The management of the Fund has from the beginning been vested in a Board of Trustees. This board at the outset consisted of four persons: Mr. Rosenwald and three members of his immediate family. At the re-organization of the Fund in 1928, the board was enlarged and now consists of eleven members chosen from the nation at large. The board is an autonomous body with full responsibility, within the laws of the State of Illinois, for the management of the corporation, including the election of succeeding trustees. (A list of present and past trustees of the Fund is given on page 52.)

In organizing the Fund, Mr. Rosenwald incorporated a provision which is unusual in such a trust: namely, that the endowment should not be treated as a perpetuity but might be expended at any time in the discretion of the trustees and must be entirely expended within twenty-five years of the founder's death. Mr. Rosenwald was suspicious of the bureaucratic and reactionary attitude that easily develops in the trustees of large endowments held in perpetuity. He was opposed to the influence of the dead hand in philanthropy or in other human affairs. At the inauguration of the en-larged Board of Trustees in 1928, Mr. Rosenwald wrote to them as follows:

> I am not in sympathy with [the] policy of perpetuating endowments and believe that more good can be accomplished by expending funds as Trustees find opportunities for constructive work than by storing up large sums of money for long periods of time. By adopting a policy of using the Fund within this generation, we may avoid

[3]

those tendencies toward bureaucracy and a formal or perfunctory attitude toward the work which almost inevitably develop in organizations which prolong their existence indefinitely. Coming generations can be relied upon to provide for their own needs as they arise.

In accepting the shares of stock now offered, I ask that the Trustees do so with the understanding that the entire fund in the hands of the Board, both income and principal, be expended within twenty-five years of the time of my death.

No act of Mr. Rosenwald's life aroused more interest and discussion than his stand against perpetual endowments. More comment, even than upon the creation of the foundation itself, was caused by the stipulation that the Fund should expend its total resources—principal as well as income—upon current needs and should exist for not more than one generation. This principle of using funds while needs were clear and interest fresh Mr. Rosenwald maintained in his own giving not only but urged as national policy in many speeches and articles, particularly in two papers published in *The Atlantic Monthly* respectively in May, 1929, and in December, 1930*.

FINANCIAL PROBLEMS

The problem of dissolving endowments is not as acute today as it was nine brief years ago when Mr. Rosenwald stipulated a short and vigorous life for the Fund. Crashing markets, limits on credit, and appalling human needs have shattered endowments, have aroused a surging public opinion in favor of using as contrasted to hoarding, and have offered so many crying appeals for philanthropic funds that there is no difficulty in

*Reprints of these articles, as of other pamphlets issued from time to time by the Fund, will be sent free to anyone on application to the Secretary, Julius Rosenwald Fund, 4901 Ellis Avenue, Chicago.

[4]

expending all that is available. The pendulum has swung so far to the other extreme that the question now is as to conserving endowments—especially those of universities, hospitals, and such permanently needed institutions—so that there may be some continuity of program and of leadership.

In the case of the Julius Rosenwald Fund, the reorganized Board received its commission from its founder just as the market was in the midst of its tremendous upswing and when financiers and statesmen were prophesying a permanent new era of prosperity. During this period, with the vigorous approval of the founder, the Fund expanded its programs and greatly increased the size and scope of its appropriations. Still, during 1928 and 1929, we could not keep pace in our spending with the rapid rise in the market value of our securities—let alone begin to make any inroads upon our capital values. During the eighteen-month period from April, 1928, through September, 1929, the trustees appropriated over five million dollars; yet during the same period, in addition to cash income currently received, the market value of our securities rose from $20,000,000 to $35,000,000, an increase on paper of three times as much as we had appropriated. Our donations were also largely on paper, for the great bulk of the appropriations were payable gradually over periods of five to seven years, or were payable only after fixed conditions had been met, many of these conditions requiring efforts which would necessarily cover several years.

Then came the crash and the succeeding dismal ebb of values which did not turn until the spring of 1933. Commitments which had been made when our securities had a market value of about $200 per share fell due when these same securities could be sold only at a fraction of

[5]

61

that figure. Furthermore, the needs in all the fields of our interest increased and multiplied. Unless we were to abandon institutions and movements with which we had identified ourselves, we not only had to meet past pledges but were also under obligation to continue to help in every way possible by additional resources and fresh stimulus.

It is fitting and proper even in a factual report to salute the courage and the persistent devotion to programs which the trustees showed during the dark years, especially from 1931 through 1934. At a time when the pattern was fright, timidity, rigid hoarding of whatever one might still have left, the Fund, while necessarily reducing new appropriations, did not withhold payments due, did not cut important personnel, did not cease contributing leadership and also money to the movements it was sponsoring. It is in fact probable that the Fund's influence was greater during the depression era than during any other period in its history.

It is not to be denied that during the mid-depression years a great deal of financial negotiating had to be done in order to avoid complete dissipation of resources and thus an ending of aid and influence at just the time when it seemed most needed. Here are some of the things we did.

In the case of pledges to endowments of institutions we arranged to pay not the capital but interest for a period of years until the principal could be turned over with less loss to the Fund. On such capital gifts totaling $611,583, we paid interest at the rate of 5 per cent per annum for periods varying from three to five years. (All these capital grants have now been paid, although a part of one of them, the sum of $166,667 to Provident Hospital, Chicago, was paid after the close of the fiscal year covered by this report.)

[6]

In the case of certain large pledges for current expense —as for example for county library demonstrations in the southern states—it proved convenient to the beneficiaries as well as to us to spread these payments over a longer period than originally contemplated, thus reducing the costs in the mid-depression years but not necessarily reducing the total amounts to be paid.

Two of the larger foundations in New York came most generously to the assistance not so much of the Fund as of institutions which would have suffered if continued contributions had not been forthcoming. The General Education Board, interested as we are in Negro education, made a number of emergency grants totaling $257,000 to various Negro schools and colleges, thus relieving the Fund of the need of additional grants or in some cases making possible postponement of our payments on current pledges without hardship or loss to the institution concerned. (All of those grants which were made on a repayment basis have been repaid and all of the pledges which were postponed because of the emergency grants of the General Education Board have since been paid in full.) The Carnegie Corporation, which has long had a special interest in library service, made grants totaling $200,000 in 1932 and 1933 directly to the Fund to enable it to carry on with undiminished vigor its program of library extension in southern counties.

By herculean efforts (which are pleasanter to look back upon than they were to go through) we struggled, on the one hand, to avoid sudden dissipation of our resources and, on the other hand, to avoid decreasing the total help available to institutions and causes which needed us more than ever before. We continued our full force of executive officers and counseling staff. In fact, we increased both the extent and the vigor of our

[7]

63

intellectual services since necessarily we could not increase our financial aid. But even in money our contributions were substantial right through the depression. For the five years from July 1, 1931, to June 30, 1936, the Fund paid out on account of its philanthropic activities a total of $4,207,127, an average of approximately $840,000 a year. Our payments during the past fiscal year, July 1, 1935, to June 30, 1936, amounted to a total of slightly more than one million dollars ($1,079,983).

In order to avoid sacrifice of securities, a part of our payments during these years were financed by bank loans rather than by sale of stock. These loans have now been entirely repaid.

To meet pledges and to continue active contributions the Fund has naturally had to expend a considerable portion of its capital. In addition to expending the total of our income from year to year, we have consumed somewhat more than two thirds of the securities which make up our endowment. While during the depression stocks had to be sold at unexpectedly low figures, the use of capital and the continuation of vigorous programs were in accordance with the desire and instructions of the founder as well as in accordance with the best judgment of the trustees.

With pledges paid and debts cleared the Fund enters another era with resources modest compared with the period of 1928 and 1929 but substantial when compared with the days of 1932 and 1933. As of November, 1936, the capital of the Fund in cash and securities has a value of approximately seven million dollars.

The stipulations of the founder and the judgment of the Board both look toward continued expenditure of principal as well as income. Since we must complete

[8]

our work within twenty-five years of Mr. Rosenwald's death (which occurred January 6, 1932) the possible life of the Fund is not beyond January 6, 1957, or about twenty more years. It is likely that the policies of the Board and opportunities for useful expenditures will bring the corporation to a close still earlier.

During the period of large resources the Fund carried out its programs largely through gifts to other agencies: public school systems, universities, health agencies, special organizations and committees. But during the depression years we had such small funds that outside grants had to be curtailed and our influence was exerted chiefly through studies, experiments, and consultant services of our own staff. We found these direct efforts so effective that even with enlarged resources we are continuing to make them a large factor in our programs. This policy is by no means new in foundation history. The Russell Sage Foundation and the Carnegie Foundation for the Advancement of Teaching, among the older trusts, have exerted their chief efforts through the studies and activities of their own staffs. Many of the newer and smaller foundations also have emphasized this procedure.

Foundations have a field of usefulness in America through both methods. The larger trusts are almost forced to a policy of disbursement, since it would be cumbersome and inefficient for them to organize under their own auspices staffs and services sufficient to expend the huge sums annually available to them. Furthermore, the large foundations can transform institutions and movements by the very magnitude of the new resources they are able to contribute. Rockefeller gifts,

[9]

65

for example, made possible such notable achievements as the creation of a great university in the capital of the Mid-West, the enlargement of public health facilities on a world-wide scale, the transformation of standards in medical education throughout America, the creation of a notable medical center in the Far East, the enlargement of the scope of research and teaching in the social sciences. Carnegie gifts established library service on a high plane throughout the country, greatly enriched certain medical centers, and are now enlarging the facilities of the nation in creative art and in popular art appreciation. The smaller foundations, on the other hand, cannot donate sums large enough in themselves to affect greatly the nation-wide needs of universities, research institutes, or service agencies. These smaller trusts, however, can often exert important influence by their own direct efforts.

Direct effort involves a different kind of responsibility from a program of disbursement. In giving away money a foundation need only assure itself of the general soundness and effectiveness of the recipient institutions; responsibility for all action and operation is left to the agencies which accept the gifts. But when a foundation makes its own studies and experiments, when it promotes demonstrations or publishes findings and recommendations under its own name, it assumes a heavy and direct responsibility. It must assure itself not only of the integrity but also of the wisdom and incisive intelligence of its staff and its operating agencies. This is an obligation which foundation trustees are usually willing to delegate to other organizations.

There is, however, a good deal to be said for direct effort. Foundations as organized in America have been peculiarly free of political pressures and private jeal-

[10]

66

ousies. They should be in a better position than most other agencies to study problems objectively and to promote fresh attacks on social complexes. Such studies can also be conducted by universities, but foundations can more readily help to translate research into action. Foundations can quickly and effectively assemble wise groups of investigators and consultants. They can with least risk to themselves or to society make carefully controlled social and educational experiments. They are in a strong position to promote demonstrations and to urge consideration of new methods of handling public problems which otherwise are in danger of being obscured by tradition, prejudice, and vested interest.

The choice between the two policies is not so much a question of the superiority of one method over the other as of expediency and effectiveness for the given foundation. The educational and social institutions of the nation are greatly enriched and strengthened by the magnificent donations which after careful study are bestowed by the larger foundations. The public weal can probably also be advanced by a continuation of the studies, experiments, and consultation services carried on under the direct responsibility of independent trusts.

While the Julius Rosenwald Fund will not cease to make grants to other agencies, its trustees have voted to continue "aggressive programs of investigation, experiment, demonstration, and stimulation" in the several fields in which it works.

[11]

67

V. NEGRO HEALTH

The general strategy of the Negro health program as conducted since 1928 includes:

(1) Enlisting the facilities and prestige of the United States Public Health Service (through a member of its staff designated as the Fund's consultant in Negro health) to arouse and extend the interest of southern health departments and other agencies in Negro health needs and in practical steps toward meeting them; also enlisting other important national agencies such as the National Tuberculosis Association and the National Organization for Public Health Nursing to supplement the Public Health Service.

(2) Aid in developing a limited number of hospitals for Negroes, conducted as demonstrations of high standards and as training centers for Negro physicians, nurses, and administrators.

(3) Encouraging the use in health departments and voluntary agencies of Negro physicians and nurses, particularly public health nurses, and assisting in establishing satisfactory training for them.

(4) Developing practicable methods of health education for school teachers, school children, and communities, according to policies and levels of expense suited to southern conditions.

The greatest amount of our contributions has gone into the development of sixteen hospitals and clinics widely distributed throughout the North and the South. The most notable single institution is Provident Hospital, Chicago, which in direct affiliation with the University of Chicago has built up a remarkably fine Negro medical staff and is in a position to offer post-graduate instruction and experience to physicians and health workers generally.

The employment of Negro public health nurses has proceeded by leaps and bounds and is now an established practice in southern counties and northern cities. The campaigns against the great scourges of tuberculosis and syphilis have proved that it is possible and financially feasible to control these plagues. With the enlargement of public health appropriations which are already apparent, campaigns against these diseases are likely to be put into effect increasingly. In the control of contagious diseases it is especially clear that the well-being of the whole population is dependent upon the health of each group.

[37]

68

VII. MEDICAL SERVICES

Throughout the eight years of the work in medical services, the chief aim has been to make good medical care more widely and easily available to persons of moderate and low incomes. To this end we have studied and encouraged (1) plans which make it possible for people to budget the uneven and unpredictable costs of sickness through insurance or taxation, (2) plans which will reduce the costs of medical care and improve its quality through better organization of professional services. Methods by which we have pursued these ends include the following:

1. Studies of the economic, administrative, and social aspects of medical services.
2. Studies and appraisals of new plans and experiments in group payment and in organized medical services.
3. Advisory and consultant service to professional groups, community agencies, and medical institutions with respect to existing or proposed plans.
4. Financial aid to a few selected plans or experiments.
5. Dissemination of our own studies and reports, and of information concerning the social and economic aspects of medical service to physicians, other professional groups, and to the public.
6. Consultation and conference with other agencies active in this field to promote coordination of work and an effective division of labor.

The Fund's officers (a) took a substantial part in the initiation, organization, and researches of the Committee on the Costs of Medical Care (to which the Fund contributed $90,000); (b) in cooperation with other foundations and agencies, gave wide distribution to this committee's studies and reports; (c) participated with the American Hospital Association in the recent development of voluntary insurance for hospital care ("group hospitalization") now established in some sixty cities; (d) carried on studies in the financial and community aspects of hospitals through the American Hospital Association and in education in hospital administration through the University of Chicago; (e) made studies and carried out practical programs in public health, rural hospitals, and public medical care through participation in the work of the President's Committee on Economic Security, the United States Public Health Service, and voluntary agencies; (f) served as coordinating influences in the work of foundations and other organizations interested in medical economics.

[41]

THE NEW PHILANTHROPY

The activities of the Fund described in these pages are more or less unrelated and as the years go on, the dispersion of the objects of our interest may increase. A survey of almost any of the large foundations will disclose an absence of close associations among its activities. So far as the Julius Rosenwald Fund is concerned, we are not occupied exclusively with the South, with persons of limited means, with schools, libraries or health or with any single class, race, region or cause. While, in order to accomplish measurable results, we shall naturally concentrate our efforts from time to time on a few objectives, we conceive it our duty to engage our resources wherever we believe they will count most toward our broad chartered purpose, "the well-being of mankind."

Whatever the specific activities, there is underlying all of them a common philosophy, which we believe to be the essence of modern philanthropy and the antithesis of traditional almsgiving. To any one imbued with the ancient ideal, ours will seem strange philanthropy. Our aim is to give as little as possible for as short a time as possible. Should any of our projects become permanently dependent upon our help, we should feel that we had failed.

A moment's reflection will disclose why we do not give alms for the temporary relief of suffering humanity. It is not for lack of sympathy nor is it because we fear the exhaustion of our funds–for the donor of the Fund has authorized the trustees to expend capital as well as in-

[4]

71

terest at any time they think best, and has required that the Fund must be entirely disbursed within this generation. The reason for our attitude is that we wish to make the Fund count for permanent gains for mankind.

The new philosophy is well illustrated in the work of the International Health Board of the Rockefeller Foundation. That Board demonstrates to communities in many lands that hookworm and other diseases can be eradicated at small cost and with immense profit, both in health and in economic well-being. As soon as the demonstration has been made, the Board prepares to withdraw, leaving the continuation of the task to public agencies. Similarly the Julius Rosenwald Fund has been proving to both races in the South that Negro schools are worth all they may cost the tax payer. Once built, the schools are maintained from taxes, and as time goes on the Fund may withdraw from this whole program with assurance that the schools will go on and multiply. In building apartment houses the purpose has been not to care for a few hundred families but to point the way to safe investment of private capital on a business basis in modern housing. In medical services we plan to make a series of demonstrations, confident that after an initial period pay clinics will prove self-supporting and other types of medical care will enlist whatever public support they require.

Foundations recognize that inertia and human contentment with things as they are often prevent or postpone new movements, though these movements may promise much for the welfare and happiness of man.

[5]

Our chief contributions are in getting new enterprises started and in proving to society that these proposals are desirable and feasible. George Bernard Shaw was one of the first exponents of this philosophy of giving. In an essay entitled "Socialism for Millionaires" published in the Contemporary Review in February, 1896, and reprinted as a Fabian tract, he pointed out in trenchant style the futility of giving to causes already accepted. "A safe rule," he said to his millionaires, "is never to do anything for the public, any more than for an individual, that the public will do for itself." He urged the use of funds not to satisfy existing "social appetites" but to create new appetites. "Never give the people anything they want," he said; "give them something they ought to want and don't." Thus he claimed benefactors could create energy in the only fundamentally possible way: by creating fresh needs and by getting these new needs recognized by the public.

There is another way of creating social energy which the new philanthropy has seized upon: the creation of new knowledge through research. The scientists who found a way to prevent typhoid and yellow fever created an urge in society to rid itself of these scourges. The researches of Faraday and the inventions of Edison created new demands in a thousand directions for the application of electricity to the service of man. Pasteur's discoveries offer the supreme example of the creation of energy, which resulted in striking improvements in man's condition. There is reason to hope that scientific studies of human relations and behavior may,

[6]

in time, show the way and create the desire to abolish mental and social ills as Pasteur created the desire and the means of controlling bacterial diseases.

The new philanthropy does not want or need endowments in perpetuity. If a cause is good it can count upon current support, once its usefulness is demonstrated; if it is poor, it ought not to be bolstered up by permanent endowment. One of the obstructions to progress is vested interests in things as they are. For example, home care for dependent children advances slowly partly because of the large trust funds held in perpetuity by orphanages; endowed societies often prevent or postpone the taking over by public funds of schooling, public health nursing or other welfare activities. We may be confident that if a public need is clearly demonstrated and a practicable way of meeting that need is shown, society will take care of it in the future.

The Julius Rosenwald Fund will continue to seek out experimental fields and to cultivate them intensively for a period. If an activity we espouse proves impracticable or unnecessary, we have made a mistake though we have probably served society by making clear the futility of that particular proposal; if the movement remains dependent upon us for support we have failed; if its usefulness becomes apparent and the work is carried on and extended to other communities we withdraw as rapidly as possible and feel we have succeeded. Our success is measured not only by the judgment we show in the projects we initiate or support but also by the ease and promptness with which our help may be ended.

[7]

74

JULIUS ROSENWALD FUND

Eight Years' Work
in Medical Economics, 1929-1936

Recent Trends and Next Moves
in Medical Care

CHICAGO

1937

JULIUS ROSENWALD FUND

EIGHT YEARS' WORK
IN MEDICAL ECONOMICS, 1929-1936

WHEN the Julius Rosenwald Fund was reorganized in 1928 as a national foundation, with an independent Board of Trustees and a substantial capital, one of its first interests was the economics of medical services. Mr. Rosenwald and the officers of the Fund had been impressed with the development of pay clinics in New York as a measure which, without charity and without profit, would bring the cost of expert medical care within the purse of the man of modest income.

AIMS OF WORK

Throughout the Fund's program in medical services, the aim has been to make good medical care more readily available to persons of moderate and low incomes by reducing sickness costs or by making it easier for people to pay them. Medical care can be made better by improved personnel and by more effective organization. Medical care can be made more widely available either by reducing costs or by increasing the ability to pay them. It was recognized that costs can be reduced by prevention of sickness (public health measures) and that ability or willingness to pay can be increased through more intelligent public demand (health education). But, leaving preventive and educational measures

[3]

to other well-established agencies, the Fund made a more direct approach to the problems of sickness costs.

In the first place, the Fund acted upon the principle that the costs of a given type and amount of medical service may be reduced through better organization and administration. The principle of the coordination of specialists, recognized as essential in business and in education, has not been applied sufficiently in health services. By studying and promoting the better organization and administration of hospitals and clinics, the Fund has taken steps to reduce the costs of producing good medical care. In the second place, the ability to pay for medical services may be increased by improved methods of individual or group budgeting. Such devices as installments, insurance, and taxation permit the individual to remove sickness costs from the category of economic "hazards," and to place medical care in his budget along with other necessities. The Fund has made special studies of these methods of payment and has attempted to influence attitudes and action concerning them.

METHODS

From the beginning our methods of work have included two phases: scientific studies and the encouragement of action. A more detailed list of the methods pursued includes the following.

> Studies of the economic, administrative, and social aspects of medical services;
>
> Studies and appraisals of new plans and experiments in group payment and in organized medical care;
>
> Advisory and consultant service to professional groups, community agencies, and medical institu-

[4]

77

tions with respect to existing or proposed plans;

Financial aid to a few selected plans or experiments;

Dissemination of our own studies and reports, and of information concerning the social and economic aspects of medical service: to physicians, to other professional groups, and to the public;

Consultation and conference with other agencies active in this field to promote common planning and an effective division of labor.

STIMULUS AND SUBSIDY

Direct financial subsidy to projects in the field has occupied a minor place. The Fund's resources, even at their peak, were limited as compared with those of several other foundations. But a policy of stimulus rather than subsidy has been maintained also because of a philosophy strongly held by Julius Rosenwald, and shared by the officers of the Fund, that enterprises which were self-supporting through payment by beneficiaries, or through absorption into the permanent social structure of government, were to be preferred to those which would require continual charitable gifts or subvention. The field of medical care lent itself to such a policy, particularly the work of hospitals and clinics, the area in which the Fund's medical interests have been chiefly expressed.

For a generation or more, hospitals and clinics have brought together an ever-enlarging investment of social capital on the one side, and an ever-improving organization of professional skill on the other. While the hospital and clinic by no means include all medical service, they do represent a focal point and the future center of the community organization of medical care.

[5]

78

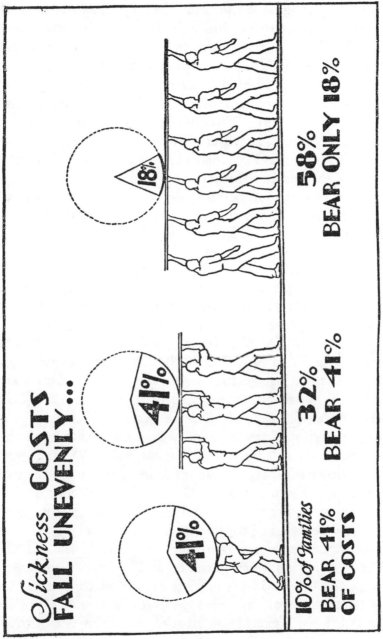

Sickness COSTS FALL UNEVENLY...

41%

41%

18%

10% of Families BEAR 41% OF COSTS

32% BEAR 41%

58% BEAR ONLY 18%

[6]

We have recognized the threat brought by institutional organization to the individuality of physician and patient alike, but we have believed that this problem can be solved by adequate administration. Its solution, moreover, is facilitated in proportion as the patient is not merely a recipient of charity but is an individual who pays his way. This is the principle incorporated in the pay clinic, in which physicians receive compensation for their services, instead of being expected to give them free, and in which patients pay the current costs of care instead of being objects of charity. Several projects will be described which involve this principle and which were aided by the Fund.

PAY CLINICS

Recognizing that a new project like a pay clinic, while it may ultimately be self-supporting, can only build up public and professional confidence gradually, the Fund as one of its first acts in the field of medical services made a grant of $250,000 to the University of Chicago Clinics, then just getting under way. These clinics are now the outstanding example of a large pay clinic in the United States. The Fund's grant, which was paid over a period of seven years, was conditioned upon the University's raising an additional $100,000 each year from other sources. These gifts, in addition to those of the General Education Board, were badly needed during the initial years and especially in the depression. The Clinics' record of progress during the "bad years" has been remarkable. A continued increase in the attendance of ambulatory patients and in the number of occupied hospital beds has been manifest through years when paying patients were declining in almost all other institutions. Several special studies of the work of these

[7]

80

Clinics have been made, one of which was financed and published by the Fund.*

Early in 1929, an active part was taken by officers of the Fund in the reorganization of another important, already well-established, pay clinic in Chicago, the Public Health Institute. The Institute had been founded shortly after the war by a group of leading business men of Chicago as a non-profit pay clinic for venereal disease, had become the largest venereal disease clinic in the country, and had accumulated a substantial surplus beyond its expenses. From the first it had utilized paid advertising in local newspapers as one of the means of informing the public concerning the dangers of syphilis and gonorrhea and of the Institute's facilities and charges for treatment. On the ground of its advertising and of "unfair competition with private practice," the clinic had been regarded as "unethical" by the Chicago Medical Society, and its medical staff was not admitted to membership.

In the spring of 1929, the Society expelled Dr. Louis E. Schmidt, a urologist of national reputation, because of an alleged indirect connection with the Institute. The accompanying fracas attracted national attention, and the advantages and disadvantages of pay clinics in general and of this particular clinic were brought into the limelight. By arrangement with the trustees of the Public Health Institute, the Fund brought to Chicago at the Institute's invitation, Dr. Harold N. Cole, Dr. Edward L. Keyes, and Dr. Thomas Parran, three physicians of the highest standing as specialists respectively

---

*Emmet B. Bay, M.D., *The Quality of Care Rendered at the University of Chicago Clinics*, 1932.

[8]

81

in syphilis, gonorrhea and public health administration. Their careful study of the Institute's professional services and policies was published in March, 1930, and while pointing out certain detailed criticisms, gave them on the whole high commendation. As the outcome of their report, a Medical Advisory Board of seven distinguished physicians of Chicago was organized by the trustees of the Institute with the participation of one of the officers of the Fund. This Board brought to Chicago two physicians of distinctive qualifications to head the two departments of the Institute treating syphilis and gonorrhea respectively. The Board also formulated policies to govern the Institute's advertising, recognizing the broad principle that medical advertising should serve as a public-health and educational measure rather than a competitive or business function.

The Medical Advisory Board's work was carried on for three years, and since it was disbanded the Institute's professional activities have continued on the same high plane which the Board established.* The use of advertising by or in behalf of medical agencies was at this time called to public attention, and the Fund commissioned Miss Mary Ross of New York to make a thorough study of the use of advertising by medical and dental societies, clinics, and other professional groups. Her extensive report was published in 1932.

The Fund supplied a small grant to help the psychiatric pay clinic of the Institute of Mental Hygiene in Philadelphia get under way in 1931-32. Another grant was made to the Union Health Center of New York, a general pay clinic maintained by the Garment

*The type of human service rendered by the Institute was reported in a study supported and published by the Fund: Bernard Regenburg, "Economic and Social Status of Patients at the Public Health Institute of Chicago," 1931.

[9]

Hospitalized Illness

STRIKES ONLY
ONE PERSON IN 15
PER YEAR

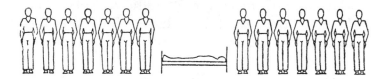

BUT IT COSTS

HALF OF
ALL FAMILY EXPENDITURES
FOR ILLNESS

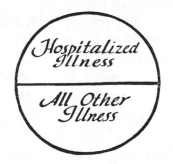

[10]

Workers' Union, to help it carry on through the depression.

The pay clinic principle, applied to hospital rather than to out-patient service, received a substantial impetus from the establishment of the Baker Memorial Hospital as a division of the Massachusetts General Hospital of Boston. By agreement between the hospital administration and its medical staff, the patient entering the hospital under the "middle-rate-plan" pays a single fee to the hospital, including both the hospital bill and the charges by physicians and surgeons for care in the institution. The maximum charge for medical and surgical services was limited to $150, by agreement with the staff. Thus, by being in a position to estimate in advance much more closely than is usually possible the total amount of his bill, the patient of moderate means is able to make much better arrangements for paying it.

The Fund pledged one-half the deficit during the first three years of the Baker Memorial, up to a total of $150,000, and actually was called upon to pay $128,571. The plan was started in Boston in 1931 at a most unfavorable time, but has steadily advanced in number of patients and in net income and is now able to utilize a sufficiently large number of beds to cover its running expenses. The abuses expected by some doubters, such as the incursion of a number of well-to-do people who sought low rates, did not develop and the income of the physicians, despite the limitation on charges, was estimated as probably larger on the average than would have been derived from similar patients of moderate economic status when doctors fix and collect their fees individually. The average total expense to the patient,

[11]

including both professional services and hospital charges, has been about half the usual local cost in similar cases.*

An endeavor was made to assist a "middle-rate-plan" in a small city, Keokuk, Iowa, in which two hospitals participated. But local jealousies among the physicians brought the attempt to a negative conclusion.**

HOURLY NURSING

A number of proposals were made to the Fund to apply a similar idea to nursing so that people of moderate means could secure nursing service in their homes on an hourly basis as required, instead of being compelled to pay for the entire time of a graduate nurse by the day or week. During 1931-33, the Fund aided an hourly nursing experiment in Chicago, at first administered by a specially organized committee, later taken over by the local branch of the Illinois State Nursing Association, which has continued it up to the present time. A report published under the auspices of the American Nurses' Association came to the conclusion that hourly nursing should be developed as part of a visiting nurses' association or general home nursing service, and has helped to dispose of the idea that hourly nursing can be conducted effectively or economically by a special organization set up for that purpose alone.

HOSPITAL RELATIONS

The policies and the public relations of hospitals are of exceeding importance not only to these institutions

---

*Two reports were published by the Fund concerning the Baker Memorial, namely: "The Middle-Rate Plan for Hospital Patients—The First Year's Experience," by C. Rufus Rorem, 1931; "How Do Physicians and Patients Like the Middle-Rate Plan for Hospital Care?" by C. Rufus Rorem, Clyde D. Frost, M.D., and Elizabeth R. Day, 1932.

**Mary Ross, "The Middle-Rate Plan for Hospital Patients—A Year's Experiment in Keokuk, Iowa," May, 1931.

[12]

themselves, but to the whole field of medical services. The Fund's staff has therefore participated actively in the work of the American Hospital Association. One of the staff has during recent years been Chairman of the Association's Council, which is advisory to the Association's trustees in studies of administrative practice and community relations, and in the formulation of broad policies affecting hospitals and the public. Another of the Fund's staff has been loaned on part time to the Association, as its Consultant on Group Hospitalization, and has also served as Chairman of a Committee on Hospital Accounting and Statistics. The report of this Committee was adopted and published by the American Hospital Association and has been widely used as a manual for the guidance of hospital administrators and accountants.

PUBLIC RELATIONS

While the depression necessarily held back new experiments which required fresh capital investment, it has stimulated experimentation in new methods of organizing and paying for medical care. Millions of people have found it difficult or impossible to purchase medical service; thousands of physicians found it hard to make a living. The years beginning in 1932 have been a period of profound ferment in medical affairs. Demands throughout the country for consultation and advice concerning new plans and experiments required extensive travel and correspondence by the staff. Many physicians and a number of local and state medical societies, hospitals, industrial executives, social workers, academic teachers and students sought advice and information. These activities led to the collection of lists of more than 350 plans and projects in voluntary sickness insurance,

[13]

THE DOCTOR and THE PATIENT

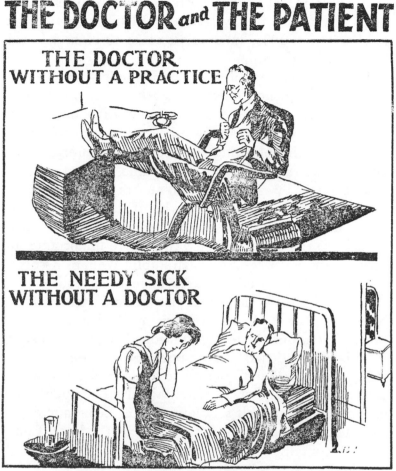

THE DOCTOR
WITHOUT A PRACTICE

THE NEEDY SICK
WITHOUT A DOCTOR

Adapted from a cartoon by Rogers in the San Francisco News.
Arranged by the National Forum.

.Before the depression, studies covering over 24,000 persons of moderate or small incomes showed that 25 to 30 per cent of these people had gone through a disabling illness—not a minor one—without any care from a physician. In California, about one third of the people studied in 1934, with family incomes under $1200, had no medical care whatever for disabling sickness.

The tradition and the ethics of the medical profession place service to the sick above financial return. But the patient must seek the doctor and the average physician spends one third of his time idle, waiting for patients.

[14]

group practice, and other methods of medical service or of paying for it. "New Plans of Medical Service," a publication of 1936, summarizes some 40 plans selected from this large group.

The dynamic state of medical economics has likewise called for frequent conferences with other foundations and with the hospital, social work, medical and public health agencies actively concerned with our field, with the aim of joint planning and economy of effort. Since 1933, public expenditures for relief and for medical care administered by governmental authorities have been greatly enlarged. Policies for the utilization of physicians, dentists, hospitals, and clinics under these auspices have therefore become vastly more important. In cooperation with the American Public Welfare Association the problems of this area have been studied and relationships between welfare and medical agencies have been formulated. As the country emerged from the depression, national planning in medical economics began to appear, particularly in public health programs. In 1934, one of the Fund's officers served as a member of the consultant staff and of the Hospital Advisory Committee of President Roosevelt's Committee on Economic Security. The Social Security Act, drafted by the latter Committee, contained provisions with important medical implications.

PUBLIC INFORMATION

These active movements were all reflected in an enhanced volume of discussion of medical economics in professional and lay circles. The medical, hospital, dental, and nursing journals carried an enlarged output of articles and correspondence on the subject, much of it ephemeral, some of it significant. A demand for general

[15]

information on the subject appeared, at first chiefly within professional circles, but subsequently from the public at large.

As the need for supplying information took on an increasingly general character, the Fund's staff prepared or secured copies of articles appropriate for distribution in professional or lay circles; printed a reading list of books and pamphlets including literature on different sides of controversial points; and made this material available through libraries and similar agencies throughout the country, besides meeting individual requests for literature.

The members of the staff were naturally called on for frequent public addresses. Articles in magazines of general circulation and in the special organs of various professional and lay agencies were prepared or their preparation arranged for. Some of the more important facts were put into chart form and issued as "A Picture-Book about the Costs of Medical Care." The illustrations in this report are from the third edition of the "Picture-Book." Altogether, during the years 1933-36, about 160,000 pamphlets and articles were distributed by the Fund, mostly on request.

PUBLIC ATTITUDES

The Fund has taken no official attitude on any legislation concerning health insurance or other matters in this field. In numerous public utterances, the staff members have expressed their views as in favor of participation on the part of the professions in the formulation and guidance of methods of medical service or of payment for it and of public recognition of the responsibility of the professions for the standards and quality of care. The present status of the medical profession, its mode of

[16]

89

practice, and financial opportunities are being continuously altered, both by advances in medical science and technique and by changing social conditions. Guidance for these changes should come jointly from the medical professions and from those who approach the problem from the standpoint of the public who pay the bills and who are recipients of service.

COMMITTEE ON THE COSTS OF MEDICAL CARE

In 1929, the Fund joined with seven other foundations in contributing to the Committee on the Costs of Medical Care, of which its Director for Medical Services had been one of the organizers. This Committee of forty-eight persons, of whom twenty-five were physicians, set for itself the task of making within five years a comprehensive survey of the economics of medical care in the United States, and the further responsibility of preparing plans and recommendations for action.

The composition of the Committee reflected the variety of interests involved in medical services. The Chairman, Dr. Ray Lyman Wilbur, President of Stanford University, a former president of the American Medical Association, was also, during most of the Committee's life, in President Hoover's Cabinet as Secretary of the Interior. Of the twenty-five medical men, seventeen were in private practive. A number of the physicians had been suggested as members by the officers of the American Medical Association. Dentists, nurses, hospital and public health administrators, economists, and men and women of the "general public" were included. Professor C.-E. A. Winslow, head of the Department of Public Health at Yale, was chairman of the executive committee, of which one of the Fund's officers was a member.

[17]

90

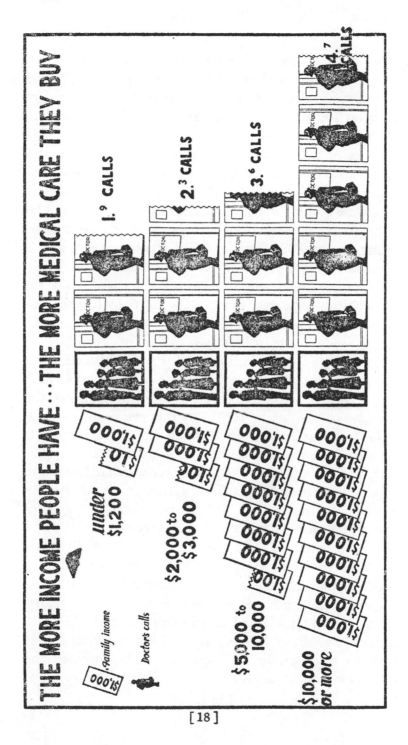

THE MORE INCOME PEOPLE HAVE...THE MORE MEDICAL CARE THEY BUY

Family income
Doctor's calls

under $1,200 — 1.9 CALLS

$2,000 to $3,000 — 2.3 CALLS

$5,000 to 10,000 — 3.6 CALLS

$10,000 or more — 4.7 CALLS

[18]

As a research undertaking, the studies of the Committee were specialized within the economic aspects of medical care. Several descriptive studies were made of existing facilities for medical service in the United States and of plans and experiments in organized medical care. The incomes of physicians and dentists were investigated with the cooperation of their national professional societies. Medical facilities, their utilization, and their costs were studied in communities of different sizes. One of the major investigations was a comprehensive survey, among nearly 9,000 families of all income groups and in all parts of the United States, of the amounts and incidence of sickness, the medical care secured, and the expenditures for care. Practically no historical or analytical studies were pursued, and only preliminary attempts were made to study quality or adequacy of service. Twenty-six volumes of special studies were published, a large summary volume of the factual findings, together with numerous minor publications and abstracts of the major technical reports.

The Committee had undertaken the highly difficult venture of requiring the same body of people to supervise a research program and also to serve as a deliberative committee to propose plans for action in an admittedly controversial field. The second task was not accomplished without dissension. A majority report signed by thirty-five members, a minority report signed by nine, and three other separate statements were included in "Medical Care for the American People," the Committee's final report and recommendations. The major dissenting group represented chiefly the American Medical Association whose *Journal*, after the recommendations had been made public in December, 1932, opposed the majority report strongly.

[19]

92

In the perspective of four years since its completion, the Committee's work now appears as of outstanding and enduring importance. The assemblage of facts has been generally accepted as the most important contribution to knowledge that has ever been available to any country about medical services and their costs. Governmental and voluntary bodies, including several state medical societies, have since pursued studies for which the investigations of the Committee had supplied the guidance as to purpose and methods. The baker's dozen of men and women trained in medical-economic research as members of the Committee's staff have, in most instances, continued investigative or administrative work in this field under governmental or private auspices. From the standpoint of social action, the very controversy precipitated by official medical opposition served to stimulate interest and to direct more attention to the subject in both professional and lay circles. Most of the numerous plans of action which have been under way since that time were recommended or forecast in the Committee's final volume.

The Fund's contribution to the Committee amounted to $90,000 during the period 1928-32, in a total of approximately $885,000 received by the Committee. Two hundred thousand dollars apiece came from three of the larger foundations. The Fund's participation in the work of the Committee, through the grant of a substantial part of officers' time, as well as through some financial aid, represents one of our most important and satisfactory contributions in the field of medical services.

When the Committee on the Costs of Medical Care went out of existence in December, 1932, the Fund accepted the Committee's request to receive and distribute its stock of pamphlets and the abstracts of its technical studies. The major publications of the Committee were issued in book form by the University of Chicago Press. The controversies due to the official medical attacks upon the Committee's recommendations greatly promoted a demand for its material. During 1933, some 20,000 of the Committee's pamphlets were requested of the Fund. Most of the remaining stock, some 40,000, has since been distributed.

STUDIES AND EDUCATIONAL WORK

All the Fund's publications concerning medical services are listed in the Appendix. Among the more interesting subjects not connected with the Fund's own projects were reviews of (1) voluntary sickness insurance as undertaken by private group clinics, initiated by physicians, (2) the industrial sickness insurance plan operated by the employees of the Standard Oil Company in Baton Rouge, Louisiana, (3) syphilis as an economic problem, and (4) the growth of clinics in the United States. Two books and several monographs by the Fund's staff were published. Assistance was given to timely studies conducted by other agencies, of medical care under the emergency relief programs.* Small grants were made to assist statistical studies in the location and mobility of physicians in the Chicago area by members of the Department of Sociology of the University of Chicago.

---

*Publications thus assisted included: "Medical Care for the Unemployed and Their Families," by Miriam S. Leuck, September, 1934; "Plans of Medical Relief in Ten Cities," March, 1936; "The Legal Basis of Public Medical Care in Twelve States," May 1, 1936. (All published by the American Public Welfare Association.) "Medical Care for Relief Clients," by the Committee on Medical Care in Community Health of the American Association of Medical Social Workers, published by the Association, June, 1935.

[21]

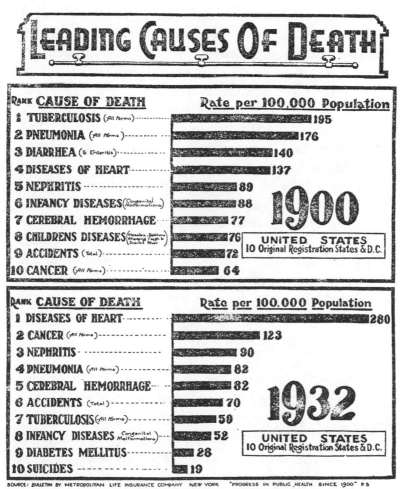

LEADING CAUSES OF DEATH

Rank	CAUSE OF DEATH	Rate per 100,000 Population
1	TUBERCULOSIS (All Forms)	195
2	PNEUMONIA (All Forms)	176
3	DIARRHEA (& Enteritis)	140
4	DISEASES OF HEART	137
5	NEPHRITIS	89
6	INFANCY DISEASES (Congenital Malformations)	88
7	CEREBRAL HEMORRHAGE	77
8	CHILDRENS DISEASES (Measles, Diptheria, Whooping Cough & Scarlet Fever)	76
9	ACCIDENTS (Total)	72
10	CANCER (All Forms)	64

1900
UNITED STATES
10 Original Registration States & D.C.

Rank	CAUSE OF DEATH	Rate per 100,000 Population
1	DISEASES OF HEART	280
2	CANCER (All Forms)	123
3	NEPHRITIS	90
4	PNEUMONIA (All Forms)	82
5	CEREBRAL HEMORRHAGE	82
6	ACCIDENTS (Total)	70
7	TUBERCULOSIS (All Forms)	59
8	INFANCY DISEASES (Congenital Malformations)	52
9	DIABETES MELLITUS	28
10	SUICIDES	19

1932
UNITED STATES
10 Original Registration States & D.C.

SOURCE: BULLETIN BY METROPOLITAN LIFE INSURANCE COMPANY NEW YORK "PROGRESS IN PUBLIC HEALTH SINCE 1900" P.5

ARRANGED BY THE NATIONAL FORUM

In 1900, tuberculosis was at the top of the list of deadly diseases; today it is seventh on the list. Many serious contagious diseases such as typhoid fever and diphtheria have greatly decreased. The diarrheas of infancy are only about one fourth what they used to be.

On the other hand, diseases of the heart were fourth among the causes of death in 1900, but are now in first place. Cancer has moved from tenth up to second place.

The great reductions in death rate have taken place chiefly by applying medical science through organized public health work.

[22]

Beginning with the academic year 1934-35, one of the Fund's staff has been Professorial Lecturer in the University, offering a course in the development of health institutions, and also developing the graduate study of hospital administration under the School of Business, with the cooperation of the University Clinics. Financial assistance was given the University for a few scholarships and for a research assistant to help in organizing teaching material. All of the 13 students of the years 1934-36 are now in administrative internships or in salaried positions. An officer of the Fund has also organized and been chairman of the Institute for Hospital Administrators, a two-weeks' "refresher course" for men and women already established in the field, which has been conducted by the American Hospital Association for the past three years on the campus of the University of Chicago.

EXPENDITURES

The financial statement in the Appendix shows that a total of $848,071 was expended during the eight years 1929-36 for the program herein described. Throughout the period, and particularly during its later years, grants to other agencies have been secondary to the central activities of studies, consultation and conference, administered by the Fund's staff. The smallness of the expenditure for information service is accounted for by the policy of utilizing existing periodicals as vehicles for publication and distribution, except for a few major studies and reports which were issued directly by the Fund. Excluding the few large outside grants, the essential work of the whole program was conducted for an expenditure of between $40,000 and $50,000 a year.

[23]

The field of medical economics is an area infused with emotion because of its intimate relations with the welfare of individuals, and involves interests which have been made to appear conflicting, whether or not they really are so. In this field it was necessary to develop methods of constructive action. It was necessary to promote, among the professional and the lay public, a belief that the problems of sickness and of its costs are capable of solution by organized action. It was necessary to cultivate the habit of depending upon facts, of securing facts through research, and of using the results of research as the basis of decisions concerning action.

Hence, the few experiments subsidized during the early years of the program; hence, active participation in the major research program of the Committee on the Costs of Medical Care, followed by development of other studies and of plans for training personnel; hence, promotional activities among the professions and the public, moving always, so far as possible, towards those methods of conference and discussion which promote thought and reduce heat.

PROVISIONS FOR THE FUTURE

The depression greatly accelerated a practical interest in medical economics among millions of the public, among many thousands of physicians, dentists and nurses, and among hospitals, public health and social welfare authorities. Before the turn of the depression had arrived, it had begun to be apparent that the need of promoting interest and action, which had been especially prominent in the Fund's work during 1932-33,

[24]

was becoming less and less important. The very sharpening of opposition from certain quarters proved again and again one of the most satisfactory evidences of a real forward movement, arising from deep-seated forces. Emphasis during the last two years of the Fund's program therefore gradually focussed upon the advancement of research in this field and upon the encouragement of group hospitalization as one specific line of action.

In 1936, the decision was reached that it would be practicable for the Fund to turn over these two lines of work to other agencies. A grant of $165,000, to be used over a five-year period, was made to the Committee on Research in Medical Economics. This Committee was recently incorporated in New York, under the chairmanship of Michael M. Davis, who from the beginning has been the director of the Fund's work in this field. The other members of the Committee are Robert E. Chaddock, Professor of Statistics, Columbia University; Henry S. Dennison, President, Dennison Manufacturing Company, Framingham, Massachusetts; Walton H. Hamilton, Professor of Law, Yale University, and Director, Bureau of Research, Social Security Board, Washington; Alvin S. Johnson, Director, New School for Social Research, New York; Paul U. Kellogg, Editor, The Survey Graphic, New York; Harry A. Millis, Professor of Economics, University of Chicago; Fred M. Stein, retired banker, New York.

The Committee will have an Advisory Council, to be enlarged as required, the following physicians now being members: Eugene L. Bishop, Knoxville, Tennessee; Samuel Bradbury, Philadelphia; Alfred E. Cohn, New York; Alice Hamilton, Washington; Ludwig Hektoen, Chicago; and Franklin C. McLean, Chicago.

This Committee, with headquarters in New York

[25]

98

City, will conduct and assist studies in the economic and social aspects of medical care; will train personnel for this field; and, in cooperation with the medical profession and other agencies, will furnish information and consultation services in behalf of making medical care more widely available to the people at costs within their means.

A second grant of $100,000, to be used over a five-year period, was made to the American Hospital Association for the study and advancement of group hospitalization and related problems. The Association has appointed Dr. C. Rufus Rorem as executive officer of a Committee on Hospital Service which, under the Association's trustees, will direct this program in future. Dr. Basil C. MacLean, Medical Director of Strong Memorial Hospital, Rochester, New York, is Chairman of this Committee, the other members in addition to Dr. Rorem being: Dr. R. C. Buerki, Director of the University Hospital, University of Wisconsin, Madison; Dr. S. S. Goldwater, Commissioner of Hospitals, New York City; and Mgr. M. F. Griffin of Saint Philomena's Church, Cleveland, a trustee of the American Hospital Association.

With these grants, the Trustees have terminated the Department of Medical Services, believing that these two agencies will carry forward effectively the Fund's long-standing and successful work in medical economics and that this action should result in the ultimate maintenance of needed activities in this field under permanent auspices.

[26]

The Commonwealth Fund

PROGRAM FOR CHILD HEALTH

Only preliminary steps toward the organization of this enterprise, authorized by the Board of Directors in June 1922, had taken place when the annual report for the year ending September 30, 1922 was written and nothing more than a brief forecast was then possible. It was stated, however, that three demonstrations, each for a five year period, would be established, one in the MiddleWest, one in the South and one probably in the Far West in the hope that if successful, they might exercise a national influence; that they would include complete educational and preventive child health activities from the prenatal period through school age; and that the specific activities undertaken would be modified as might be necessary to insure the flexibility required for adaptation to the needs of the communities chosen.

The program has advanced in accordance with this original plan. Fargo, North Dakota was chosen as the site for the first demonstration, and operations were begun in that city in January 1923. Several months were devoted to the selection of a location in the south with the result that a two-fold enterprise will be established there, an urban demonstration in Athens, Georgia, and a rural one in Rutherford County, Tennessee. Conditions in the south are such that the greatest progress can be promoted, it is believed, by a clear distinction between the urban and rural problems. The location for the third demonstration has not yet been chosen.

Administrative Organization

The organization of the American Child Health Association from the amalgamation of two societies, each of which had covered a portion of the field of child health, has, as was anticipated, greatly simplified the administrative organization. The entire enterprise is conducted under the authority and general supervision of the Child Health Demonstration Committee, affiliated with the Fund and representative of both the Fund and the Child Health Association. Mr. Courtenay Dinwiddie, Director of the Association, serves this Committee as Director of Demonstrations. Under a contractual agreement between the Fund and the Association, the staff of the latter organization conducts the necessary administrative, statistical and publicity work under Mr. Dinwiddie's direction. The staffs of the demonstrations themselves are employed directly by the Demonstration Committee and are responsible to it.

POLICIES AND ULTIMATE PURPOSE

The widespread interest that has been aroused in this program warrants a more complete statement than has heretofore been made regarding certain questions of fundamental policy. As indicated above, the Demonstration Committee is not committed to any fixed method of procedure; adaptability to local conditions has been regarded as a prerequisite of success. Nevertheless the work has progressed sufficiently to make it possible to state with some assurance a number of important principles which have governed the undertaking from the beginning.

RELATION OF CHILD HEALTH TO GENERAL COMMUNITY HEALTH

Will the demonstrations deal with child health as a separate unit or in relation to matters of general community health? It appears perfectly clear that whether a health demonstration concern itself primarily with children or with some other feature of health work is very largely a matter of emphasis of the point of departure. The health of children in any community is so inextricably bound up with the whole problem of health in that community that it cannot be treated as a separate entity; any adequate constructive effort for the benefit of children must necessarily deal

104

with many matters which greatly, however indirectly, affect the child's own opportunity for healthful living. The community which has a bad tuberculosis situation, which has an infected water supply, or dirty milk, in which typhoid or venereal disease is rife, may establish the best of direct effort for the health of its children and still accomplish little or nothing unless these underlying conditions are dealt with. The program therefore, while devoting its direct efforts to child health as such and placing the emphasis there, fully recognizes the necessity and responsibility that rests upon its administrators to leave no stone unturned to the end that such general measures may be taken in the community as shall make successful work for children possible.

Evaluation of Results

One of the great responsibilities which rests upon health workers as well as upon social workers in general is the necessity for accurate measurement of the results of their work. This is discussed at some length later in this report in connection with the Program for the Prevention of Juvenile Delinquency. The problem has been an important consideration at all times and is stated clearly and briefly by Dr. George T. Palmer, Director of Research of the Child Health Association who is in charge of this side of the work for the Demonstration Committee. In this connection, Dr. Palmer states:

"It is to the interest of all health workers in the country that the results of these demonstrations be carefully and accurately measured. If at the end of the five-year period no concrete evidence of advancement can be shown, we shall witness a reaction against further health work that will extend far beyond the demonstration centers. On the other hand, if there is well considered statistical evidence forthcoming of the changes that have been effected in the communities in question the reaction will be distinctly favorable and the further demonstrated fact that public health is purchaseable will go far to convince those who are withholding support because of a lingering doubt as to its worth."

105

Every effort will be made by Dr. Palmer and a special staff to develop means of accurate measurement and thus secure a real evaluation of results as the demonstrations progress.

Cost of the Demonstration Method

A question commonly asked concerning the demonstrations under this program as well as concerning others in the health field is whether the expense involved is not greater than could be wisely incurred by the local community. This matter received careful consideration in the preparation of the program. It was estimated at that time that exclusive of administrative charges incident to headquarters the total expense of any demonstration would not exceed two dollars per annum per capita of population. Actually, the expense of the demonstration in Fargo to September 30th has been approximately $1.30 per capita for a population estimated at 27,000, including all expenditures, whether for local work of a permanent character or incidental to administration or to evaluation of the demonstration as an enterprise of national interest. The maximum expenditure entailed at any time for this demonstration will not exceed two dollars per capita, and the maximum plus all activities of the local health department will not involve a per capita in excess of $2.66.

Such an expenditure for health facilities might well be considered justifiable, even though it were all chargeable to local activities, although admittedly few communities expend so much at present. Health is quite comparable with education in importance to the community generally. Fargo for example expended for education exclusive of capital outlay $14.80 per capita in 1922-23. Similar comparisons for other communities are possible. If a health program can be operated in a manner to affect the entire community to anything like the degree to which the average educational program does, an expenditure of $2.66 per capita would not be excessive. Actually however, the per capita cost of the demonstration is considerably greater than would be required to carry on the essentials of the work permanently at local expense. There are included in a demonstration costs for local supervision, for recording, measuring and interpreting the work done, for experimental service and for a type of administrative organization which, although necessary to the demonstration itself, should not be charged to the cost of the permanent enterprise. A careful analysis of the costs of the demonstration will be made. Present information strongly indicates the possibility of a complete and adequate program at a cost which most communities of that size can well afford and far below the maximum cost of the demonstration now in operation.

The Private Practice of Physicians

Whatever be the merits of state medicine, the Commonwealth Fund is not lending its influence to anything of the sort. It has no desire to interfere with the practice of private physicians; on the contrary, their cooperation has been sought and freely offered. An educational and preventive program of this character far from decreasing the need of the physician's service should increase it. Absolutely no remedial work is or will be done; while the influence of the demonstration staff is constantly exerted in educating people to make use of the physician's services in order not alone to get well but to keep well.

Objectives; Financial Responsibility

The objective of the program is to produce and operate a practicable plan of health work which may (1) benefit the particular community served and (2) add to our knowledge of sound methods; and which may ultimately (3) assure a higher health level in the particular community through the permanent establishment of the essential features of the work and (4) encourage other com-

107

munities to adopt similar methods. Obviously the cost of the permanent enterprise, as indicated above, must be kept within bounds to accomplish either of these two ultimate purposes; but beyond this, the Demonstration Committee believes that any community desiring a demonstration should clearly recognize from the outset a certain degree of financial responsibility. It may be desirable to repeat here the statement of the Committee's position as publicly announced some time ago.

> "The Committee in charge of the Commonwealth Fund demonstrations has been granted an appropriation estimated as sufficient to cover three five year demonstrations in three different communities of the United States. The sum to be spent in each community is not a fixed one but will depend almost entirely upon the extent to which the community is prepared to carry on permanently work which may be initiated by demonstration funds. The Committee is willing to finance the beginning of any type of work which is sound and is definitely for the health of mothers and of children of any age, provided this is considered as a first step toward the community taking over a supervisory and financial responsibility for such work within a reasonable period.
>
> "It is clear that it would be unwise for the expenditures for the demonstration to be too largely from the demonstration fund during the five-year demonstration period, and for the community at the end of that time to be faced with the question of whether it would or would not take over the work and financial responsibility for it. This means that the community's responsibility should begin at the beginning of the period and should increase steadily and fairly rapidly from year to year, until at the end of the five-year period it is carrying practically all the permanent work which has been initiated. The expenditures from the Committee funds would probably reach a maximum during the second or third year of the demonstration and decrease steadily thereafter. If the community wished to assume greater responsibility than that suggested, it would be welcomed by the Committee."

THE FARGO DEMONSTRATION

Fargo was selected as representative of the upper Mississippi valley region from thirty cities applying. It is distinctly a commercial center with a population in 1920 of 22,000, now estimated at 27,000. It is not in the registration area and the best figures available indicate an infant mortality rate of ninety per thousand live births for 1921. Its chief assets for health were an excellent water supply, a beginning of control of the milk supply, a limited nursing service, good hospital facilities,—and more important for the future than any of these—an intelligent public sentiment toward health and a cooperative and able group of physicians. A careful study of the situation appeared to promise every reasonable opportunity to cope successfully with a real problem of child health.

The work began with the organization of a general citizens' committee from which an executive committee of eleven was elected. This committee has participated actively in the conduct of the demonstration and no important step has been taken without its knowledge and approval.

DEPARTMENTS

Under the guidance of this committee and of the Director, Dr. William J. French, the organization of the work under four departments was accomplished within four months. These departments with their chief functions are as follows:

Executive: General administration; including statistical and research work.

Medical: In charge of Dr. Lester J. Evans, pediatrician; operation of health station for well babies and pre-school children; examination of school children; consultation service on request of physician.

Nursing: In charge of Miss Edith B. Pierson; community and school nursing on the district plan including children, prenatal cases, tuberculosis and contagious diseases; calls for the Health Department; birth registration calls. Staff of six nurses.

Health Education: In charge of Miss Maud A. Brown; health education including both public and parochial schools; supervised summer playgrounds.

Work Done to Date

Under the direction of Dr. French, a cooperative interplay of service between departments has resulted in the development of the work as a composite whole in an unusual degree. Scarcely a single step has been taken that has not involved more than one department and it is therefore somewhat difficult to differentiate the achievements as between departments. The outstanding accomplishments very briefly stated are as follows:

Medical: Two hundred and ninety-one babies and pre-school children and 168 school children have been examined at the center; and 1,162 children in the schools. Cases have been referred to private physicians wherever remedial treatment has been recommended and consultation service has been given to any physician upon request. Only dietary and similar advice has been given directly at the time of examination. In cooperation with this department, the dentists of Fargo examined the teeth of 1124 children last spring and 88 per cent were found to have carious teeth. The nurses are still doing follow up work in this connection and a large number of children have received dental treatment. Complete statistical results regarding this and other remedial treatment resulting from the work of the department are not yet available. In conducting this work, Dr. Evans has endeavored at all times to stimulate the public to expect and seek from their physicians advice along preventive lines and the giving of such advice by the physicians. School examinations have been closely correlated with the nursing service and the program of health education.

Nursing: The nursing service is conducted on the district plan, each nurse being responsible for all cases in her district and having certain schools assigned to her. Children absent from school because of illness are promptly visited. Those in school who need attention are looked after, frequent class room inspections are made and all children are regularly weighed and measured. After completion of the school work, home visits are made and considerable general nursing is thus supplied. One of the most important duties of the nurse has been to follow up children who have been advised to go to a physician or dentist and see that they do not neglect to do so. The department began work on March 15th, and to September 30th, six nurses have visited 2,475 individuals, or about ten per cent of the total population.

Health Education: The work of health education in the schools includes direct instruction in health and hygiene, correlation of health teaching with other subjects in the curriculum, constant though varied effort to inculcate correct habits among children, covering diet, sleep, amusements, etc., and special attention and encouragement to underweight children. Health plays, demonstrations in the preparation and value of certain foods from time to time, instruction to mothers, etc., are featured. No nutrition classes are operated, but nutrition is not neglected. The work has received the enthusiastic interest of the children and the hearty cooperation of teachers and parents. The children are encouraged to keep a health record covering essential points of healthful living and this procedure has proved both useful and stimulating. There is every evidence of remarkable progress, though results of this type will be especially difficult to measure. Marked improvement in underweight children, however, has been observed. During the summer, two organized play centers were conducted in the city parks with an attendance that reached 400 at its maximum. This particular undertaking, financed during the past summer by the demonstration, has been adopted by the Rotary Club. The department has also arranged to assist in courses in health education for students of the State Normal School.

Administrative: This department in addition to the general direction of the demonstration is devoting much attention, now that the work is well under way, to statistical recording, and is assisting in the provision for the accurate measurement of results.

SIDE LIGHTS AND SPECIAL FEATURES

Among the especially encouraging features has been the unusual degree of interest and cooperation on the part of the citizens of Fargo. Physicians, school officials, both public and parochial, civic and philanthropic organizations, business men's clubs and citizens generally have done everything to assist. Already, too, the people of Fargo have shown a desire to assume financial responsibility. Adequate quarters with heat and light have been furnished by the Board of Education. The city has recently engaged a full time city health officer in the person of Dr. B. K. Kilbourne, and under his direction an active health department has been established. This department is working in close cooperation with the demonstration, with offices adjacent, and has already attacked the milk control problem, the control of contagious diseases, and the problem of the unscreened toilet. The Board of Education has from the beginning paid the salaries of two of the nurses, the Red Cross pays for a third, and the Rotary Club as stated above has taken over the summer playground project. There seems every reason to believe that Fargo intends to do its part to make the work a complete success. Particularly interesting points are the following:

By order of the Board of Health, common colds have been ruled contagious and children having them are excluded from school. The experiment thus far has been successful and should mean much to the health of school children.

By an improvement over the method of dental examinations employed last spring, all dental work will be done by the dentists of Fargo and no dental clinic will be established.

A special agreement was drawn up in the beginning between the demonstration and the Cass County Medical Society. In this manner all possibility of misunderstanding on the part of physicians was avoided, the functions of the demonstration from a medical point of view were clearly defined and the support of the medical profession assured.

It would be unfair to close this brief statement regarding the demonstration without mention of the ability shown by Dr. French in the organization and direction of the work as well as the remarkable spirit of the staff he has gathered about him. It is rare indeed that such a devoted and enthusiastic group may be observed.

ATHENS AND RUTHERFORD COUNTY

These two communities were selected from more than forty applying for the southern demonstration.

Athens is situated in Clarke County in the northeastern part of Georgia and had a population in 1920 of 20,075 of which approximately forty per cent was colored. It is the center of a fairly prosperous agricultural county. Chief industries are the manufacture of textiles, yarns, hosiery, cotton oil, and agricultural implements. Industrial employees number about 1600 of whom nearly half are women. There is very little child labor. The city is progressive, shows an unusual interest in health and social activities, and is the educational center of the state being the home of the University of Georgia, the Georgia State College of Agriculture, the State Normal School and the Knox Institute (colored). The outstanding factors in the selection of the city were the assured cooperation and interest of state departments and officials including the Governor, the State Board of Health, Superintendent of Education and the State Council of Social Agencies, all of whom urged the selection of a Georgia community and promised complete cooperation; also the certain assistance and cooperation of the educational institutions located in Athens. A progessive and improved school system, an active Board of Health with a full time officer, and a real interest together with a desire to carry on the work of the demonstration permanently were additional favorable factors. On the other hand, the most reliable figures for 1922 indicate an infant mortality rate of 124. The health officer reports a serious tuberculosis problem and very little has been done along the lines of maternal or child health work. Nothing more than the ground work for a health program has been laid, and there is need for definite health measures not only for the health of children but for general community health, particularly in the field of sanitary control.

Rutherford County is an agricultural county situated in the central part of Tennessee with a population in 1920 of 33,000 of which less than one-third is colored. Murfreesboro, the county seat, one hour from Nashville, has a population of 5,000 and has factories employing about 600 people. The county is, however, predominantly agricultural and eighty-five per cent of the population is engaged in farming.

There has been very little development of health activities. The county has had no health board and what little public health work has been done, has been through the nurse of the American Red Cross. The vital statistics of the county are entirely unreliable, but it is known that the typhoid and tuberculosis death rates are high and the same is probably true as to infant mortality. There is thirty-one per cent of illiteracy, a not unusual condition in a rural southern community. The situation offers opportunity for a constructive health undertaking and excellent results are to be expected owing to numerous favorable factors. In the first place, there has been intense interest both in the county and among representative citizens throughout the state, and this has taken practical form in the voting of an appropriation of $4,000 by the state and an additional $4,000 by the county to provide for a full time health officer and an adequate health department. This action indicates the intention of the people to do their part. A num-

114

ber of the leading citizens organized a local public health association and have guaranteed the carrying on of the work permanently at their own expense should that be necessary. The interest and cooperation afforded by various state bodies, particularly the Department of Health, Department of Education and the State Medical Association have been unusual. The state has recently adopted a new code of school laws which provides for physical education in the public schools and for courses in health education in the state colleges and normal schools which train teachers. Finally the International Health Board is planning to undertake the establishment of county public health boards in ten Tennessee counties (not Rutherford County however), sharing the expense with the local authorities. This action has stimulated the entire state to increased health activities and it is clear that the two enterprises will be mutually helpful.

Work will be begun in these centers about January 1, 1924.

By-Products of the Program

The work in Fargo has already exerted a far wider influence and aroused a greater degree of interest throughout the state than had been anticipated. Numerous instances of this might be given. In the process of choosing Fargo, it was found that a keen interest was aroused in child health in the majority of the communities applying from the upper Mississippi valley region. In most instances it was the first time there had been any general consideration of the whole question by the leading groups of the community in unison. In at least six communities the definite statement was made that it was well worth while to have applied for the demonstration because of the increased general interest in child health needs, even though the community failed in its application. During the study preceding the choice of the two southern communities, there has been observed the organization of seven local public health associations, as a result of the competition for the demonstration. This to an extent has crystallized the aroused and organized interest in child health in these communities. In one instance, an immediate appropriation of $1000 for health work was made by the community.

Although this program has been in operation less than nine months, the progress so far achieved gives great hope of future results. The Fund desires here to acknowledge its appreciation of the able administrative work of Mr. Courtenay Dinwiddie, Director of Demonstrations.

DIVISION OF RURAL HOSPITALS

As the first project in the Rural Hospital Program, a fifty bed general hospital is under construction in Farmville, Virginia, this community having been chosen as the result of a preliminary study discussed in the 1925 Annual Report. The study, completed early this year, was undertaken to determine the advisability of inaugurating a program through which the Fund would assist rural communities in establishing hospital facilities, and resulted in the setting up of a Division of Rural Hospitals on March 1, 1926. The Division is prepared to cooperate with selected rural communities by. contributing two-thirds of the capital cost involved in build-

[61]

117

ing a hospital, in addition to furnishing building plans and specifications, advising in the selection of equipment and in the organization of the institution for operation. Provision for two such hospitals per year on the average is contemplated.

Farmville having been selected for the location of the first unit under this scheme, a somewhat detailed description of that community and of the building under construction there will serve as a description of the points of emphasis of the program as a whole. Farmville is located in the south-central part of Virginia, a thoroughly agricultural section. Though small, it represents a growing community, which has increased in size from 1,500 to 4,000 in the past six years, and, as the county seat of Prince Edward County, is the trading and transportation center for a considerable surrounding area. It is, in fact, the largest urban center in a completely rural area of thirty-five mile radius, which the hospital is to serve and which embraces in addition to the one whole county, parts of eight adjoining counties—an area not served by any existing medical institutions, although it includes a total population of 60,000 with 27,000 negroes. Two educational institutions, one within the town and one six miles away, increase the need for hospital facilities and at the same time are a factor in influencing public sentiment to an appreciation of the importance of improving the present inadequate health provisions. A part-time health officer and a sanitary engineer, together with a single public health nurse, employed by a private organization, represent the only attempts at community health control. There are no organized hospital facilities nearer than Lynchburg, fifty-eight miles west, and Petersburg, seventy-five miles to the east. Although there is sufficient wealth and appreciation of the need of a hospital to make possible the raising of a substantial part of the total

[62]

cost involved, the community could not assume the full cost of establishing a modern, fully equipped institution.

The community seemed, on the whole, thoroughly representative of those the Fund aimed to reach, not only in its need and its strategic location, but in the assurance given of professional support, of general cooperation, and of ability to guarantee the current operation of a first class institution. This opinion was at least partially borne out by the ready response of local citizens, as soon as decision was made in favor of Farmville. Funds were secured by organized local effort sufficient to meet the cost of the hospital site and one-third of the anticipated cost of building and equipment. The Fund then, on a contractual basis, assumed obligation for building plans and specifications and for the remaining part of the cost of building and equipment, the local residents, through a permanent organization incorporated under the State laws for charitable purposes, retaining full property rights and full responsibility for the construction and operation of the hospital.

The plans for the institution, to be known as the Southside Community Hospital, were prepared by the New York architects, Henry C. Pelton and James Gamble Rogers, Associated, who have been retained by the Fund for its hospital program. The building is to be of red brick, fireproof in construction, of the southern colonial style of architecture, and is planned to meet all reasonable demands of the community for general hospital care, including maternity and out-patient service. All facilities and activities are housed under one roof, including the service departments and adequate X-ray and laboratory facilities for a comprehensive range of clinical procedures, with provision for the separate care of colored patients, and space reserved for nurse training and for staff meetings. Although the initial bed capacity is to be

[63]

119

fifty, the structure has been so planned that when conditions require, this may be doubled at a relatively small cost, by removing the nurses' dormitory and the power plant and laundry to separate units, and utilizing the space thus vacated for additional beds and extension of out-patient activities. The services of the hospital are to be maintained according to approved professional and administrative standards, and will be available to all residents of the area, regardless of economic status, race, color, or creed. The facilities generally will be open to the practice of all ethical physicians of the area. An organization of the medical profession co-extensive with the hospital area has been formed, and steps are being taken to secure the cooperation of related social and health agencies in the utilization of the institution as a center of preventive and educational health activities.

Two principal considerations prompted the Fund to the adoption of the program of which the Farmville hospital represents the first activity: the obvious and widespread lack of accessible hospital facilities of general character in rural districts, and the accumulating evidence of the disadvantage of rural communities as compared with urban in the matter of health, as shown in many instances both by their higher morbidity and mortality rates, and the higher proportion of defects among rural school children. While this is partially attributable to differences in measures for sanitary control, it seems safe to assume that the increasing disparity between urban and rural health hazards is due also to the limited health facilities available in rural sections. This, of course, is not merely a question of hospitalization alone, but involves as well the scarcity of public health activities and of medical and nursing personnel. The Fund, however, has selected the hospital as an avenue of approach to the problem because of its basic relationship to the other health needs of

[64]

a locality and in the belief that the development of first class hospital facilities in any community will serve as an inducement to medical men not otherwise willing to consider rural practice. The present disproportionate distribution of physicians between the cities and rural areas has long been a matter of concern. It is obvious that the comparative economic potentialities of city and country and the comparative opportunities for keeping professionally abreast of the times are chief determining factors in the physician's choice of location. The presence of adequate hospital facilities, laboratory and X-ray, has a very obvious bearing in the latter connection; also the evidence indicates a potential increase in the practice of the rural physician through the availability of a good hospital, by enabling him to do better work, to do more work through centralization of the serious cases, and to avoid the necessity of sending certain types of cases to distant cities because facilities are lacking on the spot. There is general agreement that the provision of such facilities in rural areas should exercise a positive influence in attracting and holding a more adequate supply of medical men.

A second consideration entering into the selection of the hospital as an approach to the rural problem is its importance in any community health program and the opportunity it offers as a center for development and correlation not only of remedial but of educational and preventive health activities as well. Its obvious benefits to the community give it a strong appeal and a definite assurance of local cooperation.

The essentiality of hospital facilities to a community health program was brought forcibly to the attention of the Fund in connection with its Rutherford County Child Health Demonstration in Murfreesboro, Tennessee. With no adequate hospital facilities nearer than Nashville, thirty-two miles away, the work of the demonstration has been con-

[65]

121

stantly handicapped by the difficulty of securing the correction of physical defects discovered or other necessary medical care. To meet this situation the Fund made an appropriation for the erection of a fifty bed general hospital, located in Murfreesboro but serving the whole county area. The hospital, which is now nearing completion, is to be administered locally on much the same basis as those made possible under the Division of Rural Hospitals, and although not regarded as a part of the Hospital Program, is fairly representative of its underlying purposes and illustrates the intimate relationship between the hospital, remedial medicine and an educational and preventive public health program, such as it is hoped will be developed in each community to the greatest degree practicable.

In broad terms, therefore, the program aims first of all to stimulate the establishment of approved general hospital facilities in rural districts, and, second, to demonstrate the practicability of integrating the hospital in a comprehensive local health program involving the active cooperation of all forces at work in the community. These hospitals, strategically located in various sections of the country, it is believed, will in time influence neighboring communities to establish similar facilities out of their own resources, and will help to break down the tradition that the hospital is purely a rehabilitative institution.

After seven months of operation, construction of one of the hospital units is actually under way; decision as to the location of the second is pending;[1] and initial steps have been taken for the third. The local experience with the first hospital so far as it has progressed, the general public interest evidenced in the large number of appeals received from thirty-four states, the approval of the project by many

[1] Second unit awarded to Glasgow, Kentucky, November, 1926.

[66]

authorities in the several branches of the health field, and the degree of cooperation already offered, promise the achievement of worthwhile results.

CHILD WELFARE

Five years ago the child health program was inaugurated with the organization of a child health demonstration in Fargo, North Dakota. That initial demonstration has now nearly run its course, and the city has chosen to adopt as its own all the essentials of the demonstrated program. The fifth demonstration year in Fargo is the fourth in Clarke County, Georgia, and Rutherford County, Tennessee; the third in Marion County, Oregon. In the time remaining before the seven-year project is completed, the emphasis will naturally fall on the consolidation of the public health positions already staked out in the three communities where Fund activities continue, on the full transfer to the local authorities of responsibility for further child health work,

16

125

and on the task of gathering up, comparing and interpreting the results of seven years' experimental effort.

The past year has shown some new peaks in service, and but few changes in program. In Fargo the final take-over of demonstrated activities has proceeded smoothly and a staff dentist has been added to the public health personnel. In Clarke County public attention was focused on dental hygiene, with the notable result that the children in the five white elementary schools were able to attain one hundred per cent correction of dental defects according to the records of the local dentists. In Rutherford County a new high level of immunization against communicable diseases was reached, and sanitary activities were greatly strengthened by the addition of a deputy health officer and a second sanitary inspector to the county health unit. In Marion County interest in school health has taken a long stride under the special stimulus of an "honor roll" campaign. The Child Health Demonstration Committee has secured a complete appraisal, by the staff of the American Public Health Association, of public health performance in all four communities,[1] and has begun a publishing program which has placed informal reports of the demonstration in the hands of approximately 12,000 readers.

The results of an intensive demonstration of child health services may be expected to fall roughly into three groups. The most immediate, and the easiest to measure, is the building up of a definite public health program, incorporating adequate services to mothers and children, in the hands of suitable personnel and supported by a sufficient appropriation of public funds. Each demonstration has in effect been an in-

---

[1] Since the use of the City Appraisal Form in Fargo and Athens was reported in 1926, the Committee on Administrative Practice has developed a County Appraisal Form which has been similarly applied to the rural demonstrations.

17

formal contract between the Commonwealth Fund and the community, by virtue of which the Fund undertakes to show at its own expense what good public health work for children is, and the city or county undertakes to provide—so far as the demonstration is convincing—for the continuance of the demonstrated activities at its own expense. These contracts are being fulfilled by the gradual assumption of increasing financial responsibility in each community; and the appraisal of public health activities in each center shows a steady gain in their scope and extent.

A second group of results, more difficult to measure, but of underlying importance, relates to the health status of the group directly served. Vital statistics are of clear import in this connection only when a long period of time shows genuine trends as distinct from temporary fluctuations, and are to be trusted only when the body of cases on which rates are computed is large enough to outweigh the effect of accidental variations. In a five-year period in a community of 50,000 or less, only slight indications of health progress can be expected from such vital statistics as can be made available. If full and dependable records of sickness could be secured, they should show more quickly and clearly than the death rates the results of some phases of demonstration activity, but with present possibilities of record-keeping, the difficulties of getting information of this sort have proved insurmountable. Quite beyond the reach of present methods of measurement lie what in the long run may be the most important results of public health effort for children; the upbuilding of individual vitality; the better adjustment of growing children to school and family; the better preparation of children for economically productive maturity; the release of energy, through robust physical health, for the tasks and opportunities of citizenship.

18

A third group of results will be found in the community attitudes—primarily in the demonstration centers but also elsewhere—which follow from the educational work of the demonstrations. On these attitudes both public health services and private health progress are ultimately dependent. At a given moment irrelevant political considerations may cause the health budget to lag behind public opinion, or even to anticipate it, but over a period of years, within economic limits, it will rather accurately reflect the wishes of the taxpayers. There is evidence that the demonstrations are already proving their case, not alone with the officials, but with the sound business sense of the community. The full measure of this effect must be looked for five, ten, even twenty years after the close of the demonstrations. Equally significant are the attitudes that find expression in the home, the school, the physician's office. No one member of the circle involved in health promotion—the parent, the child, the physician, the teacher, the nurse, the health officer—can enforce health. A desire for health, in the child; a recognition of the value of health supervision, in the parent; an understanding of constructive health service, and a desire to give it, in the physician; a realization by both health officer and citizen of their mutual responsibility and their opportunities for teamwork—all these attitudes are being cultivated by the demonstrations because they are recognized as being essential to full-rounded health progress. Here too the full story can be told only after a generation, perhaps, has made clear how firmly and permanently these attitudes have been developed.

In the meantime there are waymarks of progress in each of these three directions. In the matter of direct stimulus to public health planning and service, the experience of Fargo is the most complete and hence the most instructive.

19

Six years ago, before the demonstration, Fargo was typical as a prosperous small community, burdened by no unusual health deficiencies, which had never become awake to the need and value of systematic public health service. The functions of a health department were divided between a part-time health officer, a sanitary inspector, a state employee in a branch of the state university laboratory which happened to be located in Fargo, a school nurse, and a Red Cross nurse. Such health work as was done—subsequently rated in accordance with the City Appraisal Form of the Committee on Administrative Practice at 320 points out of a possible 1,000—was scattering and quite uncoordinated. The community budget for public health, including the maintenance of an isolation hospital, was not low as compared with prevailing small-city standards—eighty-eight cents per capita—but sixty cents of this went for the hospitalization of communicable diseases and only twenty-eight for preventive work and health promotion.

The first direct effect of the demonstration begun in 1923 was that the city, in order to do its share, employed a full-time health officer. At that time less than 40 per cent of all American cities (of 10,000 or more population) had taken this primary step. Around the health officer the demonstration then built a carefully planned structure of health services—the Board of Education, the Red Cross, and later the Tuberculosis Association sharing in the cost, and the city gradually increasing its stake in the program. The community found these services good, and in the fiscal year 1927-8 Fargo will be served by a full-time health officer, a sanitary and food inspector, a part-time school physician, a school dentist, six public health nurses, a director of school health education, and two clerical workers—the entire staff being carried on the public payrolls with the exception of the

20

school dentist, whose salary is temporarily subsidized by the Red Cross. The budget for public health activities has risen to $1.51 per capita; and while the appropriation for the isolation hospital has fallen to 38 cents per capita, $1.13 is devoted to the general purposes of the health department and of health education in the public schools. With this development, the volume and standard of public health services have also increased so rapidly that the American Public Health Association appraised Fargo's performance in 1926 at 814 points out of a possible 1,000.

While such "take-over" is still incomplete in the other centers, local appropriations for health have gradually increased in each of them. During the past year a significant indication of the drift of public opinion in Rutherford County was seen in the vote of the County Court, by a large majority, to levy for the year 1928 a tax of five cents per hundred dollars of valuation for the health unit to replace the three-cent levy fixed in 1926. In Athens the school board, already carrying the major part of the salary of the director of school health education, made room in its budget also for an oral hygienist whose value had been dramatically shown by the achievements of the last school year above recorded. An interesting illustration of the way in which a demonstration may serve as the nucleus around which varied efforts for public health gather is found in Marion County, where the organized dentists of Oregon have helped to finance an experimental program in dental hygiene which is already well established in the county and has begun to influence public health dentistry in other parts of the state.

The inference from such practical endorsements is that the staff workers sponsored by the demonstration have succeeded in serving a sufficiently large part of the community to influence public opinion and have commended themselves

21

130

to those who have been served. Although no one of the demonstrations has thought it wise (in view of local resources) to provide nursing service in the ratio which is considered theoretically desirable—one nurse to 2,000 people—it is interesting to note that in Fargo, in 1926, the staff nurses visited children or adults in approximately half of all the families in the community; in Clarke and Rutherford Counties, about a third; and in Marion County, with a working area of a thousand square miles, nurses are reaching ten per cent of all families. An exceptionally complete job has been done by the staff dentist in Marion County, who in 1926 actually inspected the teeth of nine out of ten children in the schools of the entire county.

Since the program has been directly focused on the health of mothers and children, it is fair to ask whether the service given to these special groups has been at the expense of the balanced development of public health. The fundamental purpose of the demonstrations was to secure a wider acceptance of maternal and child health services as an essential part of a complete public health program. It was clearly recognized from the start that only when the more familiar routines of the health department were competently performed could such specialized services be added with any hope of success. The Child Health Demonstration Committee has therefore supported to the best of its ability— first by moral and then, in the rural demonstrations, by financial aid—the full range of health department services. How well these services have fared is indicated by the chart on the opposite page, in which by averaging the performance[1] of all four communities, for the corresponding pre-demonstration and demonstration years, in three major groups of public health activities, a comparison is shown between child health progress and that of communicable

[1] As rated by the American Public Health Association on its Appraisal Forms.

22

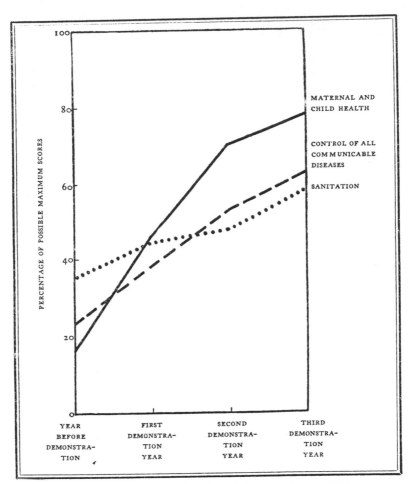

MATERNAL AND CHILD HEALTH

CONTROL OF ALL COMMUNICABLE DISEASES

SANITATION

TRENDS IN PUBLIC HEALTH PROGRESS IN DEMONSTRATION AREAS

As rated for certain groups of activities in appraisals by the American Public Health Association. Average of ratings for four years in Fargo, Clarke County, and Rutherford County, and for three years in Marion County.

disease control and sanitation. Child health services, beginning at a relatively low level, have bettered at a more rapid rate, but a comparable gain has been registered by the other groups of activities. It seems fair to conclude that the intensive promotion of child health in these four communities

23

INFANT MORTALITY RATES FOR RESIDENTS
OF DEMONSTRATION AREAS

DEATHS UNDER ONE YEAR PER 1000 LIVE BIRTHS

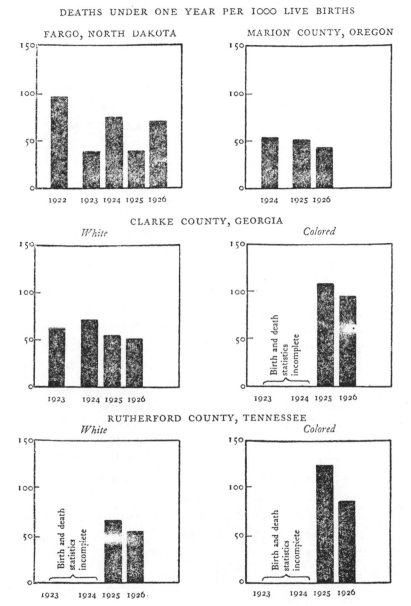

FARGO, NORTH DAKOTA

MARION COUNTY, OREGON

CLARKE COUNTY, GEORGIA

White

Colored

Birth and death statistics incomplete

RUTHERFORD COUNTY, TENNESSEE

White

Colored

Birth and death statistics incomplete

Birth and death statistics incomplete

24

has been accompanied by substantial progress all along the line in public health.

When an attempt is made to measure progress by vital statistics, a familiar difficulty is found. Before sound health department practice is begun the recording of births and deaths is usually so meagre and inaccurate that there is no firm basis for "before and after" comparisons. When the demonstrations began only Marion County was in both the birth and death registration areas; Fargo came into the birth registration area with North Dakota in 1924; Tennessee has been admitted only this year; Georgia is still outside it.[1] Particularly among the colored population of Clarke and Rutherford Counties has reporting been fragmentary and undependable. Yet, with due reserve, it is worth while to examine the infant mortality rates for Fargo and Clarke and Marion Counties for the pre-demonstration year and each succeeding year to 1926 (1927 figures are not available as this is written.) It appears from the chart herewith (p. 24), that there has been a slight decrease in infant mortality in Marion and Clarke Counties. The exceptionally low figures for Fargo in 1923 and 1925 show a fluctuation which is greater than would be expected even with so small a number of cases and are thus far unexplained. Rutherford County rates and those for Negroes in Clarke County are given to show the present favorable situation, although the lack of adequate records prior to the demonstration makes it impossible to attach much importance to the trend. It is interesting to note that in Rutherford County in 1926 only 3 per cent of the 478 infants under observation by the nursing service died in their first year, as compared with 14 per cent of the 250 not receiving this service.

The emphasis of the demonstration is on preserving and

[1] Since this was written the state has been admitted as of 1928.

25

building up the health of the so-called "normal" child. In an effort to determine, if possible, the broad outlines of the health history of the group of children served in Fargo, an exhaustive study is being made of the records of health center and school medical examinations, weighing and measuring, throughout the demonstration. The accompanying graph represents a summary of some early findings.

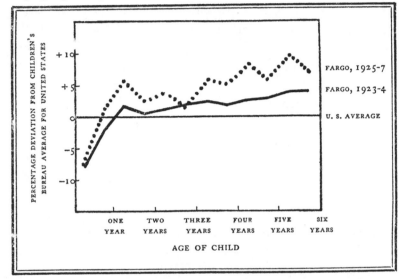

WEIGHT IMPROVEMENT IN FARGO INFANTS AND PRE-SCHOOL
CHILDREN DURING THE DEMONSTRATION PERIOD

As shown by 5642 measurements of 2096 children examined at health centers

When the weights of infants and pre-school children under observation at the health centers early in the demonstration are compared with later weights (taken during the past three years), and with the average for children throughout the United States, a clear-cut gain for Fargo children is indicated. Further study of these figures in comparison with clinical findings is of course necessary and will be made before final conclusions are drawn.

26

Studying and evaluating group attitudes is one of the most fascinating and least satisfactory—because the least exact—of all forms of social inquiry. The experience of the demonstrations appears to point strongly toward one conclusion: that it is possible to set up, in a relatively short time, an attitude on the part of school teachers which gives health a radically different status in the schoolroom, and so in the minds of growing children, from that which it has previously held. The four school health educators have all succeeded to a marked degree in developing a genuine interest in health teaching among the public school teachers in the elementary grades and this has been reflected in a quick response on the part of the children, who have espoused health habits, kept daily health records, submitted cheerfully to the ministrations of doctor and dentist, and joined eagerly in a variety of competitive and individual tests of their health achievements. Naturally it is not only the child in school who benefits by this emphasis on simple daily health habits. An amusing illustration of the impact of the new teaching on conditions in the home may be gleaned from this paragraph, taken from a composition written by a youngster hailing from one of Fargo's foreign-born families:

I have three sisters and two brothers. My biggest sister and I never ate food when we were babies like the four other children. Mamma didn't know the difference.

How I am now mamma says is from oatmeal and milk. Ever since the Health Records came out I have tried to keep them up. My weight is 60 pounds. I am 10 years old. Mamma didn't care for it at first but now she likes it. Our home is much cleaner. We had it clean before, but Oh! there is so much difference now.

To a very considerable extent this progress in health education has been accomplished not by the importation of made-to-order methods, but by personal leadership and

27

136

sound planning on the part of the director which has stimulated the teachers, often inexperienced and hesitant, to
create their own technique by the application of sound
pedagogy to sound facts, and to play an understanding part
in a unified effort to build up the health of their pupils. In
Fargo, a compact and homogeneous city, this process has
been carried through more consciously and consistently,
perhaps, than has been possible under the confused conditions—racial diversities, scattered rural schools, irregular
school terms—of the other demonstrations, but a similar
approach to the problem has been evident in all. The
Fargo teachers not only have learned how to deal with the
individual child's health problem with unusual directness
and clarity, but have united in drawing up a course of health
instruction covering the first six grades, which has been
adopted as standard procedure. The response of the teachers
to such leadership has nowhere been more spectacular than
in Athens, where the teachers of one elementary school,
attended chiefly by the children of millworkers, took the
initiative in setting up a revolving loan fund from which
parents could borrow the cost of needed medical and dental
work for their children, and pushed through to a successful
conclusion a campaign for dental corrections which eventually spread throughout the city schools.

The immunization of children against diphtheria, smallpox, and typhoid, is an important piece of public health
strategy and a contribution to the health of the individual
child. It is significant also as an index to the development
of an attitude toward preventive medicine which is not the
least of the gains to be looked for from the demonstrations.
In Rutherford County—which before 1924 knew almost
nothing of any such measures except smallpox vaccination—
there have been 3,345 completed inoculations against diph-

28

theria, 7,687 smallpox vaccinations, and 8,21 completed typhoid inoculations in a span of about three and a half years. These numbers have been swelled considerably by the blue ribbon campaign in the schools, which has aroused mounting enthusiasm in 1926 and 1927—blue ribbons being awarded only to children who had qualified by receiving all three immunizations as well as by the correction of physical defects and a satisfactory observance of health habits. In Marion County, 3,112 diphtheria inoculations were given in the first eight months of 1927 as the direct result of a county-wide campaign of education led by the deputy health officer. In 1926 there were thirty-one in the entire year. When children voluntarily troop to the doctor for long-range protection against communicable diseases, an attitude of far-reaching importance has been fostered. A similar attitude generally shown by adults would powerfully affect public health progress.

Another community attitude that is somewhat measureable is the willingness of lay men and women to take personal responsibility for a share in public health work. In Fargo, where an executive committee representing leading groups has collaborated with the demonstration, a public health association is planned, to act as a voluntary citizen group in support of the health officer. In Clarke County a local committee has been especially active in a campaign for the take-over, and "block mothers," working under the auspices of the Parent-Teacher Asssociation, have been notably successful in promoting the medical examination of children about to enter school. But it is in Rutherford and Marion Counties that the volunteer health worker comes most clearly into the picture. Fourteen communities in Marion County have organized health councils which form a link between the technical workers of the demonstration

29

and the community at large; eleven of them maintain separate health centers to which the pediatrician and nurse come on regular schedule, the other three uniting at one center in Salem. The missionary spirit which some of these groups show is illustrated by the expedition organized by four ladies from a mill town 40 miles from the county seat who went to a timber town 22 miles farther out to show the folks there how to set up a health center. In Rutherford County a somewhat more recent development has been the organization of health committees, now seventeen in number, which perform a similar function, except that it has not seemed wise to establish permanent health centers outside Murfreesboro. The outline of what one small group of sixteen Rutherford County women has done since its organization in January, 1927, is a homely but illuminating record of genuine community participation in health work. These women have secured for their local school two portable sanitary drinking fountains; have made it possible to serve a hot lunch to the younger school children twice a week; have assisted in weighing and measuring children at the health conference held in their schoolhouse; have helped with the arrangements for school medical examinations; have completed a loan closet for sickroom or maternity use; have reported to the demonstration office cases needing nursing care; and have been active in spreading announcements for the inoculation clinics. Even when the problem is the delicate one of improved home sanitation a similarly cordial response to health department leadership is evident: parent-teacher workers and local magistrates in Rutherford County are taking the lead in bettering their own sanitary arrangements as a step toward changing the somewhat primitive conditions which prevail throughout the rural part of the county.

30

In all such community organization the immediate goal is no more important than the ultimate change in the standards which are accepted and enforced by public opinion. The heart of the demonstration job is after all to make public health, particularly as it concerns children, interesting and thus desirable. A straw in the wind which points toward success in this direction is that in Fargo, Athens, and Marion County commercial organizations have begun to include the local health work among the advertised assets of the community. The newspapers, too—even the scattered local weeklies of Marion County—give evidence that health news has become a matter of general interest. In a word, the public mind has been opened to a new range of ideas; the service of doctors, nurses, and teachers has given the new ideas practical form; and the skilful promotion of community organization has made the resulting health progress a matter for local pride and the object of local effort.

Closely allied to this popular demand for health services is the attitude of the local practitioner toward health supervision. The medical societies in the four communities have officially endorsed the demonstration program as a whole. Individual practitioners have gone further in indicating that they recognize and welcome the aid of the demonstration in promoting preventive medical service. In a group of doctors who were recently asked to state their impression of the results of the community health program as reflected in their own practice one called attention to "better response in supervision of well infants," another to "more attention to nose and throat and eyes of apparently healthy children." Another reported, "Am seeing more children in my practice than formerly," still another, "Women report well for pre-natal and post-natal observation." Another physician in the same community has called attention to the fact that the

31

sound medical and nursing procedures of the demonstration tend to strengthen the position of the well-trained practitioner in competition with the cultist and faddist. As a corollary to an increasing desire for health supervision, the physicians in the demonstration communities have responded cordially to special opportunities for improving their own preventive practice—attending institutes on preventive pediatrics, calling the demonstration pediatricians into consultation, and in one case at least voluntarily suggesting special clinics to prepare themselves for increasing participation in the community health program. Such attitudes on the part of both patient and physician should result in definite betterment of the health of the growing generation.

It is too soon to speak definitely and finally of these somewhat intangible factors in community life, but the indications point strongly toward the conclusion that the demonstrations are not merely building up public health apparatus, but are helping to create the public opinion which, in years to come, will make it possible for that apparatus to function effectively.

32

THE DIVISION OF RURAL HOSPITALS

The rural hospital program has maintained, during the past year, its experimental character. No new hospital awards have been made; building construction in the five communities already selected[8] has proceeded according to schedule, with some progressive modification of plans; postgraduate fellowships for physicians and nurses have been gradually developed; medical and nursing institutes have been held; continued study has been given to the question of nursing education; public health organization has been tentatively and very modestly begun.

The program is and should be experimental. Even if it were merely a building project, the task of designing, financing, and equipping the most suitable hospital plant for rural use would call for untiring technical investigation and continuing study of plans and building costs. But it is more than a building project; it is an effort to attack from a fresh angle the difficult problem of medical and public health service in small towns and the open country. It is an effort to change the community standard of living in respect to the care of the sick, the prevention of disease, the protection of health. As such it presents so many new and complex situations that progress must be slow and staff workers must proceed carefully step by step.

The hospital district itself is an anomaly. Within a travel radius of something over an hour by automobile—an obviously practicable unit of territory for hospital and public health service—there are, for example, in the Farmville district nine counties, in the Glasgow district ten, which the hospital is expected to serve. Like the regional planner, the hospital board in such a case must draw financial and moral

[8] Farmville, Virginia; Glasgow, Kentucky; Farmington, Maine; Beloit, Kansas; Wauseon, Ohio.

42

support from a congeries of unrelated political divisions. How are the geographical unity and the governmental disunity of such an area to be reconciled? How are the prestige of the trading center and the independence of the outlying farm communities to be kept in balance? How are established habits of social action to be modified to permit effective team-work in a new population grouping?

The problem of community budgeting for health purposes, touched on in connection with the child health report, arises also when hospital and health unit begin to function side by side. It is clear that they are important to each other: the hospital is needlessly burdened if it must care for the victims of inadequate maternity service, neglected childhood, and faulty sanitation; and the health officer is at a considerable advantage if he can look to the hospital for aid in certain diagnostic problems and in the correction of serious defects in children, for dependable service to the sick and competent assistance in the preventive and educational field. Yet the parallel development and financial adjustment of these activities in a community which is unfamiliar with both, and which has limited resources, may be a puzzling task for the local leaders of public opinion.

Such problems and many others of equal delicacy, make it clear that it is not enough to build a hospital in an accessible town and expect it to work automatically. It is necessary, to be sure, to determine with care what sort of plant is technically appropriate and economically feasible; but it is also necessary that public and professional thinking reach a clear understanding of the purpose of the hospital; that the medical staff grasp firmly the opportunity which it offers for professional progress; that the ways in which the hospital can serve a growing constituency be made clear; that a reasonable course of public health development

43

144

adapted to the community be worked out; and that board and staff adopt sound standards of performance. None of these results can be secured through any rigid adherence to preconceived theories. They call for a genuinely experimental attitude.

For further study of such problems as these the staff of the division has been enlarged during the year by the addition of Lester J. Evans, M.D., formerly associated with the child health program of the Fund, and Alma C. Haupt, R.N., formerly assistant director of the Division for Austria. The staff has been thus constituted in order that each step in the development of each hospital project may be considered from the four-fold point of view of hospital technique, finance, and general administration; of medical standards and policy; of public health organization; and of nursing technique. The aim is to provide for the local administrative authorities, so far as they desire it, the technical knowledge and growing experience of a trained staff, in the solution of the many new and perplexing problems which arise.

The selection of physicians for the post-graduate fellowships, and the planning of their work, have been matters of personal contact with the local medical group. Increasing effort is made to fit the available training into the individual physician's own needs and into the medical situation of the community from which he comes. Care has been taken to see that men from the outlying rural districts as well as the larger towns are included: out of a total of twenty-five fellowships awarded thus far, nine have enabled physicians from the smaller villages and open country to spend three or four months in city medical centers. The physicians who have completed their periods of study and have returned to practice are unanimous in their testimony that the experience was a valuable one. During the year a beginning has been

44

145

made in extending similar opportunities for post-graduate study to nurses associated with the hospitals, and in several cases appointees to executive positions have been given special courses in preparation for dealing with the somewhat unusual professional problems which these hospitals present.

The most interesting experiment of the year has been the formation of the Southside Health District surrounding the hospital in Farmville, Virginia. The nine counties which are roughly circumscribed by the 35-mile circle used to define the hospital area have a population of 111,000 of which nearly half is colored. Hitherto their local personnel for public health has been limited to a sanitation officer and a nurse in Prince Edward County, a Red Cross nurse in Nottoway, and a sanitation officer in Powhatan. The other five counties have been without public health service except as it was supplied by traveling workers from the State Health Department or the Red Cross. The State Health Department, with the aid of the Fund, has now linked these nine counties into a public health district and staffed a district unit with a health officer and nurse, both on full time. The function of the unit will be to coordinate the services of the county health workers already on the job, to stimulate the employment of a minimum health staff in each county, and to introduce such district-wide services as prove possible. The health officer, for example, turned his attention immediately upon taking office to a malaria epidemic in one county. The nurse, in addition to organizing local activities and doing a limited amount of instructive visiting, will arrange for the follow-up of cases referred from the hospital for after-care.

The first step in setting up the district health plan was to form an advisory committee which includes the state health officer, the director of nurses in the state department of health, the president and superintendent of the hospital, the

45

chairman of its Women's Auxiliary Board and a representative of its medical staff, the district health officer, a representative of the state Red Cross and representatives of the Commonwealth Fund. While not an executive body, this committee hopes to assist in shaping a health program in which the district unit and the hospital will reinforce each other as agencies for preventive service, and to aid in the difficult task of community budgeting for all health work. A quarterly bulletin will be circulated through the district to interest and inform the public.

The nine counties are all in the dark tobacco section of the state where an unfavorable market for several years has had a depressing effect. It is a question how far any one of them could go alone at present in financing an adequate public health staff. There is, however, as is usual in Virginia, a considerable amount of community organization for educational and health work: the Community Education Association is represented by many local school groups; there is a home or farm demonstration agent, or both, in all but one of the counties; there are eight county Red Cross chapters and a number of tuberculosis associations; each county has a colored rural school supervisor. It should be possible, under state leadership and with the cooperation of a well-equipped hospital, to test pretty thoroughly the utility of this novel form of public health organization.

Except for the county health unit which preceded the building of the Rutherford Hospital in Murfreesboro, Tennessee, there is as yet no comparable development in any of the other communities where the hospital program has been introduced. In Beloit, Kansas, and Wauseon, Ohio, where contracts have just been let for hospital construction, the program is in an early state. No appointments have yet been made to staff positions; no medical or nursing fellowships

46

have been awarded; and no definite public health projects have been worked out. In Farmington, Maine, and Glasgow, Kentucky, building construction is about half complete, and the hospitals are expected to open their doors in the spring of 1929. Some fellowships have been awarded in Glasgow, and superintendents have been appointed by the hospital boards to take office before the opening of the hospitals. Public health activities are still in the stage of preliminary planning with official and unofficial agencies.

In Farmville, however, the program is in full operation. One institute for physicians and one for nurses have been held, and both were warmly received by the local professional groups. Both physicians and nurses have been given fellowships for post-graduate study. The district health officer and his nurse assistant are at work. Utilization of the hospital is increasing. By an interesting coincidence, the first service given within its walls after the formal opening in November, 1928, was a public health clinic for the tuberculous, conducted jointly by state and local health agencies. The Southside Community Hospital and the Southside Health District have begun a significant experiment in public health teamwork.

47

III. RURAL HEALTH AND RURAL MEDICINE

DIVISIONS OF PUBLIC HEALTH AND HEALTH STUDIES

PROGRESS in public health goes on at many different levels. During the past two decades vigorous activity has been found in the rural parts of the United States, where experiments and demonstrations of every sort, ranging from the single nurse to the fully staffed county health unit integrated with a local hospital, have been going on. The technic of serving a rural population has been pretty well worked out; the economics of providing such service is still at loose ends. There is as yet no sure formula by which the economic resources and the manifest health needs of a rural district can be reconciled; no dependable index of the amount of state or federal aid which may be reasonably and productively put into a backward community; no easy solution for the problem of great area and scattered population of counties in the West, nor of the most handicapped regions of the South. It would be unfortunate if the county health unit, which has won recognition as the norm of rural health organization, should be standardized at a point either beyond the reach of most counties or below the purchasing power of the more prosperous communities; indeed it is probably much too soon to attempt standardization of organization, and programs of work must always be flexibly adjusted to local situations.

The Fund has shared in the development of rural health service on several levels. It has aided the state health department of New Mexico to provide a bare minimum of nursing service in counties otherwise uncared for. In connection with the Southside Community Hospital in Farmville, Virginia, it

12

149

has collaborated with the state health department in setting up an organization slightly more elaborate—a small central full-time staff coordinating the work of county nurses and sanitarians, and endeavoring to fill gaps generally, in a group of nine counties treated as a health district. In connection with the Community Hospital at Glasgow, Kentucky, it has aided the state health department to establish a single county unit with a small staff. It has centered its attention, however, on the problem of enriching the service of counties already organized, or groups of towns already receiving numerous health services, in the hope of throwing light on the capacity of locally supported county or town-union health departments to render service which is reasonably complete.

This is not an easy task. The progress of public health handicaps its friends. If yellow fever threatened an American city money would be poured out for protection. But when a generally healthy group of people has set up a decent minimum of safeguards against disease, and few gross dangers seem to threaten the average household, it becomes harder and harder to prove to the taxpayer that he will get his money's worth out of larger payments for public health service. In spite of the existence of more than 500 full-time county health departments, the rural neighborhoods which have as effective a health service as they might have, considering the present state of technical information, could probably be counted on the fingers of one hand.

When the Fund undertakes to convince the people of six rural areas, and through them rural citizens everywhere, that the best in public health is not too good for them, it is necessary first of all to define what is "best" for a given community. The health staff which cramps its work because of bad judgment, limited imagination, or inadequate personnel is an

13

expensive luxury just as truly as one which is overgrown. The lone nurse serving 20,000 people, while she helps scattered individuals, may actually retard the health progress of her county if she permits the public to unload on her harried shoulders responsibilities which they should find other means of carrying. The purpose of immunization against diphtheria is, obviously, to cut down the incidence of the disease, but if too few young children are reached, according to a recent study,[1] the expenditure of time and money produces no measurable effect in that direction. On the other hand, though the danger is not alarming under present conditions, it is possible for the health department to accumulate—as other governmental bureaus have often done—so large a staff that the public becomes disgusted with its extravagance and reacts sharply against the whole program. It is certainly possible for one part of the health department program to absorb so much of the funds and time available that a lop-sided piece of work is done, essential fields are neglected, and thoughtful citizens lose confidence in the health officer's leadership. Most rural health departments are now so sadly understaffed that the practical problem is to build them up. But there was never a time when it was more important to plan shrewdly for maximum output with a limited staff, in order to hold the ground already gained and clear a path for future advances; and present economic pressures make it imperative to stick close to essentials.

While sound plans must be hammered out on the field, there are some resources—a few more each year—for a systematic approach to the task. The methodical analysis of health department functions, stimulated years ago by Dr. Charles V. Chapin of Providence, has been for a decade the

[1]"Study in the Epidemiology of Diphtheria in Relation to the Active Immunization of Certain Age Groups," by Edward S. Godfrey, Jr., M.D., *American Journal of Public Health*, March, 1932.

14

chief concern of the Committee on Administrative Practice of the American Public Health Association. The urban and rural appraisal forms[2] worked out by this committee, while they do not profess to be based on optimum standards, furnish useful specifications for balanced activity. A special study of rural health work, recently completed by Dr. Allen Freeman of Johns Hopkins University under this committee's auspices, draws a base-line from which progress can be measured and indicates where special effort is necessary. Recent investigations of field experience with immunizations against diphtheria,[3] made under the direction of the same committee, help the health officer to keep his feet on the ground. The Commonwealth Fund has assisted in these projects and continues to share in similar undertakings through its Division of Health Studies.

But it is possible to overdo standardization, and we are far from being sure enough of ourselves in public health to say how much of any standard program is universally applicable. One of the tasks of the Fund's Division of Health Studies has been to assemble all the relevant information about each of the areas where the Division of Public Health is at work, so that local programs can be tailored to fit the community in question.

Six Problems

Six rural health departments are at present receiving subsidy and counsel from the Fund: those in Lauderdale and Pike Counties in Mississippi, Gibson and Sullivan Counties in Tennessee, and the Southern Berkshire and Nashoba town-unions in Massachusetts. Study of the topography, population, economic and cultural situation, and vital sta-

[2]*Appraisal Form for City Health Work*, third edition, 1930; *Appraisal Form for Rural Health Work*, second edition, 1932; New York: American Public Health Association.
[3]See page 14.

15

tistics of these communities indicates clearly that no single formula can be applied to the solution of their health problems or to the measurement of their accomplishments.

Three areas—the two Mississippi counties and Gibson in Tennessee—are warm, flat, and occasionally marshy: all show a yearly incidence of more than 1,000 cases of malaria per 100,000 population. The other three are hilly and well-drained; malaria is negligible in all of them. The largest area, Lauderdale, with 700 square miles and 52,911 people, has more than twice the size and population of the smallest, Nashoba, with 287 square miles and 21,917 people.

The Massachusetts areas have a static population, with a substantial minority of foreign-born whites, a few Negroes, and a high average age. In Nashoba, for example, almost half the people are over 35 years old and one out of ten has reached the age of 65. Gibson County in Tennessee, and the two Mississippi counties, are growing at a rate roughly comparable with that of the states in which they lie, have less than one per cent of foreign-born whites, and have Negro populations ranging from 21 to 45 per cent. Their population is younger than that of Massachusetts. Sullivan County stands by itself. Shortly before 1920 a planned industrial city, Kingsport, was built and opened for settlement. Young workers poured into it from the Appalachian highlands, and the county as a whole grew 41 per cent in the last decade. The population is almost entirely native white (0.3 per cent foreign-born, 3.5 per cent Negro), and it is a young group; less than 29 per cent are 35 or over, and only one out of every 28 citizens has seen his sixty-fifth birthday. One might speculate at length on the differences in temper and outlook which would be found in a settled, aging community in the North, a shifting, young, homogeneous community in Tennessee, and a community split almost in half by the color line

16

in Mississippi. Marked differences appear in the vital statistics; for example, the Mississippi counties have double the birth rate of Nashoba and the Southern Berkshire area, and the mortality rates for cancer and heart disease are half again as high in Massachusetts as in the other areas. The health department in Sullivan County has 1,200 babies under one year of age to care for; Nashoba and the Southern Berkshire area together can marshal less than 500.

Economically the six areas show still another grouping. Nashoba, Pike, and Gibson are essentially rural and agricultural, but farmland and buildings are worth $248 per acre in Nashoba and $24 in Pike. Lauderdale has a large urban group; Sullivan and the Southern Berkshire area have important industrial interests. The spendable money income per capita in Nashoba in 1929[4] was estimated at $1,091; in Gibson $246. Per capita savings bank deposits in Massachusetts are from five to fifteen times as great as in the other areas. Less than 3 per cent of the adult population in the Massachusetts areas is illiterate; the Tennessee counties show 6 and 7 per cent; the Mississippi counties 11 per cent.

Disease incidence varies widely. In the ten-year period ending with 1930, there was no case of smallpox in either Massachusetts area. In the last four years of this decade Sullivan showed 37 cases per 100,000 population. In Massachusetts typhoid fever occurs rarely, and the problem is to handle the infrequent outbreaks resulting from the activity of a carrier. In the other areas the typhoid death rate[5] varies from 9.9 (Sullivan) to 17.8 (Gibson). In diphtheria, while the downward trend is general, the southern counties show a perceptible lag behind Massachusetts. Tuberculosis is less menacing in Massachusetts than in the southern counties

[4]*Sales Management Magazine*, September 27, 1930. The Middlesex County figure has been used for Nashoba.
[5]For the period 1926–1930.

17

where the incidence among Negroes is heavy: Lauderdale has a rate[6] of 108.6 as compared with 31.3 for Nashoba. Such comparisons might be carried on almost indefinitely, but those already made suggest how necessary it is to plan an individual approach to every district.

The Field Units

In its public health program the Fund tries to strike a balance between sound general principles and the strategy which is dictated by the needs and psychology of a given community. One of the most effective tools for strengthening both plan and performance is the field unit which has been set up in each of the three states. This unit, an innovation in rural health organization, consists of a team of carefully selected workers—a physician trained in public health, a nurse, a sanitarian, and a clerk. Singly and in combination, these workers act as intermediaries between the state health officer and the local health department, bringing the former accurate information and a skilled interpretation of local situations, advising the latter, stimulating better technic in individual tasks, and helping to map the strategy of local service.

In Mississippi, before the organization of the field unit, the state health department ordinarily made a field contact only when it was necessary to save a budget by intensive effort, to adjust differences of opinion, to cope with an epidemic, or to stiffen a drive for elementary sanitation. The field unit set up in the summer of 1931 has already visited every one of the 28 organized counties in the state to establish working relations with the local staff, has made complete factual studies—the first ever attempted—of the work of 24, and has given in-

[6] For the period 1926–1930.

18

tensive care to Pike and Lauderdale Counties. Stress has been laid on budget planning, betterment of routine practices, communicable disease control, nursing, and general balance of program in accordance with local needs. Records have been studied and suggestions made for their standardization. The field unit has helped local personnel to think objectively about their work. In one county where the health officer, interpreting his local situation too casually, was complacent about the conditions relating to diphtheria, the field unit cut through to the facts of the case with the result that 3,056 immunizing treatments were given in four months as compared with 272 for the preceding ten years!

Of the 95 counties in Tennessee 42 have full-time health departments, either singly or in two-county units. With substantial help from the United States Public Health Service, the Rockefeller Foundation, the Commonwealth Fund, and, on special problems, the Rosenwald Fund, the state health officer has brought full-time county health work to a pitch where it is probably better organized and better supervised than in any other state. Even here, however, the time of the supervisory force, prior to the organization of the field technical service, was given mostly to promotion and to personnel matters. The new unit has been found to be a definite asset in improving the quality of local performance, and has been enlarged. Dr. E. L. Bishop, state health commissioner, comments on the field unit as follows:

My opinion is that no service we have ever developed in this department has a more profound influence in the development of both better quality and better quantity of public health activity. In this connection, I am sure you will also be interested to know that Alabama, one of our neighboring states, has developed a very similar service and a unit of personnel closely comparable to ours. This has been done on the state health department's own initiative.

19

The administrative situation in Massachusetts differs sharply from that in either of these southern states. Of the fourteen counties in the state only one has health service organized on a county basis; public health responsibility is diffused among a great number of separately incorporated cities and towns; and the state health department wields only so much authority as it can earn for itself by persuasion and manifest technical leadership. Distances are not so great as in the typical southern states, and the staff of the state health department is more readily on call. The field unit here, therefore, plays a less important role than in Mississippi or Tennessee, confining its attention to the two town-unions aided by the Fund and to Barnstable County on Cape Cod, which has its own full-time department. But it has proved useful in laying the foundation for a uniform record system, working out problems with the local health staff, referring knotty questions to the state department, bringing back decisions on policy, and helping to translate these into action. Members of the field unit have substituted for local workers in emergency and the sanitarian, in particular, has been indispensable in getting local sanitary programs under way.

The Mississippi Counties

In Lauderdale County, on the eastern border of Mississippi, the Fund is supplying 53 per cent of a $42,300 budget (78 cents per capita) for county health service. A full-time department in this county jogged along comfortably from 1928 to 1931; in the summer of that year new personnel and a new concept of health work quickened its pace. The health officer has been stimulated to plan and carry out a balanced program. The nursing staff has been increased and strengthened. A perfunctory milk-meat inspection service has given

20

way to the aggressive work of an inspector with a veterinarian's diploma; the percentage of the city milk supply which is pasteurized has been almost doubled. Two typhoid carriers have been discovered, one of whom may have been responsible for a widespread epidemic in 1923. The appointment of a dental hygienist has been followed by a school campaign in which 3,500 out of 4,000 city school children were certified as free of dental defects. Two chest clinics are being held each month; old and new cases of tuberculosis are being followed up; and there is marked improvement in the tone of communicable disease control generally.

Three separate efforts had been made in Pike County to launch effective health work before the establishment of the present service late in 1931. With the budget of $29,250 (89 cents per capita), of which 62 per cent comes from the Fund, the county now has a full-time staff of ten persons. Communicable diseases are systematically investigated and recorded. Growing use is made of the public health laboratory. A thoughtful attack is being made on sanitary problems. A considerable number of school children have been examined. Infant and preschool conferences have been begun, and 98 per cent of the children attending them have been immunized against diphtheria. The development of competent service during the past year has been matched by a striking shift of public opinion from indifference or hostility to cordial support of the health department. This was dramatically revealed when a few food-handlers attempted to block the department's work. The editor of the McComb *Enterprise*, a leader in the campaign for better health service, found the whole community up in arms and marshalled a demonstration before the county Board of Supervisors which resulted in a clear-cut endorsement of the new unit.

21

Gibson County was the first unit to begin operating under the Fund's present public health program. In 1930 a full-time county health department, dating from 1922, was expanded and reorganized; in 1932 it had a staff of eleven and a budget of $29,231 (62 cents per capita), of which the Fund supplied 40 per cent. The health officer, an enthusiastic clinician, has established genuine leadership among the physicians, has kindled their interest in prenatal and obstetrical problems, and has built up an aggressive program for venereal disease control. One or two physicians, accepting scholarships for postgraduate study soon after the program was launched, caught the idea of collaboration between general medicine and public health and have led their colleagues to make liberal use of health department facilities. While the program as a whole has been less evenly developed than in some of the other counties, there has been a high level of achievement in the fields which especially command local interest. Prenatal cases have come to the nursing staff in such numbers that the health department has found it hard to carry them. Medical supervision was established before the fifth month of pregnancy in 23 per cent of the prenatal cases visited by the nurses in 1931; before the seventh month in 57 per cent; and before the ninth month in 96 per cent. The growth of this service is shown in the following table:

EXTENT OF NURSING SERVICE FOR EXPECTANT MOTHERS
AND FOR INFANTS, GIBSON COUNTY

	1929	*1930*	*1931*
New prenatal cases under nursing supervision	32	321	400
Ratio of cases under prenatal nursing supervision to total births, in percentage	3.8	35.5	41.9
Infants under nursing supervision	151	420	584
Ratio of infants under nursing supervision to live births, in percentage	18.9	47.6	62.5

22

159

Sullivan County has had full-time health department service since 1928. The Fund now contributes 51 per cent of a budget of $23,526 (43 cents per capita) which provides a staff of nine persons. Of two school nurses employed by the industrial cities of Bristol and Kingsport one has been and the other shortly will be attached to the county nursing staff in the interest of unified planning and supervision. The story here is of methodical, uneventful progress in rounding out and building up an adequate county health service. In 1929, before Fund aid was given, the work done in vital statistics, venereal disease control, tuberculosis control, maternity, infancy, preschool, and school hygiene scored below 50 per cent of the standards established in the Appraisal Form for Rural Health Work. In 1931 all but one of the fields of work specified in the Appraisal Form showed ratings above 60 per cent. Improved technic in communicable disease control, steady pressure for immunizations against typhoid fever and smallpox, increased nursing service for the tuberculous, the establishment of three venereal disease clinics, the development of prenatal and infant care by the nurses to a point where a third of the expectant mothers and more than half of the newborn infants come under supervision, the successful introduction of the blue ribbon plan of stimulating school hygiene—all these changes have contributed to the attainment of a total rating for the department of 700 points out of a possible 1,000. For the past two years deaths from diarrhea and enteritis under two years of age have been so greatly reduced that the average rate for 1931-1932 is less than half the rate for the two preceding years.

The Massachusetts Town-Unions

In the four counties already discussed the public health problem, though difficult enough, is not complicated by ques-

23

tions of jurisdiction and organization. The county health unit is accepted as the normal vehicle for rural service. In Massachusetts the situation is quite different. The county is an unimportant agency of government; the town is an independent political entity and jealous of its independence. Health jurisdiction rests in the town in spite of the fact that it is usually too small either to find funds for full-time health service or to exercise any significant control over sanitation and communicable disease. The towns, the schools, and voluntary agencies have provided a considerable body of health service—part-time health officers, part-time school physicians, visiting nurses, milk inspectors—and have spent a good deal of money in doing so. The sixteen towns which now form the Southern Berkshire health district, before they came together, were finding approximately $1.78 per capita per year for such purposes; the fourteen towns in the Nashoba district, $1.10 per capita per year. It is doubtful whether they were getting their money's worth, because there were too many separate and uncorrelated jobs. But neither poverty nor indifference to health values is the major obstacle to progress: the first need is to clear the channel for thrifty and efficient use of the community's existing resources.

This requires an approach which is quite unlike the typical demonstration of health services in undeveloped or underdeveloped territory. The individual towns must first be led to share their health responsibilities; means must be found to permit the actual pooling of their appropriations; workers on the job must slowly be brought to recognize the advantage of staff team-work; the services of established societies must be respected; public and private activities must be fitted gradually into a pattern which will justify itself both to the professional worker and to the voter, who holds through the town-

24

161

meetings a close grip on the public purse. This calls for imagination, tact, and patience on the part of the health officer. He must find a way to render service which his part-time predecessors could not render, and so demonstrate the value of the unit; he must also stay his hand when action would antagonize a group which is not quite ready to give up its isolated position.

Such a process has been going on in the Southern Berkshire area since the end of 1930. The boards of health of fifteen towns surrounding and including Great Barrington agreed to appoint a single health officer as their common agent, and one hesitant partner, a mountain town with sixty residents, joined the group a year later. An "advisory" nurse, two staff nurses, and a clerk were placed on the district unit. The sanitarian of the field unit was assigned to the district to organize an inspection service; after a year of effort, the immediate problem was neatly solved by spreading the service of two existing inspectors, one employed jointly by the towns of Lee, Lenox, and Stockbridge, the other employed by Great Barrington alone, to cover all the remaining towns in the district. Still later, an important step toward unified nursing service was taken when the Great Barrington Visiting Nurse Association, already serving five towns besides Great Barrington, agreed to federate with the district health unit, with the director of the Association as supervising nurse. Under this arrangement the health unit has the added advantage of being able to use as its headquarters the endowed house, centrally placed, which belongs to the Association. Meanwhile the unit has given nursing service to towns in need of it and has set up a dental hygiene service, using half the time of a state worker and correlating the efforts of the local dentists and parent-teacher associations. These de-

25

velopments have done much to translate the elusive concept of inter-town cooperation into the kind of reality that can be seen and talked about by the average citizen.

The Nashoba district, centering in Ayer, had a little less in the way of health service to begin with. Two staff nurses have been assigned to unfilled territory; a district sanitary inspector has made good progress in securing tuberculin tests for local herds; and the health officer has carried on immunization campaigns in seven towns. A diagnostic service for tuberculosis has been tentatively launched and plans are in order for the beginning of well-child conferences at which a skilled pediatrician from Boston will demonstrate the technic of examination and health teaching to the local physicians. Further study will be needed before a wise adjustment can be made of nursing service throughout the district, but the ten nurses employed locally are already accepting in some measure the leadership of the district "advisory" nurse. The laboratory set up a year ago in cooperation with the Community Hospital in Ayer is well regarded by the physicians. The unit has the advantage of well-informed, aggressive leadership on the part of the business man who heads the Associated Boards of Health and should continue to grow in usefulness during the coming year.

The Financial Outlook

There comes a time in such projects when it is fair to test their success by the willingness of the community served to assume, up to the limit of its power, the cost of health service. These six units, still in the period of early development, can hardly be said to have reached that stage. The subsidies from the Fund are still serving, therefore, as a bulwark for the new activities; yet since these subsidies are proportionate to the funds supplied by local and state appropriations, the

26

163

fate of each piece of work has definitely rested with the state and county or district concerned. The six projects have fared well so far. There have been no crippling reductions in budget, and the states have proved their faith in the experiment by keeping up their share of the cost even in the face of severe fiscal stress. In Mississippi, for example, where the state health department suffered the loss of a full third of its income in 1932, there was no decrease in the state appropriation or in local funds for health work in Pike County. In Lauderdale County local appropriations were one-third greater in 1932 than in 1931. In Tennessee, where the state health department shared in a horizontal cut of 11¼ per cent applied to all state services, the state maintained its share of the costs of health work in Gibson and Sullivan Counties. The local tax levy for health in Gibson County was cut 14 per cent, slightly more than the general tax rate but less than the school tax rate. In Sullivan County, though the general tax rate was cut 24 per cent, the lump-sum appropriation for health was increased 20 per cent. In Massachusetts there was only a nominal reduction in the state budget and none in the local budgets for the Southern Berkshire and Nashoba areas.

Some further light on the current financial outlook for public health work of an advanced type comes from the experience of Rutherford County, Tennessee, and Fargo, North Dakota, where child health demonstrations were carried on prior to 1929. Both budgets have been reduced for the year beginning July 1, 1932, by 20 per cent in Rutherford and by 18 per cent in Fargo. In both instances the schools took a larger cut, and in Rutherford the situation was gravely complicated by bank failures which had embarrassed the whole community. In Marion County, Oregon, a drastic cut was made, but there a fundamental weakness in the health

27

department may fairly be held jointly responsible with the depression.

So far as the contacts of the Fund indicate, public health holds its own by comparison with other governmental services and the loss of income which health departments must naturally share with other public agencies has not reached the point of disaster. The present project in rural public health is still young, but the Fund has no reason to change its belief that if public health work is soundly planned and capably administered, with full recognition of local needs and capacities, and if the health officer keeps the public abreast of what he is doing by intelligent and persistent educational leadership, small cities and rural communities will do their part toward providing an adequate health service. The task of the Divisions of Health Studies and Public Health is then to help define and illustrate adequate health service for rural districts, and to show the health officer the way to carry his public with him.

THE DIVISION OF RURAL HOSPITALS

In spite of the close relation between public health and the broader field of medicine, much more attention has been paid in this country to the development of public health service for rural communities than to the betterment of their basic medical service. The rural hospital program of the Fund is an attempt to provide, through the construction of general hospitals and the operation of special educational services in connection with them, a means of overcoming something of the lag which rural medicine shows by comparison with the highly developed structure of medical practice in the cities. Its immediate objectives are not only to make a place where those grievously ill can be competently cared for, but to set up higher standards of therapy

28

and preventive care which will color the everyday home-and-office practice of the physician.

One of the most obvious indications of this rural lag in medicine is the fact, often noted in recent years, that the men to whom the farmer and villager must turn for help in sickness are an older group than their city colleagues and that as they drop out of practice there are few well-qualified young men to take their places. It is not impossible to make a good living in the rural practice of medicine, but it is easier to make a large return in the city, and it is far easier to practice modern medicine in the city than in the ordinary small town. The Fund believed, when it began its rural hospital work, that the presence of a well-equipped hospital, with a diagnostic laboratory, convenient x-ray facilities, and good nursing care, would help to make rural practice more attractive to young physicians, and this belief has been justified by the experience of the six communities where such hospitals have been built.[7] Five young men have opened offices in Farmville, Virginia, since the hospital there was projected. Four men who had seen service in the local hospital as residents—two in the Beloit district, one each in Wauseon and Glasgow—have hung out their shingles somewhere in the area served by the hospital. A senior medical student at Vanderbilt, required to visit the Rutherford County Health Department and Rutherford Hospital as part of his instruction, has decided to settle in a Rutherford County hamlet. All sorts of personal reasons may influence the choice of a place to practice, but some of these young men say definitely that the hospital has been a deciding factor in their own cases. They will be useful reinforcements for the thinning line of medical service.

[7]Murfreesboro, Tennessee; Farmville, Virginia; Farmington, Maine; Glasgow, Kentucky; Beloit, Kansas; Wauseon, Ohio.

29

The bulk of the practice in these and other communities, however, will be done for many years, and properly so, by physicians of riper years. It is not easy to find objective measurements for changes in the character and quality of medical practice, though the Division of Rural Hospitals is at present feeling its way toward the formulation of such measurements. But much may be inferred from the informal, intimate contacts with local physicians which representatives of the Division make in the course of their advisory service to the hospitals and the hospital communities, and the burden of evidence in all of these six areas is that the men who lead their profession locally are conscious of a general improvement in the kind of medicine that is being practiced. The records kept of cases in the hospital show in many instances a consistent use of sound diagnostic procedures which would have been difficult if not impossible for most of the physicians in the absence of a hospital. In several communities the hospital has furnished a convenient link between the local practitioner and a medical center; some of the local physicians find that the resident, a youngster fresh from training, is also a valuable co-worker.

While out-patient service develops slowly in these hospitals, for reasons which have been outlined in earlier reports, it changes the medical picture significantly in those communities where it is firmly established—chiefly Farmville and Rutherford. The sight of three or four doctors working together in a clinic, comparing their observations, discussing a case with genuine professional interest, is a gratifying one when it is recalled that some of these same doctors would have found little opportunity a few years ago to meet on such a footing. Something of the same spirit has grown up about the x-ray service in Farmington, and if competitive rivalries die hard in some of the hospitals, the very

30

167

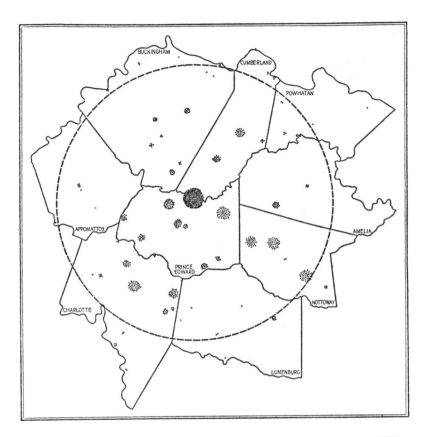

WHERE SOUTHSIDE HOSPITAL PATIENTS CAME FROM IN 1931. THE
CIRCLE HAS A THIRTY-FIVE-MILE RADIUS FROM FARMVILLE

urgency of the current economic situation tends to bring
staff members into some degree of partnership.

The expectations of the Fund have been met in another
phase of hospital experience. Farmville offers an interesting
illustration of the validity of the scheme which governed the
original choice of hospital areas. It was assumed, when the
plan was drafted, that a sufficient clientele to make economi-
cal use of a fifty-bed hospital was likely to be spread over a

31

168

service area with a radius of thirty-five miles or less from the hospital, and that such an area would send cases to the hospital if the institution was conveniently placed with reference to established lines of trade and communication. The circle describing the service area of the Southside Community Hospital at Farmville sweeps over nine counties, and with due allowance for breaks and bulges due to the pull of hospital centers outside the area, the actual spread of service, as the accompanying map shows, tends to fill out the circle. More than half the in-patients, in 1931, came from outside the central county, Prince Edward. Detailed study of the distribution of service shows several outlying towns from which patients have come in growing numbers year by year. Sometimes this cumulative evidence of confidence in the hospital seems to link up with the attitude of a local physician who has been away for postgraduate study and is trying to practice better medicine. It is of vital importance for any program of rural hospitalization that just such habits of using a hospital should be formed, for it is hard to find a firm economic base for hospital service within the compass of a single small town.

The six hospitals in which the Fund is interested have shared with similar institutions throughout the country the severe handicaps caused by the lowering of the general income level. It is common experience that fewer patients can pay the usual rates for hospital service and that the demand for free or part-pay service is relatively increased. Average occupancy in these six hospitals, which in almost every case was climbing slowly upward until the past year (for the effect of the depression seems to have been much more obvious in 1932 than in 1931 in these rural communities) has declined, the decreases ranging from 7 per cent in Farmville to 42 in Glasgow. It has been necessary for the local boards to

32

169

cut expenses and in some instances to let staff vacancies go unfilled. But not one of these six hospitals has closed its doors or suspended service for a day, and there has been reassuring evidence that these communities will not willingly relinquish the advantages which the hospital has brought them.

The experience of Farmville is particularly enlightening, since this hospital was opened before the depression, almost met with disaster, and has won some degree of stability in spite of the fact that the region which it serves has been handicapped for many years by low prices and poor crop conditions in its staple product, tobacco. In its first full year of operation, 1928, it gave 5,820 patient-days of service; in 1929, this total fell off slightly; in the next two years the count rose steadily to a peak of 7,580. If the experience of the first nine months of 1932 (to the end of the period covered by this report) is maintained throughout the year the annual total will be 7,267—a decrease, but not a disturbing one. Cash receipts from patients, however, tell a somewhat different story, rising gradually from $23,766 in 1928 to $27,429 in 1930, declining in 1931, and falling back to $23,966 as the estimated total for 1932. The reason for this drop is evident when the economic classification of patients is recorded:

CLASSIFICATION OF PATIENTS, SOUTHSIDE COMMUNITY
HOSPITAL, 1929–1932

	PAY PER CENT	PART-PAY PER CENT	FREE PER CENT
1929	41.5	52.3	6.2
1930	35.7	50.3	14.0
1931	23.2	54.1	22.7
1932 (nine months) . .	18.1	55.6	26.3

33

There is a notable and consistent decline in pay work with a corresponding rise in free work, with the part-pay group comparatively unchanged. Presumably patients who would formerly have been able to pay in full have moved over into the part-pay classification, and others who might have paid something are now receiving free service. Not all this change can safely be attributed to shrinking personal incomes; the hospital has developed an out-patient department during this period, which tends to increase the volume of free care, and the influence of the Fund has been exerted to persuade the local board to permit a reasonable expansion of free work. But after allowing for both these factors, it seems clear that, under existing arrangements, the public is unable to pay as much for hospital care as was the case two or three years ago.

Yet the average occupancy and the total service, as measured in patient-days, has declined very slightly, and public and private contributions have met the deficit. One is tempted to infer that this community, accustomed to economic handicaps, has established in five years the habit of using hospital facilities and the conviction that the community must and can find some way of meeting their cost. It can hardly be doubted that a better level of medical service to the community as a whole results from this habit and this conviction. If the depression persists, the picture may change, but the experience of Farmville is heartening to the other hospitals, which were established more recently and had little opportunity to develop a stable financial plan before the present economic situation multiplied their difficulties.

All six of the communities have adopted thus far entirely conventional methods of meeting the operating deficits of their hospitals. In Farmington, voluntary contributions carry the budget; in Murfreesboro, public appropriations; all the

34

other hospitals have relied on a combination of private and public funds, the latter being provided either as direct subventions or in the form of per diem payments for the care of indigents. In several areas whose economic life has been seriously disarranged by existing conditions these resources have barely sufficed to maintain the hospitals, but it has not seemed wise to the Fund to step in and relieve the community of its responsibility. Until the public faces squarely the issue whether it will or will not keep the doors of the hospital open, it is never going to learn what the hospital is worth, and until opinion on this point is crystallized the hospital is never going to exert its maximum influence on standards of medical care. Glasgow, which has suffered most during the past year, seems to have reached just this critical point; after an anxious interval public opinion has rallied to the support of the hospital. Here the local board has begun an experiment with a family membership scheme. This provides for the payment of a small fixed sum in semi-annual or monthly payments for a term of five years, with the understanding that such payments will be credited against hospital bills if any member of the family needs hospital service within the five years. The principle of spreading the costs of hospital care as widely as possible over the community seems sound. The Fund is now studying the mechanics of such types of hospital financing, in the hope of making an experiment in the near future in the application of the fixed-charge or voluntary insurance plan to a new rural hospital.

35

The Milbank Memorial Fund

MILBANK MEMORIAL FUND

QUARTERLY BULLETIN

NEW YORK
HEALTH AND TUBERCULOSIS DEMONSTRATIONS

| VOL. I | JANUARY 1924 | NO. 4 |

MEETING OF THE ADVISORY COUNCIL

THE Advisory Council of the Milbank Memorial Fund held its second annual meeting in New York City on November 15, 1923, with almost its entire membership present. The purpose of the meeting was to review the progress of the demonstrations in Cattaraugus County and in Syracuse and to consider a tentative plan for the proposed New York City demonstration, which as shown in a later section (p. 39), had been carefully developed by the Technical Board and submitted in advance to the members of the Advisory Council for their individual criticism. While it is not possible to present here all of the interesting and inspiring suggestions brought out in the discussion, this issue of the Quarterly Bulletin has been enlarged to include extracts and summaries of some of the speeches.

The members of the Advisory Council were welcomed on behalf of the Fund by Edward W. Sheldon, president of the Board of Directors. The meeting was presided over by the Chairman of the Council, Dr. William H. Welch, Dean of the School of Hygiene of Johns Hopkins University. A tribute to the late Dr. Hermann M. Biggs, former Commissioner of Health of the State of New York, and member of the Fund's Advisory Council and Technical Board, was presented by Dr. T. Mitchell Prudden and adopted as a minute of the Council.

SUMMARY OF THE PROCEEDINGS

EDWARD W. SHELDON, *President, United States Trust Company of New York:*

Mr. Albert G. Milbank, who presided at the first meeting of the Advisory Council, has asked me to express, on behalf of the Directors and Officers of the Milbank Memorial Fund, a welcome to you tonight and our most cordial greetings. I like to feel that all of us, hosts and guests, are thinking of that noble woman whose gracious hospitality we are now sharing and who devoted her life and her talent variously and constructively to the great cause of making the world a better place for other people to live in, and to whose prescient judgment our gathering here tonight owes its cause. I shall always treasure in my heart, with grateful pride, the faithful and inspiring friendship with which she so long honored me, and may I ask you to rise and drink to the dear memory of Elizabeth Milbank Anderson?

     *   *   *   *   *   *   *

Since our last meeting a year ago, this Council and the whole State of New York has suffered a tragic loss in the death of Dr. Hermann M. Biggs, one of the original members of this Council and of our Technical Board. Dr. Prudden has kindly consented to prepare for our minutes a tribute to Dr. Biggs. Owing to the condition of his voice, he feels unable to read this himself, so the secretary will present it to the Council. . . .

HERMANN M. BIGGS, since its organization a member of this Council, died on June 28, 1923. Born at Trumansburg, N. Y., in 1859, of English descent, he graduated from Cornell University in 1882 and in the following year from the Bellevue Medical College. After his interneship in Bellevue Hospital and a year of medical study abroad, he was made Director of the Carnegie Laboratory in New York and for several years was a teacher of various phases of science relating to medicine, and finally became Professor of Medicine at the Bellevue School.

For twenty-two years he served on the Department of Health of the City of New York.

It is difficult for those who did not live through the period of great enlightenment which the new knowledge of bacteria and their significance in infection ushered in, to realize how utterly changed was the outlook for helpful service in the prevention and treatment of disease, and how fundamental and far-reaching were the problems crowding in upon the pathway of medical research. It was in this period, back in the closing years of the last century, that Dr. Biggs found many of the sources of his inspiration, and framed his steadfast purpose to bring as speedily as might be the new acquisitions of science to the service of mankind.

In all the phases of sanitation and disease control and prevention in the great city, to which the new outlooks in science gave promise of help, Dr. Biggs, as an officer of the Health Department was ready with new projects for advance just as soon as the fitting hour arrived.

In 1892 he organized a Division of Pathology, a new feature in health administration. He established a Municipal Laboratory for the early detection on a large scale of infectious germs, the first in the world, which presently became a model.

He initiated the crusade for the prevention of tuberculosis and set about the education of the people and the medical profession, almost as soon as the tubercle bacillus had been discovered. Visiting nurses were secured for tuberculous patients; the Otisville Sanitarium was created; the Riverside Hospital was adjusted for the hopeless, and finally after some years of constructive pioneer educational work, notification of tuberculosis came without a murmur, even from the scores of eminent physicians who at first would have none of it. And his eager interest in the rescue of mankind from the universal scourge never wavered, his sturdy efforts never flagged.

The Bureau of Child Hygiene took form and grew under his inspiration; he initiated milk inspection; he was a helpful member of the Advisory Board at Quarantine. He early recognized the importance of the antitoxin for diphtheria and started its manufacture in the new laboratories, so that it might be available at moderate cost.

In 1902, Mayor Seth Low called Dr. Biggs to fill a new office in the Health Department, that of General Medical Officer, which he held for eleven years.

When finally Dr. Biggs laid down his tasks in the service of the City of New York he was called by the Governor of the State to assist in the preparation of a new Health Law under which he was presently appointed Commissioner of Health and Chairman of the newly organized Public Health Council.

The Health Department of the State was speedily reorganized. It swung abreast of the new currents in science, entering a period of active and far-reaching usefulness. A new and remarkable *esprit de corps* sprang up in the Department and spread to all phases of its activities, and the Health Department of the State of New York soon became an example for many commonwealths. Great laboratories materialized, reaching in their ministrations every corner of the State. New forms of service developed, the old took on new life.

But the vision and activities of Dr. Biggs had a wider range than the purlieus of the great metropolis or the health interests of the State. He wrote or inspired many scientific papers on subjects relating to the public health. He was a leader in organizations for the promotion of human welfare the world over. He was a member of many learned societies. He ministered to the poor and friendless in several hospitals. He received high honors and wide public recognition of his service from many sources. He was head of a Commission sent by the Rockefeller Foundation to study tuberculosis in France. He was a member of the Foundation's War Relief Commission. He was for a time Medical Director General of the League of Red Cross Societies in Geneva.

And withal he was a successful and well beloved practicing physician.

New projects in the interests of health seemed always forming out of the wide reaches of his knowledge and experience. If the summons to advance sometimes seemed audacious to his associates, sooner or later they usually realized that he had chosen wisely the occasion and the hour. His judgment of public opinion was sound. He was not readily baffled by opposition. But he could always wait. The potent and varied forces of education seemed

179

ever in his consciousness and formed the basis of the great forward movements in public welfare which he dreamed of or carried to triumphant conclusions.

He knew human nature; he readily won unswerving loyalty; he was trustworthy, far-seeing, wise. And his devotion to his fellow men, whether as public administrator, educator or physician, was untiring.

He cherished an eager interest in the establishment of the Milbank Memorial Fund. He shared generously in the counsels of its officers and friends. Here as elsewhere his great knowledge, his experience, and the wide range of his vision, gave to his service as counsellor a priceless value.

He was a great leader, a good citizen, a steadfast friend, a benefactor of mankind.

MR. SHELDON: We have all listened to this beautiful and discriminating tribute to Dr. Biggs. Those who are in favor of adopting it as read, and spreading it upon the records of the Council, will kindly manifest it by rising. . . . The minute is unanimously carried.

*   *   *   *   *   *   *

I cannot refrain, on behalf of the Directors of the Fund, from uttering a word of admiration and gratitude to the individual members of the Advisory Council who have so generously promised to give us the aid of their experience and the benefit of their criticism in developing and carrying on this interesting experiment in humanitarian effort. Mr. Kingsbury has been good enough to prepare a memorandum setting forth the roles of the Advisory Council, the Technical Board, and the Directors, and he has, I think very wisely, had it printed so that each member may take a copy with him.[1] You are all so highly experienced in so many fields of social endeavor that we are embarking confidently on this new voyage of discovery in search of perhaps a fairer golden fleece. Now I have the satisfaction of yielding the floor to your distinguished Chairman. Several years ago I remember that I had the advantage of his wise counsel in connection with another important effort for the well-being of this city, so that I feel tonight deeply convinced of the privilege I have in sitting at his feet now.

WILLIAM H. WELCH, M.D., *Dean of the School of Hygiene, Johns Hopkins University,* Presiding:

I was unfortunate in not having been able to attend the meeting a year ago, when I was elected Chairman of the Advisory Council. I esteem it a very great honor, indeed. Speaking in behalf of the membership of the Advisory Council, Mr. President, I am sure that every member of the Council considers it a very great privilege to be permitted to serve on this body. While it is a pleasure to be able to contribute what we may in advice, many of us here who are active in the cause of public health and social endeavor shall, I am sure, derive as great a benefit from, as we can possibly bring to, the deliberation and work of this great undertaking.

I have been asked to say a few words on "The Significance of the Health Demonstration." It seems needless before this audience to dwell upon this theme. It is a natural expression of the thoughts and activities of the founder of the Milbank Memorial Fund, Elizabeth Milbank Anderson. A woman of very broad vision, she was

---

[1] This memorandum appears on p. 35, under the title "The Advisory Council."

convinced that the best philanthropic activity is preventive and constructive, not merely palliative, relief-bringing and meeting only the emergency of the moment. I doubt whether any enterprise could have been conceived which is more in harmony with her thoughts than this one.

The methods which are to be adopted, or have already been adopted in carrying out these demonstrations, will serve as a model for similar undertakings. No new machinery is being created. The work is being done through the cooperation of the constituted health authorities and existing agencies. A demonstration such as this, which has as one of its main objects to show how public and private health endeavors can with effective results be coordinated to a common end, is well worth while even if nothing more come of it.

Of course, no one can, at this early stage, entirely predict the significance of these demonstrations. Whether large results are to be achieved is not problematical. Much has already been shown by the Framingham Demonstration. It is very fortunate that we have had the services of Dr. Donald B. Armstrong, executive officer of that demonstration, as a guide in entering upon this one. Again, in the anti-tuberculosis activities of the New York Association for Improving the Condition of the Poor there is enough to give a sure basis for undertaking this step. What at first may seem very incidental, even by-products of an undertaking, often turn out to be in some way the most significant. While in the anti-tuberculosis movement, for example, the emphasis lay primarily upon the control of tuberculosis, we now see that this is fundamentally a general health problem, and that it cannot be treated successfully as an effort directed solely toward the prevention of this one disease. While we can be sure of very significant results, we can be equally confident that they will be in directions which no one at the moment can fully realize. While I should not venture to predict, I feel quite certain from all experience in public health efforts that these results—accessory, if you like, incidental, if you like—will loom very large when the work is completed. I have every confidence that the demonstrations are going to be successful.

Those interested in the prevention of disease and the promotion of health are heartened that such men as those which constitute the Board of Directors of the Milbank Memorial Fund have lent an ear to the appeals of public health men that an opportunity be given to apply the knowledge which we now possess to the prevention of disease, and the improvement of health. This is the first effort made on a varied and large scale, in which there is going to be anything approaching an adequate application of existing knowledge about the problems of public health. And how many open problems there are, upon which light surely will be shed by these demonstrations!

That great results are to follow from this work, which will serve as a model, advancing greatly the cause of public health, not merely in New York State and in America, but in the world—I essay to speak in behalf not only of the members of the Advisory Council, but I think I may speak also for those interested in public health (and particularly public health officials) the world over.

We are to have the opportunity of hearing reports on the rural and urban demonstrations that are now under way in Cattaraugus County and in Syracuse, and on the proposed New York City Demonstration. The up-state demonstrations are under the general operating agency of the State Charities Aid Association, and it gives me great pleasure to present Homer Folks, who will tell something about the progress there.

HOMER FOLKS, *Secretary, State Charities Aid Association:*

The up-state demonstrations are now ten months old in the County of Cattaraugus, and about six months old in the City of Syracuse. It was fundamental, in the philosophy and planning of this undertaking, that whatever was done should be thoroughly grounded in the institutions and the life and public affairs of the community in which the work was to be done, and should not be regarded as a strange something imported into the community. I shall try, in the short time allotted me, to indicate what has been done in these localities towards securing a sound basis, sound basic machinery for what other public health activities may thereafter be built upon it, leaving it to the representatives of these localities to speak of the more particular things which have thus far been done.

In the development of the public health policy of New York State and in the State's health work since 1913, it has become increasingly evident that a single community, town or village, is too small to permit a health administration isolated therein to be effective. Step by step we have moved toward the possibility of a larger unit; and two years ago we passed in this State a permissive law by which a county might establish its own health board and have its own health officer. It was in our thoughts that at some future time, in some perhaps distant and indefinite period, some county might be moved to take that step as an example to the other counties. It has been the good fortune of this State that the first step taken in the development of this demonstration in Cattaraugus County has been, as you know, to act under that permissive law and to establish a County Board of Health there. A County Health Officer has been appointed there also, the only county health officer in the State of New York, and we have him with us here.

A very important phase of public health work is that connected with the schools. In aproaching this problem in Cattaraugus County, we were confronted with the individual school district, the logical unit of school health work, but one which is still smaller than the town or village.

Although there was a crying need for a wider unit for the school health work in the rural districts, no provision was made by the law for either an individual district unit or a larger one. As a result, without having any law, warrant or authority, or anything at all except the good offices of the Milbank Memorial Fund and some of its resources, there was created in Cattaragus County an office of county superintendent of school health. Without any legal status, this official called together a few months ago the trustees of all of the rural and village schools in the county, and invited them to establish a County Council of School Health. Under this Council, the trustees were to see that every child received an adequate medical examination. Fifty-three hundred of these children, living in the least accessible parts of the county, have already been examined; and letters have gone to their parents telling of the defects discovered. For the first time in this State, we have here really effective county-wide harmonious administration of the health of school children.

No less apparent, as far as we could see, was the primary

necessity for the co-operation of voluntary organizations of citizens. There was a County Tuberculosis and Health Association in Cattaraugus County (one of a sisterhood of sixty-four such county units in this State) with an excellent history of accomplishments to its credit, but unable with its limited resources really to effect a firm vital connection with every hamlet, every village and every school district there. By providing for that organization a very efficient, competent, mature executive secretary, who also serves as the county public health education official, this wide contact has been made possible.

Now, passing a moment to Syracuse. The ·situation there is quite different because in that city of 175,000 people we have had for years a well-organized division of school health in the department of education, and also we have had a county health association. There are difficulties, however, even in our cities. It is the habit of New York municipalities to elect a new mayor every two years and it is the rule and not the exception to change them. It is, I am sorry to say, the rule and not the exception for an incoming mayor to select a new health officer. With no guarantee of continuity of office and without adequate remuneration, it has not been possible, therefore, to get full-time health officers in our cities. That was the condition in Syracuse, but there we have at least helped to build up the basic machinery by providing as an aid to the health officer, the full-time services of an administrative assistant.

The chief work in Syracuse has been to build up the particular services (tuberculosis, contagious diseases, public health education, the work for children of pre-school age, etc.), of which Dr. Thomas P. Farmer, Dr. John L. Heffron and others will speak. It has been a pleasure, too, to help the Department of Education there round out its program and to demonstrate how a more complete service of nursing and of home visitation can benefit school children in such a city.   Here, too, a public health education expert has been added to the staff of the local Onondaga County Tuberculosis and Public Health Association.

In both of these localities (fully in Cattaraugus County and largely in Syracuse, but in the process of further development there), we have secured in a short period of time the basic machinery upon which may be established, as rapidly as the communities can assimilate new ideas and new methods of work, every phase of public health activity which may be desired of the public health authorities, school authorities, or volunteer agencies.

DR. WELCH: I can't imagine anyone more interested in these demonstrations than a health officer in whose province they are going to take place and I am sure that the Health Commissioner of the State of New York fully appreciates his good fortune in that regard.   It is a very great satisfaction to introduce Dr. Nicoll, who will speak to us on "The New York State Health Department and the Demonstrations."

MATTHIAS NICOLL, JR., M.D., *Commissioner of Health, State of New York:*

These demonstrations come at a very opportune time in the progress of the work of the State Department of Health.   As I have said on many a previous occasion, it is my personal opinion that under the present organization we have about reached our limit in the methods of control of disease and the improvement of health in the State of

New York. It has always been necessary to administer the affairs of health in the fifty-seven counties of the State, practically from Albany. That was very important in the beginning but, as I say, we have reached the limit of results by any such method. I think we who have had any experience in rural public health work, are agreed that the only way to accomplish efficient work is by moving the direct unit of control nearer to where the work is to be done. In other words, to establish the county unit. We were making very little progress until this opening, which is but one of the benefits of this demonstration, was brought to us and resulted in one of our progressive rural counties adopting the step which Mr. Folks has described.

I am glad that he emphasized the inspection of the schools. It is not only the finding of defects but the taking of steps to remedy them that is important; and there is nothing which will result in more good from this county demonstration than the proper inspection and thorough physical examination of school children, with attendant provisions for correcting defects.

Through its Director of the Bureau of Vital Statistics, Dr. Otto R. Eichel, the State Department of Health has been, I am glad to say, of some assistance to the demonstrations in doing statistical work. The Department has loaned one of its epidemiologists to assist the Syracuse Commissioner of Health, Dr. Thomas P. Farmer, as his deputy, and one of his nurses to aid the Cattaraugus County Health Officer, Dr. Leverett D. Bristol. We have done what we could and are ready to do as much as we possibly can to further this work. We are agreed that it is the most important step that has been taken in the State for the advancement of public health.

I think we are rather prone to speak of a demonstration of this kind as accomplishing results which can be measured statistically—by taking out a slide rule and figuring out death rates. I doubt very much whether at the end of four or five years our statistics will show any surprising number of lives saved in Cattaraugus County, for example. But there are many things that cannot be measured by a statistician, which make for the health, welfare and happiness of the community, county or city, which has a good health administration. We must take that into account and not be discouraged if, as the months go by, we cannot determine very definite results in the lowering of the incidence of disease and of deaths from disease. I do not mean to say that these results will not show, especially in the cities. If Syracuse, for instance, does not eradicate diphtheria within five years, I shall be very much disappointed. I feel that very strongly and would like to make a prophecy that it will come about.

I look forward with a great deal of hope and assurance to the success of these demonstrations. They will succeed because they must succeed. I cannot conceive of any greater disaster than the lack of their success.

DR. WELCH: We are now to hear about the Cattaraugus County Demonstration. I was much interested to learn that Dr. Leverett D. Bristol, Commissioner of Health of the State of Maine, had been willing to transfer his activities from a state commissionership to a county in the State of New York. That shows what county health work in New York, as contrasted with that of states in other parts of the country, holds in the way of opportunity for progressive health officers. It is a great personal pleasure to present Dr. Bristol.

LEVERETT D. BRISTOL, M.D., *County Health Officer and Director of the Cattaraugus County Health and Tuberculosis Demonstration:*

In the first place, let me say that the demonstration is being received with whole-hearted anticipation and favor by the people of Cattaraugus County. The clinical services, for example, have developed a very marked appreciation, some clinic visitors voluntarily traveling as many as thirty or forty miles for examination. Our records show that the clinics were first attended chiefly by persons brought in by the nurses, but as the clinics have become established, people have come to them largely as a result of publicity.

Again, in the County Board of Supervisors we have a splendid spirit of co-operation. The Board has under consideration the increase of its 1923 county health budget of $9,300 to $16,000 in 1924, and there are encouraging prospects that they will take this action.[2]

We find also that the President of the County Medical Society and most of its members are in harmony with the Cattaraugus County demonstration, as is the medical profession generally throughout the county. The Secretary of the Society is a member of the County Board of Health. As a result of sending three local physicians to the Trudeau School of Tuberculosis at Saranac Lake, a small group of the younger medical men are meeting monthly for the discussion of health problems.

That the local authorities in the towns of the county are

---

[2] Since this meeting, the Board of Supervisors of Cattaraugus County have granted this appropriation. See p. 44.

co-operating in the work is shown by the fact that quarters for three of the six district stations that have been established have been provided rent-free. In one or two of these localities we anticipate that we will receive local financial assistance in the maintenance of the stations located there.

With such local co-operation as these instances indicate, we fully expect the Cattaraugus County demonstration to be a success. We expect that our work will demonstrate that the county is the logical unit for carrying on rural health work. Meantime, we hope to inaugurate many activities for the promotion of the general health of the county. To mention but one or two of our many objectives, we hope to develop courses for the local health officers, post-graduate courses for physicians, and a unit for the training of nurses in rural public health nursing. A course for special training in rural public health nursing is particularly needed.

DR. WELCH: We are now to hear about the Syracuse demonstration and I will first call upon the Health Commissioner of that city, Dr. Farmer.

THOMAS P. FARMER, M.D., *Commissioner of Health, Syracuse, New York:*

First of all, I feel that, as the official head of the Health Department of Syracuse, I cannot let this opportunity go by without expressing on behalf of the official city government and of the City itself, our appreciation to all here that the demonstration for a middle-sized city was located in Syracuse. I wish to assure you that the City is greatly interested in the project. We feel also that it is a great privilege to be invited to participate in a movement which has had its origin in the work and interest of the philanthropic woman who has been so beautifully described by Mr. Sheldon, and which has received official direction from a man who had such noble ideas about public health and welfare as he whom Dr. Prudden has described.

As Mr. Folks has remarked, the Syracuse demonstration has been going on for only six months and we are just beginning to make progress. Our chief work thus far has been with tuberculosis. Several nurses and doctors have been added to the personnel of the Tuberculosis Bureau, and by opening new clinics we have been able to reach a larger number of people than heretofore. Clinics held in various foreign sections of the city, under the auspices of the Onondaga County and Public Health Association, have been very well attended and have brought to light a number of cases of tuberculosis which were unknown before.

At the present time, we are conducting in Syracuse a course of instruction given by prominent specialists on tuberculosis. This course consists of two hour clinics at the Onondaga County Tuberculosis Sanitarium, followed by a lecture given elsewhere.

We are making great improvement in our methods of record keeping in the Department of Health. Previous to the establishment of the demonstration, this has been one of the weak points of the health administration. Recently, we sent a representative of the Department to study the methods of recording used in the State Department of Health and in the New York City Department, as one step in bettering our record keeping routine.

It is, of course, important that the Department of Health be assured that patients in the community suffering with communicable diseases are receiving adequate medical attention and supervision. The Department can have this assurance about patients who are being treated by private physicians, only when these physicians report on such cases periodically. It is not so difficult to get a doctor to report such a case in the first instance as it is to get him to continue to report on it. To prompt his co-operation in Syracuse, we have adopted the procedure of telling the physician that if at the end of any two-week period he has not kept the Department informed that such a case is still under his care, we will assume that he is no longer controlling it and that he is willing to have a public health nurse visit the patient. In such instances we assume, of course, that if the patient has changed doctors, the new attending physician will have reported the case to the Department.

Dr. Nicoll has said that he wants us to eradicate diphtheria from Syracuse. We have already cut it down to half the rate it was last year. We hope that our newly adopted milk code will be a model for other cities in the State. We have put into it everything the New York City milk code has and, I believe, a few improvements besides.

Dr. Welch: There is nothing more characteristic of the modern public health movement than its progress in the public schools. It is very important that we should hear from a representative of education and I have pleasure in calling upon Mr. Hughes.

Percy M. Hughes, *Superintendent of Public Instruction, Syracuse, New York:*

Dr. Farmer has expressed the appreciation of the City of Syracuse for this demonstration. May I say to the

Board of Directors of the Milbank Memorial Fund that we in the schools esteem most valuable the work which has been done there through the public schools. Our corps of medical attendants has been increased by the addition of a supervisor of health education, a chief medical inspector, an assistant inspector, five nurses, and by dental hygienists. We are getting a teacher of hygiene and sanitation, who will teach health principles to the children in the schools.

A day and a half after school began last fall, all of the children in the grade schools of Syracuse, 19,670 of them, had been given medical examinations, and 141 cases of more or less serious contagious disabilities had been discovered. During the month of October, 1923, the nurses visited 937 homes of school children, whereas during the corresponding month of the preceding year we had been able to visit only 574 homes. Through the instruction of the children and through the influence of the nurses in visiting the homes of parents, we believe that we are reaching also the children of pre-school age, and that this work of reaching the younger generation of the City of Syracuse will have its fruitage in the years to come.

DR. WELCH: Nothing is more important in this demonstration than that it has the sympathy, interest, understanding and support of the practitioners of medicine, the general medical profession. I think, therefore, we are very fortunate in the opportunity of hearing from a distinguished representative of the medical profession in the City of Syracuse. I take pleasure in presenting Dr. John L. Heffron of the Medical School of Syracuse University.

JOHN L. HEFFRON, M.D., *Dean Emeritus, Medical School, Syracuse University:*

I think that no memorial could be devised that should so signally honor the memory of a great and good woman as one devoted to the betterment of the health of the public. The members of the profession of medicine in Syracuse are profoundly grateful that the City was chosen for a health demonstration. We are unanimously behind the work of our Department of Health; and we are to a man behind this demonstration. Our most difficult problems have grown out of the lack of financial resources. The assistance of the Milbank Memorial Fund has put courage into our hearts. But we shall have to proceed slowly; not attempt too many things at once; and not push improvements faster than they can be assimilated.

Commissioner Farmer has told you some of the things we have done. He has not told you, however, what I think you ought to know. He feels, and so do all of us who consult with him, that there should be in Syracuse a Director of the Demonstration, who has such a reputation for thoroughness of training and for successful administration of health work that he will command the respect of the members of the profession of medicine in Syracuse. Dr. Farmer has given much time to this demonstration. He has and will administer the regular work of his office in a way to meet the full approbation of his confreres. But a special director is needed, who with the advice of the Technical Board, will inaugurate new measures and suggest improvement in present methods. He is needed to co-ordinate these measures and methods with those already functioning in the department of health; he is needed to lead in the health education of the people; he is needed to

keep our volunteer organizations and our people in touch
with the progress of the work of the Demonstration; and
he is needed as a method of communication with our neighbors concerning the accomplishments of our demonstration.
I believe that no expenditure could be made that should
insure so certainly the success of the Syracuse Demonstration.

DR. WELCH: It has been gratifying to hear these reports on the rural and the urban demonstrations. We are
eager to hear about the proposed New York City demonstration, which, complementing these, makes this project
national in application and significance. The experiences
of those who had been active in the Framingham Demonstration and in the work of the New York Association for
Improving the Condition of the Poor were among the
influences which led the Board of Directors of the Milbank
Memorial Fund to enter upon these demonstrations. Bailey
B. Burritt, the General Director of this Association, has
contributed a great deal in thought and effort to the fram-
ing of the plan proposed for the New York City demonstration. I have great pleasure in introducing him to you.

BAILEY B. BURRITT, *General Director, New York Association for Improving the Condition of the Poor:*
From the first, it was felt that New York City offered
a great opportunity for a health demonstration. Its problems are typical of those in many large urban areas, where
lives a sizable percentage of the population of the United
States. The rest of the country is in the habit of looking,
more or less, to this city for leadership in different avenues
of its life—and because New York City and New York

State have been so peculiarly leaders in this field, I think
it looks here, in part, for guidance in its health work. Most
of the public health movements that are expressed in voluntary national health organizations have had their origin in
and are located in New York. Then, too, there are here
a number of well developed local voluntary organizations,
with activities already well co-ordinated with the work of
the public health authorities. For reasons, of which these
are but a few, we decided that, although there were many
obstacles to overcome, it was well worth while to undertake a demonstration in New York City.

Careful consideration has been given to the question of
where in the City the demonstration should be held. Several months were spent in analyzing the situation, studying
social and statistical data pertaining to ten areas in the
Boroughs of Manhattan and the Bronx. A study was also
made in the Borough of Brooklyn. These surveys led us
to the conclusion that the area bounded by 14th Street
and 63rd Street, Fourth Avenue and the East River presents the greatest opportunities for a successful metropolitan demonstration.

This district has a population of 216,000, of which 37
per cent. are foreign born, as compared with 35 per cent.
foreign born in the Greater City. The two largest foreign
racial groups in the area are the Italians and the Irish; the
former constituting 25 per cent. of the foreign born population, and the latter, 19 per cent. Our studies show that
the age grouping in the district is fairly typical of that in
the entire city. There is also in the district quite an interesting distribution of income ranges, including those whose
families are among the poorest and the richest. The birth
rate is practically identical with that of Manhattan. The

death rate is somewhat greater than that of this Borough, being a little over 17.6 there as against 14.3 in all of Manhattan. Infant mortality is similarly higher and the death rate from tuberculosis somewhat greater than in the entire Borough.

The district's social service facilities are fairly well developed and it presents exceptional opportunities for medical training—a factor which is considered very important by the Technical Board of the Milbank Memorial Fund, which originally recommended the selection of this area.

The plan outlined for the development of the demonstration in this district presupposes that all of the activities there of the volunteer organizations and of the public health department can be co-ordinated and concerted towards the ends in view. If the plan doesn't mean this, it fails to meet the purposes we have in mind. It is a pleasure to report that in what contact we have had with the heads of the local official health department and the volunteer organizations, we have found a sympathetic interest in the plan and a responsive determination to co-operate in making it a success.

DR. WELCH: In listening to what the various speakers have told us about these demonstrations, a great many questions may have arisen which one would like to have discussed. I think that it is a very wise provision that an item appears on the program entitled "General Discussion." I am going to ask Dr. James Alexander Miller to open this part of the program.

JAMES ALEXANDER MILLER, M.D., *President, New York Tuberculosis Association:*
It was with a very peculiar pleasure that I have listened

to Mr. Burritt and realized how far we have progressed
since last year, when it was my privilege to speak at the
first meeting of this Council. I have come more and more
to the belief that there is no place in this country, and
perhaps no place in the world, where a bigger success can
be made of a health demonstration than in this City. It is
heartening to realize that we are now actually to start on
the undertaking.

There occur to me certain advantages which will come
from this New York City demonstration, and which might
be emphasized at this time. A project of this kind must
be thought of largely in terms of co-operation. We have
found that co-operation has already been given in the
rural county and in the urban demonstrations. There is
no place where this is more necessary and more difficult,
and withal more possible, than in New York City, where
we have already come to learn, in part, how to co-operate.

One of the broader aspects of the metropolitan demonstration is that it will afford extraordinary opportunities
for a training school and educational center, for those who
are actively engaged in public health work and for those
who are students in it.

There is no place where better facilities are at hand to
offer training and field work to physicians themselves, and
to health officers, social workers and medical students.

Again, careful consideration will need to be given to
the interpretation of results as they are attained in these
demonstrations. We expect to have very accurate book-
keeping, and in interpreting the facts recorded, the Advisory Council can no doubt be of very material aid. This is
a very important part of the demonstrations because it is

thus that their findings will be made most useful to the entire country.

One of the opportunities in these demonstrations, and particularly in that in New York City, is offered in showing not only how far we can successfully apply methods known to prevent disease and to promote public health, but how far we can progress in attaining new methods—how far we can apply what we know, and how very materially we can widen the horizon of the knowledge we now have. In other words, we have here an opportunity for good organization. If we are also to have expert direction, we must realize the necessity of depending upon scientific medicine. That will mean research, not only in the medical laboratory but in the broader social laboratory which such a district as the one chosen for the metropolitan demonstration will especially offer.

* * * * * * * *

After this discussion of the plan for the proposed demonstration in New York City, which had been submitted to the members of the Advisory Council before the meeting, the body adopted the following resolution, introduced by Dr. William H. Park, Director of the Bureau of Laboratories of the Health Department of the City of New York:

RESOLVED, That the following expresses the consensus of opinion of the Advisory Council in relation to the proposed New York City Demonstration:

1. That the plan of organization as revised by the Technical Board in the light of criticisms and suggestions submitted by the members of the Advisory Council is soundly conceived and meets with the approval of this body.

2. That it is desirable to undertake the proposed demonstration as soon as satisfactory co-operation of public and private agencies concerned is definitely assured; a detailed scheme of organization, which guarantees unity of operation, is developed and subscribed to by the co-operating organizations involved; and effective leadership is known to be available.

*   *   *   *   *   *   *   *

DR. WELCH: We are to listen now to one who, I think, delights in criticism, but who has been one of the great forces in furthering public health movements in America. Dr. Lee K. Frankel, who has organized the health activities of the Metropolitan Life Insurance Company, has, I think, introduced a new and very important idea in life insurance. Dr. Frankel is also Chairman of the National Health Council, a very promising and already very active and potent organization.

LEE K. FRANKEL, PH.D., *Third Vice-President, Metropolitan Life Insurance Company:*

This is one of the occasions on which I have absolutely no criticism to make. There have been times possibly when I have questioned whether New York State, with its tremendous health organizations, was the state in which a demonstration of this kind should be carried on. If I ever questioned that, my doubt was dispelled yesterday when, coming down on a train, I happened to be reading one of the Rochester papers, one I believe of considerable standing in the community. In that one issue I must have seen from fifteen to twenty advertisements of patent medicines and proprietary articles, representing every imaginary cure for every imaginary disease. It struck me that that was rather indicative of the type of health education to which the great public, even in the State of New York, is now too much subjected. It strengthened my conviction that those who constitute this public are, after all, the ones who must be reached and gotten back of any health movement. I think that one of the primary objects of these demonstrations will be to bring the subject of health right down to the people, to show them in their own terms what scientific medicine means, what the health movements are, and, in other words, to cultivate a health habit among them. I am delighted that the project is going along so nicely in these three different sections.

The Framingham Demonstration is now in its last year. Probably nothing is more significant in the result there than that practically every activity undertaken in the demonstration, and every suggestion made, will be taken over next year as a part of the community's current practice.

DR. WELCH: Probably no one is in a position to get a better perspective of the national significance of these demonstrations than the head of the Public Health Service. I think it is most gratifying that the chief of that Service, which has come to occupy a position of primacy among welfare agencies in the country, is one who represents the cause of public health so effectively and so worthily. I take pleasure in presenting Dr. Cumming, the Surgeon General of the United States Public Health Service.

HUGH S. CUMMING, M.D., *Surgeon-General, United States Public Health Service:*
There has never been, I think, such an opportunity for

forwarding the public health movement in this country as is that now presented by these demonstrations. Such a provision of counsel, composed of leaders in the several forms of public health activity, has not before been brought together on a similar project. ThePublic Health Service will follow particularly the county health movement to learn from it lessons which, by application to their own problems, may help other states.

The demonstration in the area selected in New York City will be looked upon with great interest by the other large cities of the country. A great deal has already been in evidence which might be applied to cities of less than metropolitan size. The plans have been well thought out; there are very definite objectives; there is co-operation with the official health organizations, and there is counsel from leaders in all of the avenues which combine to make a comprehensive public health program.

These undertakings have been well called demonstrations, for with such guidance they could hardly be called experiments. Yet they are to be more than demonstrations, because if they are simply manifestations of problems already thought out, they are more or less failures. I feel particularly gratified that I am to associate with others on this Council in undertaking the pioneer health work, which is also to be a feature of these projects.

DR. WELCH: I do not believe that Dr. Livingston Farrand can make a greater contribution to public health in this country than he has made through his pioneer work in tuberculosis. He is to address us on the subject of the demonstrations.

LIVINGSTON FARRAND, M.D., *President, Cornell University:*

I hope that sight will not be lost of the great significance of this choice of activity by the Milbank Fund. After all, as I understand it, the Trustees of this Fund were not hampered as to the lines along which to direct that particular benefaction. It was only after the most careful thought on their part and after getting all the advice they could in all related fields, that they finally chose this series of health demonstrations as promising the greatest contribution to the welfare of humanity which they could see within the lines of their broad trust. Now, that fact would lead one to imagine that this was about the last word to expect in the way of promising results in this field, but as I have been sitting here thinking of what it was that led to this decision, it seemed to have been quite inevitable that we should have come to the agreement that what was needed was the application and demonstration of existing knowledge.

It seems to me that we are dealing here with a profound principle of education. It is not only a fact that public health, human vitality, lies at the very basis of our modern civilization; it is an admitted fact that following the war the problem of human vitality became an absolutely fundamental problem in the economic rehabilitation of society. That has, of course focused public attention upon the importance of this particular problem. Moreover, in the development of modern civilization, it has come to be equally apparent that about the most difficult thing with which the world has to contend is the lack of application of knowledge which is already in possession of the experts. Our enormous advance in scientific knowledge of every kind has been the great characteristic of the last fifty years.

There is no field in which that has been more strikingly evident than in the fields of medicine and of medical science. When we view the technical advances that have been made since the days of Pasteur, when we see, as we do, what would result if these discoveries were fully applied, and when we recognize that practically the only obstacle in the way of that application is recognition on the part of the public of those facts and of the possibilities of their application—then we begin to see why demonstrations of this kind were recommended, after sober consideration by the best counsel obtainable, as being the most promising way of attaining results in human welfare to which a trust, like the Milbank Fund, could be devoted.

We are primarily interested in the field of health, but I do not think that we want to lose sight of the fact that what we are doing here reaches far beyond the simple problems of health and the prevention of disease, and even the building up of human vitality. Any demonstration that can make good in this particular is going to reverberate far beyond its particular technical field. It is going to be felt not only in the field of health and in the whole field of social work, but it is going to be a tremendously effective factor in the maintenance of stability in the somewhat tottering situation in which the world finds itself today. There is no greater contribution, to my mind, that could possibly be made in any field by any trust, than this new undertaking by the trustees of the Milbank Fund.

Dr. Welch: As the last speaker, we are to hear from Dr. Haven Emerson, former Commissioner of Health of the City of New York and now of the College of Physicians and Surgeons, of Columbia University.

HAVEN EMERSON, M.D., *College of Physicians and Surgeons, Columbia University:*

We in the medical profession are nowadays getting far enough away from disease to think in terms of the preponderating group of healthy persons and to bend our efforts to make life consciously, instead of accidentally, successful for them. It is not death rates, but health rates, that we are concerned with. Nobody is really interested in death rates; people are interested in life. We can influence mothers with our education because they are interested in the life of their children. We can interest children because they are intensely interested themselves in whatever happens to their own careers. We can teach the sick when they are sick, we can teach communities when they have contagious diseases, but the average healthy person is not interested in health as long as he has it.

I believe we should estimate the results of the work that is under way not in terms of reduced death rates, reduced sickness, but in the certainty and continuity of family life. We see now, it seems to me, the family and the maturing child as our goal. The studies of the New York A. I. C. P. and the results of the anti-tuberculosis work in New York has shown that family life, upon which our whole civilization depends, has been made more secure by health. A demonstration of our confidence that science can save the family is one way, in addition to those which have been shown, of practicing our faith in the knowledge at hand. I should like to suggest that we make a study, so far as possible, of the extent of family breakdown. We can measure our health work, as we will, by the number of families that we prevent from breaking up. Certainly the first thing sickness brings into the household is the risk of breaking down the family and if we have so diminished the hazards of sickness that a smaller number of families in Syracuse and in Cattaraugus County and in New York City are broken down temporarily or permanently, we have accomplished something more than the reduction of disease.

Dr. Prudden has referred to the clearness of Dr. Biggs' vision, when he conceived the possibility of eradicating diphtheria. We are approaching the threshold of the elimination of other diseases. We are looking forward, as we believe, to the elimination of tuberculosis. If this can be done, and we think we can accomplish it in this particular way, it is worth buying, worth spending money for.

In these demonstrations, we must have certain indices of our results that are not expressed in entirely the way that we have been accustomed to in measuring success in health work. As Dr. Nicoll has said, it is not the immediate results we must promise ourselves. It is the more remote, the more intangible, the ancillary results—not only the reduction of sickness, but the protection of family life, the securing of education and the development of character. The objective of school health work is not only to remove and reduce defects, but to deliver healthy children at the school to learn. I should say that the measure of success of this new effort will be determined by our ability to eliminate all of those elements that go to prevent the child from attending school because of low vitality and from receiving effective training while there.

We should measure our results also by the reduction in the annual bill for the purchase of the patent medicines to which Dr. Frankel has referred. If we haven't reduced these sales in the next five years, we will not have corrected those present vicious and malignant forces in the community which use the power of advertising to prey upon ignorance and stupidity.

Again, I suggest that these demonstrations will have failed unless the people in the communities where they are conducted are taught to do as much for the protection of their own health as is now done for them. By that I do not mean merely the taking over of this work by the community, as is being done in Framingham. I should like to see more individuals in these communities take care of their health as they would a private investment. I should like to see them willing to spend as much on the health of their children as they are ready to spend on their own, to do as much for their children's health as the school systems and health departments will have done.

A radical change is needed in the common attitude towards public health service. It has been thought of as something which chiefly concerns our public and private health agencies. It must be made a part of our annual personal budgets and not be left entirely to the makers of the municipal, county and state budgets.

Our health departments, moreover, must be kept nonpartisan. We shall not have succeeded entirely within these communities until they are convinced of the necessity of keeping their public health activities as much out of politics as they have their departments of education.

Finally, as I have suggested before, our problem in no little degree is to develop character. It was Dr. Osler, I believe, who in commenting upon the treatment of tuberculosis said that it is what is in the head more than what is in the lung that determines the outcome of the individual case. In any health activity we undertake, we must constantly deal with character, with the reaction of the individual to the possibilities of life. I cannot think of the vision and faith of Mrs. Anderson and of the support that she gave to the A. I. C. P., in which she was so much interested, without believing that she would wish us to consider this not only a movement of science, but one of religion, an attempt to alter American character, to make a permanent impression upon the manner of life of our nation.

The Advisory Council

The Advisory Council was created by resolution of the Board of Directors of the Milbank Memorial Fund, May 22, 1922. Invitations to serve on this Council were issued to thirty-one men and women—recognized leaders in public health and social work, prominent business men and economists interested in improvement of public health and promotion of the general welfare.

The Council held its first meeting at the Hotel Commodore, November 16, 1922, with Mr. Albert G. Milbank of the Memorial Fund in the chair. It organized by electing Dr. William H. Welch chairman and John A. Kingsbury secretary.

With the maturing of the plans and the broadening of the demonstrations program, which originally dealt largely with tuberculosis, this Council has been increased until it now embraces a body of forty-two advisors, representing every important field of public health. In creating this body, the Board of Directors stated that the Council would be called together occasionally for criticism of the program and of plans and procedure, and that to its members would be submitted from time to time reports of progress for such suggestions as they might offer.

In other words, the Board of Directors does not intend to make great demand on the time of the members of the Council nor expect them to attend regular meetings, but it does desire that each member take seriously the invitation to criticize the plans as they formulate and to make suggestions for the effective development of this health program.

The meeting of the Council on the evening of November 15, 1923, was the first since its organization, a year ago, when its members met to receive the report of the preliminary work relating to the selection of the county and the city for the upstate demonstrations, and to consider the program which had been the subject of months of careful study by the Technical Board, copies of which had been submitted in advance to the Council members.

Beginning with the present calendar year, a Quarterly Bulletin has been issued by the Milbank Fund for the purpose of keeping the members of the Advisory Council, and others especially interested, fully informed of the progress of the demonstrations.

Obviously it is not practical to call together so large a group as this Council for frequent conference. Therefore, a Technical Board was created which is responsible for maturing the plans for the demonstrations. This Board is expected to keep in intimate touch with the development and progress of the several demonstrations, to advise the Directors with reference to the selection of localities best suited for demonstration purposes and in regard to the designation of operating agencies, and finally to make recommendations with reference to the distribution of functions and funds to the various participating agencies, official and voluntary. Naturally, all plans are subject to the approval of the Board of Directors of the Fund for they cannot delegate their trusteeship, but the Directors look to the Technical Board for recommendations and to the Advisory Council for general criticism of these recommendations.

MILBANK MEMORIAL FUND

REPORT FOR THE
YEAR ENDED
DECEMBER 31, 1923

with an account of
The New York Health Demonstrations

MILBANK MEMORIAL FUND
FORTY-NINE WALL STREET
NEW YORK

213

FOREWORD

THERE has been material progress in the New York Health Demonstrations since April 3, 1922, when the Board of Directors of the Milbank Memorial Fund voted to concentrate a substantial part of the Fund's income in supporting this project. The sum of $325,000 a year for at least five years has been set aside by the Fund to support these demonstrations, the aim of which is to ascertain the effectiveness and cost of certain measures for the prevention and control of disease, reduction in the numbers of deaths, and for the promotion of individual and community health in rural, urban and metropolitan communities in New York State, typical of constitutent elements of the country at large.

Two communities have already been selected as demonstration centers. Work was begun in 1923, in Cattaraugus County, a typical rural district in the western part of New York State with a population of about 72,000, and in the City of Syracuse, which has a population of about 190,000. Organization of a demonstration in the City of New York and funds for its support have been authorized by the Fund's Board of Directors.

It has not seemed pertinent at this early stage of the demonstrations to attempt to measure by statistical procedure whether the increased health facilities made available as a result of these undertakings have resulted in any measurable increase in the individual and community health of the districts chosen for demonstration purposes. Because many of the services to be carried out in the program are preventive and constructive, it is not expected that they will show immediate concrete results. For this reason, the material presented in this volume pertains chiefly to the origin, objectives, methods and organization of the project.

The attempt has been made to indicate in Part II the major observations which entered into the decision to conduct the demonstrations. Important in this connection is the summary by Dr. Hermann M. Biggs, late Commissioner of Health of the State of New York, of the history of the health movement in this State, which forms the background for the general program outlined for the development of the undertakings.

It has not been possible to include in so short a space all of the data about the communities studied, which was considered pertinent in the selection of localities typical enough of representative populations in the United States to be acceptable as units of the demonstrations project. Rather than to attempt this, it was thought advisable to make available to individuals seeking additional information, the original manuscripts from which data have been selected for presentation here.

It is a privilege to express to the authorities under whose responsibility the demonstrations are progressing in each locality, to its boards of counsel, and to the staff of its operating agencies, the deep appreciation of the Board of Directors of the Milbank Memorial Fund for loyal and intelligent co-operation in forwarding these projects, through which it is hoped to forward the promotion of public health, not only in the communities where these intensive efforts are being made, but in the country at large.

John A. Kingsbury
Secretary

July 12, 1924

CONTENTS

PART I

REPORT FOR
THE YEAR ENDED DECEMBER 31, 1923

I

THE YEAR IN REVIEW

The New York Health Demonstrations   *Page 16*
Some Estimates of the Significance of the
    Demonstrations   *18*

THE NEW YORK HEALTH DEMONSTRATIONS

The Rural Health Demonstration   *Page 25*
The Urban Health Demonstration   *29*
The Metropolitan Health Demonstration   *34*
Organization and Supervision   *36*

II

GRANTS OF THE MILBANK MEMORIAL FUND

THE NEW YORK ASSOCIATION FOR IMPROVING THE CONDITION OF THE POOR

The Department of Social Welfare   *Page 41*
The Home Hospital   *44*
The New York State Ventilation Commission   *46*

GRANTS TO OTHER AGENCIES

Public Health   *Page 49*
Health Education   *50*
Child Health and Child Welfare   *52*
Special Health Research   *52*
Co-ordination of Social Effort   *53*
Probation Work   *54*
Relief   *54*

FINANCIAL STATEMENT
WITH SUMMARY OF INCOME AND DISBURSEMENTS

PART II

THE NEW YORK HEALTH DEMONSTRATIONS
Their Origin, Scope and Methods

III

THE PURPOSE OF THE NEW YORK HEALTH DEMONSTRATIONS

Past Progress in the Control of Disease   *Page 66*
The Purpose of the New York Health Dem-
   onstrations   *75*

IV

THE DEMONSTRATIONS PROGRAM

The Home Hospital   *Page 80*
The Framingham Demonstration   *81*
Demonstrations in Larger Population Units
   Needed   *81*
The Demonstrations Program   *82*
Tuberculosis   *86*
Communicable Diseases   *91*
School Hygiene   *93*
Maternity, Infancy and Child Hygiene   *94*
Social Hygiene   *95*
Mental Hygiene   *96*
Industrial Hygiene   *97*
Sanitation and Food Inspection   *98*
Health Conservation and Life Extension   *99*
General Operations   *101*
Demonstrations Extension Program   *102*

V

SELECTING THE DEMONSTRATION DISTRICTS

Selecting the Rural Demonstration District Page 110
Selecting the Urban Demonstration District   *113*
Selecting the Metropolitan District   *118*
Methods of Procedure in Organizing the
   Demonstrations   *132*

APPENDIX

Brief for Investment in Adequate Home Treat-
   ment for the Prevention of Tuberculosis—By
   Haven Emerson, M.D.   *Page 141*

ILLUSTRATIONS

Page

Locations in the State of New York of the Health Demonstrations of the
Milbank Memorial Fund.. 14

Deaths from all causes in the United States (registration area), per 1,000
population, 1910–1921.. 17

Administrative divisions, with local headquarters, of the Rural Health
Demonstration in Cattaraugus County, New York, showing the accessibility of schools to the district and field health stations.......... 26

Cases of tuberculosis, pulmonary and other forms, reported in Syracuse,
1920–1923.. 30

Clinic attendance of tuberculous patients in Syracuse, showing new admissions and revisits, 1919–1923................................. 31

Deaths of children under one year of age, per 1,000 live births (infant mortality) in Syracuse, 1902–1922, showing also the birth rate, and the
infant death rates from preventable and from non-preventable causes. 32

Major causes of infant mortality in Syracuse, 1922...................... 33

Medical and social activities in the central section of the City of Syracuse,
New York, 1924... 62

Deaths from pulmonary tuberculosis in the City of New York, per 100,000
population, 1868–1923.. 67

Number of deaths from tuberculosis in the Boroughs of Manhattan and the
Bronx, City of New York, by years, 1887–1921...................... 69

Major causes of death in the United States (registration area), per 100,000
population, 1910 and 1920.................................... 70

Deaths from typhoid fever in New York State, exclusive of the City of New
York, per 100,000 population, 1898–1921......................... 71

Deaths from cancer and from tuberculosis in the United States (registration area), per 100,000 population, 1911–1922..................... 72

Deaths from cancer in New York State, exclusive of the City of New York,
per 100,000 population, 1901–1920............................. 73

Deaths from acute respiratory diseases in New York State, exclusive of the
City of New York, per 100,000 population, 1901–1920............... 75

Medical and social activities in the Yorkville and Bellevue Tuberculosis Clinic
Districts of the Borough of Manhattan, the City of New York, 1922... 105

219

Page

Deaths from all causes in the four New York State counties considered as areas for the rural health demonstration, per 1,000 population, during the periods, 1915–1917 (inclusive), 1918, and 1919–1921 (inclusive)... 110

Deaths from all causes, of children under ten years of age (per 1,000 children in this age group), in Cattaraugus County, 1917–1921.............. 111

Deaths from pulmonary tuberculosis in the four New York State counties considered as areas for the rural health demonstration, per 100,000 population, during the four-year periods, 1914–1917 and 1918–1921.... 112

Deaths from all causes in the five New York State cities considered as areas for the urban health demonstration, per 1,000 population, during the three-year periods, 1909–1911 and 1919–1921.................... 113

Deaths from all causes in Syracuse, per 1,000 population of the age indicated, during the three-year periods, 1909–1911 and 1919–1921............. 114

Deaths from all causes, of children under ten years of age (per 1,000 children in this age group) in Syracuse, 1917–1921......................... 115

Percentage of population under and over twenty years of age in the combined Bellevue-Yorkville tuberculosis clinic districts, in other districts, and in the City of New York, 1920............................... 120

Percentage of native born and foreign born in the combined Bellevue-Yorkville tuberculosis clinic districts, in other districts, and in the City of New York, 1920.. 121

Deaths from pulmonary tuberculosis among foreign born in the City of New York, per 100,000 population in each respective group, during the four-year period, 1918–1921.. 122

Deaths from pneumonia among foreign born in the City of New York, per 100,000 population in each respective group, 1921.................... 123

Deaths from cancer among foreign born in the City of New York, per 100,000 population in each respective group, 1921.................... 124

Deaths from organic heart diseases among foreign born in the City of New York, per 100,000 population in each respective group, 1921.......... 125

Deaths from Bright's disease among foreign born in the City of New York, per 100,000 population in each respective group, 1921............... 126

Deaths of children under one year of age, per 1,000 live births (infant mortality), in the combined Bellevue-Yorkville tuberculosis clinic districts, in other districts, and in the City of New York, 1920............... 127

220

Page

Decrease in deaths from pulmonary tuberculosis in the combined Bellevue-Yorkville tuberculosis clinic districts, in the Borough of Manhattan, and in the City of New York, per 100,000 population in each respective region, 1915–1922... 130

Deaths from pulmonary tuberculosis in the Borough of Manhattan of the City of New York. Annual average death rate, per 100,000 population in each sanitary area for the six-year period, 1915–1920 132-133

PART I

REPORT FOR
THE YEAR ENDED DECEMBER 31, 1923

I

THE YEAR IN REVIEW

THE NEW YORK HEALTH DEMONSTRATIONS

II

GRANTS OF
THE MILBANK MEMORIAL FUND

FINANCIAL STATEMENT
WITH SUMMARY OF INCOME AND
DISBURSEMENTS

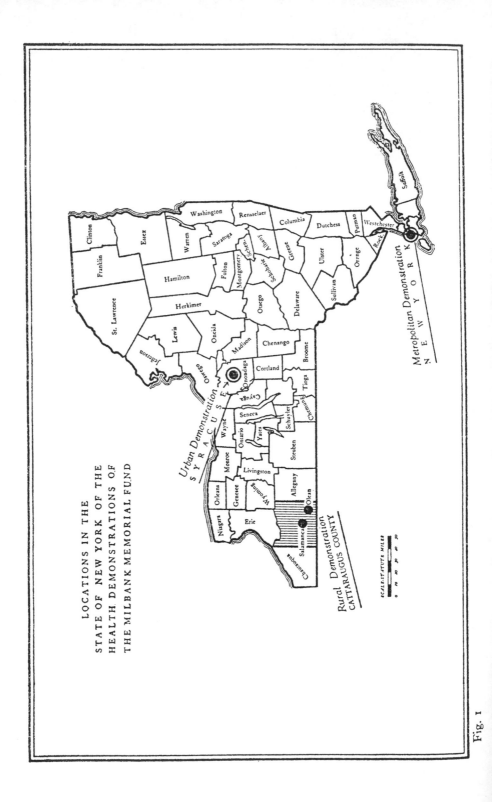

LOCATIONS IN THE
STATE OF NEW YORK OF THE
HEALTH DEMONSTRATIONS OF
THE MILBANK MEMORIAL FUND

Fig. 1

224

MILBANK MEMORIAL FUND

I

THE YEAR IN REVIEW

HE calendar year, 1923, marked the entering of the Milbank Memorial Fund upon its eighteenth year of philanthropic activity. Since its establishment by Elizabeth Milbank Anderson on April 3, 1905, the Fund's appropriations to "improve the physical, mental and moral condition of humanity and generally to advance charitable and benevolent objects" have totaled $2,440,571.80. The measures thus fostered were of immediate benefit to many specific groups—some of them in remote parts of the world, but most of them in the United States, and particularly in the City and State of New York. In accordance with its policy, an inheritance from the far-reaching insight of its founder, its philanthropy has in the main been directed at the improvement in the general level of public health and public welfare through the translation into practical usefulness of knowledge sustained by scientific research and through the demonstration of principles confirmed by experience.

During its existence, the Fund has not undertaken to set up any independent operating agencies but has sought to reach its social objectives by the utilization of existing organizations, official and voluntary, or by the initiation and temporary provision of activities where none exist but are needed. In its work, it has attempted to co-operate with, and contribute through, enterprises soundly established, of strong leadership, and of expert resources, thus capitalizing existing organization and personnel.

During the year, ended December 31, 1923, grants of $334,385.92 were made to organizations engaged in nine

225

general phases of public welfare. While it will be noted that these contributions, which are reviewed in Chapter II, reflect an interest on the part of the Fund in health education, child health and child welfare, and special health research, social welfare, general education, the co-ordination of social effort, probation work, and relief, it will be observed that a substantial part of this amount was used in promoting public health, and particularly in forwarding the New York Health Demonstrations.

The New York Health Demonstrations

As a result of the past experience of the Fund and as an outcome of studies made in 1922, the Board of Directors on April third of that year authorized the support of a plan which would attempt to demonstrate, by co-operation with three typical communities embracing a population of half a million people, whether by intensive application of known health measures the extent of sickness in the United States can be further and materially diminished and mortality rates further and substantially reduced, and whether or not such practical results can be achieved in a relatively short period of time and at a per capita cost which communities will willingly bear.

In the last half century, striking progress has been made in the diminution of disease through preventive medicine and the prosecution of public health measures. Except for the year, 1918, when, due to the influenza epidemic, the death rate was abnormally high, the general death rate in the United States (registration area) declined from 15.0 per 1,000 population in 1910 to 11.6 in 1921. (Fig. 2) Among medical men greater importance than ever before is now given to the principles of preventive medicine. To this

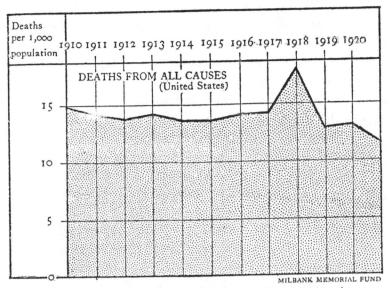

Fig. 2. Deaths from all causes in the United States (registration area), per 1,000 population, 1910–1921

interest is attributable, in part, the development of modern movements toward the conservation of individual and community health by making available to the layman the knowledge and the means for an unprecedented warfare on disease, which it is anticipated will result in the prolongation of the useful period of the average life. Enrolled in this cause are the New York Health Demonstrations, the origin, methods and objectives of which are narrated at length in Part II of this volume. It will be noted in Chapter V that the selection of Cattaraugus County for the rural demonstration and Syracuse for the urban demonstration was made in the closing weeks of 1922, so that the year, ended December 31, 1923, comprised the first anniversary of the work in these communities.

It is impossible to reiterate too frequently or to stress too strongly the fact that the demonstrations are conducted *by* and not *on* the people in the demonstration centers.

In pioneer work of this character it is necessary to consider the objectives from two somewhat different, but by no means divergent, points of view. The first involves the matter of definite health accomplishments within a specified period of time; or, otherwise expressed, the achievement of results which may be measured primarily in terms of reduced morbidity and mortality rates. It is obvious that the consideration of objectives from this standpoint introduces a large element of chance into the calculations, because the results would then become dependent upon factors over which only a relatively small degree of control could be exercised. The presence or absence in the demonstration areas of epidemics, as for example, poliomyelitis or influenza, would exert a tremendous influence upon such measurable results as are based exclusively upon morbidity and mortality rates. It is, therefore, of the greatest importance to have clearly in mind that there are factors aside from these which contribute in no small measure to the results obtained in combating disease. Measurable results of a statistical character are significant but if the demonstrations' objectives are to be practicable it is of basic importance that the program be developed in a manner and at a rate which shall not exceed the ability of the local health authorities and the voluntary agencies to take over as rapidly as the desirability and feasibility of such action on their part may be demonstrated.

Some Estimates of the Significance of the Demonstrations

At its meeting on November 15, 1923, the Advisory Council directed its attention to a final criticism of the matured program, and to a consideration of the probable benefits which would be derived from the demonstrations.* This Council embraces a body of forty-two men and women—recognized leaders in public health and social work, prominent business men and economists interested in public health work and in the promotion of the general welfare. Among its advisors are representatives of every important field of public health.

At this time, it was noted by Dr. William H. Welch, Dean of the School of Hygiene of Johns Hopkins University and Chairman of the Advisory Council, who presided at the meeting, that this undertaking represents the "first effort made on a varied and large scale, in which there is going to be anything approaching an adequate application of existing knowledge about the problems of public health."

He added that no one, at this early stage, can entirely predict the significance of these demonstrations, but that the experience of the anti-tuberculosis activities in New York City and in Framingham gave a sure basis for entering upon the work. "What at first may seem very incidental, even by-products of an undertaking, often turn out to be in some way the most significant," he said. "While we can be sure of very significant results, we can be equally confident that they will be in directions which no one at the moment can fully realize."

Dr. Matthias Nicoll, Jr., Commissioner of Health of the State of New York, also cautioned against attempting to measure statistically all of the results of the demonstrations, —"by taking out a slide-rule and figuring out death rates." There are many things, he reminded, that cannot be measured by a statistician, which make for the health, welfare and happiness of the community, county or city, which has a good health administration.

*A summary of the discussion at this meeting is given in the Milbank Memorial Fund Quarterly Bulletin, January, 1924.

"I do not mean to say that these results will not show, especially in the cities," continued Dr. Nicoll. "If Syracuse, for instance, does not eradicate diphtheria within five years, I shall be very much disappointed. I feel that very strongly and would like to make a prophecy that it will come about." But he added that even the lack of definite results in the lowering of the incidence of disease and of deaths from disease should not cause discouragement with the outcome of the project.

Dr. Nicoll said that one of the benefits already derived from the projects had been the establishment of a county health district in Cattaraugus, adding that those who have had experience in rural public health work are agreed that "the only way to accomplish efficient work is by moving the direct unit of control nearer to where the work is to be done." He pointed out that it has always been necessary to administer the affairs of health in the fifty-seven counties of New York State, practically from Albany. He expressed agreement with the fundamental philosophy and planning of the undertaking which provides, as Homer Folks, Secretary of the State Charities Aid Association, had previously pointed out, "that whatever was done should be thoroughly grounded in the institutions and the life and public affairs of the community in which the work was to be done, and should not be regarded as a strange something imported into the community." Dr. Nicoll added that those in the state health administration agreed that the demonstrations constituted "the most important step that has been taken in the state for the advancement of public health."

On this point, Dr. Welch remarked that because the work is being done largely through the co-operation of the constituted health authorities and existing agencies, and with no newly created machinery, the demonstrations will serve "to show how public and private health endeavors can with effective results be co-ordinated to a common end," adding that this alone "is well worth while even if nothing more comes of it."

"That great results are to follow from this work, which will serve as a model, advancing greatly the cause of public health, not merely in New York State and in America, but in the world—I essay to speak in behalf not only of the members of the Advisory Council, but I think I may speak also for those interested in public health (and particularly public health officials) the world over," said Dr. Welch.

Speaking of the national significance of the demonstrations, Dr. Hugh S. Cumming, Surgeon-General of the United States Public Health Service, said: "There has never been, I think, such an opportunity for forwarding the public health movement in this country as is that now presented by these demonstrations. Such a provision of counsel, composed of leaders in the several forms of public health activity, has not before been brought together on a similar project. The Public Health Service will follow particularly the county health movement to learn from it lessons which, by application to their own problems, may help other states.

"The demonstration in the area selected in New York City will be looked upon with great interest by the other large cities of the country. A great deal has already been in evidence which might be applied to cities of less than metropolitan size. The plans have been well thought out; there are very definite objectives; there is co-operation with the official health organizations, and there is counsel from leaders in all of the avenues which combine to make a comprehensive public health program."

Dr. Lee K. Frankel, Third Vice-President of the Metropolitan Life Insurance Company, observed that "one of the primary objects of these demonstrations will be to bring the subject of health right down to the people, to show them in their own terms what scientific medicine means, what the health movements are, and, in other words, to cultivate a health habit among them."

"We in the medical profession," said Dr. Haven Emerson of the College of Physicians and Surgeons of Columbia University, "are nowadays getting far enough away from disease to think in terms of the preponderating group of healthy persons and to bend our efforts to make life consciously, instead of accidentally, successful for them. It is not death rates, but health rates, that we are concerned with. Nobody is really interested in death rates; people are interested in life. We can influence mothers with our education because they are interested in the life of their children. We can interest children because they are intensely interested themselves in whatever happens to their own careers. We can teach the sick when they are sick, we can teach communities when they have contagious diseases, but the average healthy person is not interested in health as long as he has it."

"I suggest that these demonstrations will have failed," continued Dr. Emerson, "unless the people in the communities where they are conducted are taught to do as much for the protection of their own health as is now done for them. By that I do not mean merely the taking over of this work by the community, as is being done in Framingham. I should like to see more individuals in these communities take care of their health as they would a private investment. I should like to see them willing to spend as much on the health of their children as they are ready to spend on their own, to do as much for their children's health as the school systems and health departments will have done."

"A radical change is needed in the common attitude towards public health service. It has been thought of as something which chiefly concerns our public and private health agencies. It must be made a part of our annual personal budgets and not be left entirely to the makers of the municipal, county and state budgets."

Dr. Welch brought out that the demonstrations project "is a natural expression of the thoughts and activities of the founder of the Milbank Memorial Fund, Elizabeth Milbank Anderson. A woman of very broad vision, she was convinced that the best philanthropic activity is preventive and constructive, not merely palliative, relief bringing and meeting only the emergency of the moment," he said. "I doubt whether any enterprise could have been conceived which is more in harmony with her thoughts than this one."

"What we are doing here reaches far beyond the simple problems of health and the prevention of disease, and even the building up of human vitality," remarked Dr. Livingston Farrand, President of Cornell University. "Any demonstration that can make good in this particular is going to reverberate far beyond its particular technical field. It is going to be felt not only in the field of health and in the whole field of social work, but it is going to be a tremendously effective factor in the maintenance of stability in the somewhat tottering situation in which the world finds itself today. There is no greater contribution, to my mind, that could possibly be made in any field by any trust, than this new undertaking by the trustees of the Milbank Memorial Fund."

"It was Dr. Osler," said Dr. Emerson in closing the session, "who, in commenting upon the treatment of tuberculosis, said that it is what is in the head more than what is in the lung that determines the outcome of the individual case. In any health activity we undertake, we must constantly deal with character, with the reaction of the individual to the possibilities of life.

"I cannot think of the vision and faith of Mrs. Anderson," he continued, "and of the support that she gave to the New York Association for Improving the Condition of the Poor, in which she was so much interested, without believing that she would wish us to consider this not only a movement of science, but one of religion, an attempt to alter American character, to make a permanent impression upon the manner of life of our nation."

THE NEW YORK HEALTH DEMONSTRATIONS

The Rural Health Demonstration

THE rural demonstration in Cattaraugus County began in January, 1923, with the creation there by the local Board of Supervisors of a County Board of Health—the first in New York State to be established pursuant to the permissive law of 1921 authorizing Supervisors to take such action. The activities of the Board were at first administered by Dr. H. A. Pattison who, in January, was granted temporary leave of absence from his duties with the National Tuberculosis Association to undertake this work. Dr. Leverett D. Bristol, former Commissioner of Health of the State of Maine, was appointed the County Health Officer and Director of the Demonstrations in April, 1923, and in his official relations to the County Board of Health became the occupant of the first position of its kind created in the State of New York.

During the year, this pioneer health department, with headquarters in Olean, has developed its facilities to serve effectively in the six administrative districts into which the county has been divided. (Fig. 3) District health stations have been established at Olean, Salamanca, Franklinville, Cattaraugus, Ellicottville and Randolph. Each consists of at least three attractive and well-equipped rooms, one of which serves as the office of the public health nurses of the district, one as a general meeting or waiting room, and one as an examination or clinic room. Various regularly scheduled diagnostic clinics are held at the stations, and they are centers also for other neighborhood activities. For example, instruction in child hygiene is given there, and meetings of mothers' health clubs are held there.

During 1923 important advances were made in the development of a generalized public health nursing program

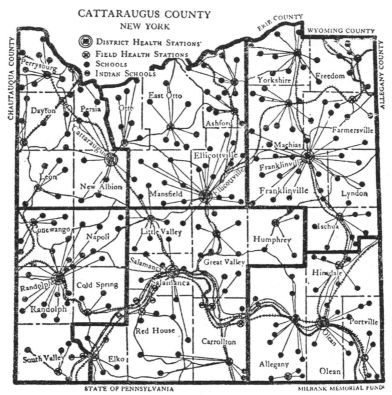

Fig. 3. Administrative divisions, with local headquarters, of the Rural Health Demonstration in Cattaraugus County, New York. Here is shown also the accessibility of schools to the district and field health stations

throughout the county. On December thirty-first, there were nine nurses on the demonstration staff. In addition, seven other public health nurses employed by the Red Cross, local boards of health and school authorities were assisting in conducting the demonstration. While consisting chiefly of visits to patients suffering from communicable diseases, and particularly tuberculosis, the nursing service has included work with health classes, such as those in home hygiene and in the care of the sick. There are, for example, in Cattaraugus County about 1,400 Indians, most of them living on the Allegany Reservation southwest of Salamanca. During the year, a study was made by the nursing staff of the apparent health needs of this group. This resulted in a definite program of education in personal and home hygiene among the Indian mothers there, and in the establishment of a limited amount of health work in the reservation schools.

It should be noted that the work of the Rural Health Demonstration is not limited to the activities under the immediate direction of the Cattaraugus County Board of Health. The school health work, for example, is an important unit of the demonstration program. In New York State, health supervision in public schools and measures for the improvement of school hygiene are made a responsibility of the school authorities and are not, except in large cities, under the direction of the health authorities. In the development of an adequate school health service in Cattaraugus County, it was decided in a conference of the local trustees and superintendents of the various school units to organize the school health work on a county-wide basis by the voluntary co-operation of the local trustees of the several school districts. As a result, an unofficial county school health service was set up, with Dr. C. A. Greenleaf as Director.

By the end of December, 6,647 children in 249 rural schools had received medical examinations, as a result of this service. In instances where examination of the pupils reveals physical defects, the attention of parents is brought to the necessity of securing medical or surgical treatment for the children, and in many instances it is suggested what care is necessary and how it may be secured. Urgent cases are followed up by the public health nurses at the district stations, and a complete follow-up of all children noted as having physical defects is planned.

Equally noteworthy is the activity of the Cattaraugus County Tuberculosis and Public Health Association, which is carrying out a county-wide program in the prevention and control of tuberculosis, the extension of popular health education, the discovery and treatment of crippled children, and in other ways. The activities of the County Health Board are administered largely through five bureaus.

Bureaus of the Cattaraugus County Board of Health

Bureau of Records and Reports at Olean, New York. Responsible for collecting, recording, tabulating and interpreting statistical information about the general health conditions in Cattaraugus County and for keeping a record of the development of the demonstration in the county. Frederick L. Thompson, Chief of Bureau.

Laboratory Bureau (Cattaraugus County, Diagnostic Laboratory) at Olean, New York. A general diagnostic laboratory service with chemical and bacteriologic examinations of water, milk and food; bacteriologic investigations of various infectious diseases, including routine diagnosis of cultures; and experimental work in bacteriology and clinical pathology. Dr. J. P. Garen, Director of Laboratory.

Bureau of Tuberculosis at Olean, New York. Diagnostic and consultation service for diseases of the lungs. Visiting nursing service and consultation clinics at district stations. Dr. Stephen A. Douglass, the Director, is also Superintendent of the County Sanatorium.

Bureau of Maternity, Infancy and Child Hygiene, being organized at Olean, New York, by a trained public health nurse loaned by the Division of Maternity, Infancy and Child Hygiene of the New York State Department of Health. To organize and supervise pre-natal and child health clinics.

Bureau of Health Education and Publicity at Salamanca, New York. Responsible for the popular dissemination of information intended to further personal health, hygiene and sanitation, and to promote the general health conditions in the county. The Director of this Bureau, John Armstrong, serves also as Executive Secretary of the County Tuberculosis and Public Health Association.

The Urban Health Demonstration

In general, the program of the urban health demonstration in Syracuse during its first year of operation has involved the development of existing facilities for the conservation and promotion of individual and community health. For some years, Syracuse has had a representative Department of Health, modern hospitals, and a number of private health agencies. Under the guidance of the local Commissioner of Health, Dr. Thomas P. Farmer, the services in the Health Department for the discovery and supervision of tuberculosis and communicable diseases were expanded; the existing facilities for public health education were increased; health services were extended in both the public and parochial schools; and special studies have been made to determine what further steps may be necessary for the protection of maternity, infancy and early child life, for the promotion of industrial hygiene and mental hygiene, and for the control of venereal disease.

Among the first definite projects to be considered were the control of tuberculosis, and the control of communicable diseases. In the preparation of the tuberculosis project it was decided that a complete program for the control of tuberculosis should not be attempted during the first year. The specific measures, recommended by Dr. H. B. Doust, Director of the Bureau of Tuberculosis, and his assistants, were the following:

1. The development and extension of the clinic service with additional hours for consultation as they become necessary.
2. An increase in the number of physicians in the clinic with service in the homes of indigent cases.
3. An increase in the number of nurses, with a more extensive home service than has been possible in the past.

4. The search for contacts and for undiscovered cases of tuberculosis and the more extensive examination of such contacts both by private physicians and in the tuberculosis clinic.

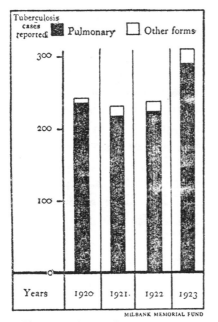

5. The examination of certain groups for signs of early tuberculosis, including undernourished school children, industrial groups, groups of food handlers, etc.

6. A careful compilation of existing records and reports and the study of these reports to determine the prevalence and distribution of tuberculosis in its relation to residence, age, race stocks, etc., in Syracuse.

Fig. 4. Cases of tuberculosis, pulmonary and other forms, reported in Syracuse, 1920–1923

It was expected that during the year sufficient information might be secured to determine with reasonable accuracy the total number of cases of tuberculosis in Syracuse and the necessary requirements in order to secure adequate treatment for every case. An intensive investigation was made of the cases of tuberculosis recorded in the files of the Department of Health during the previous ten years. The number of cases shown to have been reported annually, 1920 to 1923, is indicated in Fig. 4. A smiliar inquiry into the number of patients receiving clinic treatment for tuberculosis made it plainly evident that because of the increased facilities of the Bureau of Tuberculosis it has been possible to reach a larger number of sufferers than hitherto. (Fig. 5)

A post-graduate course in the diagnosis and treatment of tuberculosis for local practitioners was held in Syracuse during November and December. This was conducted with the co-operation of the Medical Department of Syracuse University and with the assistance of special lecturers of national reputation. That the course was popular was indicated by the fact that the applicants for registration were double the number that could be accommodated.

Over 21,600 children in the Syracuse public schools have been examined by the school nurses since the beginning of the 1923 winter term and these examina-

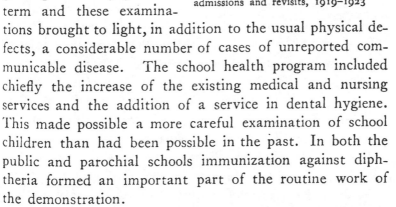

Fig. 5. Clinic attendance of tuberculous patients in Syracuse, showing new admissions and revisits, 1919–1923

tions brought to light, in addition to the usual physical defects, a considerable number of cases of unreported communicable disease. The school health program included chiefly the increase of the existing medical and nursing services and the addition of a service in dental hygiene. This made possible a more careful examination of school children than had been possible in the past. In both the public and parochial schools immunization against diphtheria formed an important part of the routine work of the demonstration.

A number of children in both the public and parochial schools has been examined and treated for goiter. The treatment consists of the administration of a preparation of organic iodide. Examinations carried out in November and December showed that 4.58 per cent of the children in the public grammar schools had demonstrable goiter and that 13.87 per cent of those in the high schools showed definite enlargement of the thyroid gland. These children are being treated for this condition either by their family physicians or by the school medical staff.

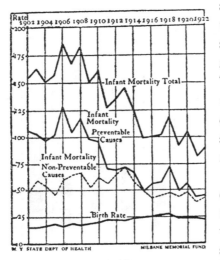

Fig. 6. Deaths of children under one year of age, per 1,000 live births (infant mortality) in Syracuse, 1902–1922. There is shown also for the same period the birth rate, and the death rates from preventable and from non-preventable causes

Studies of the annual death rates of Syracuse infants under one year of age were made for the demonstration by Dr. Otto R. Eichel, Director of the Division of Vital Statistics of the New York State Department of Health. These show that the rate of infant deaths per 1,000 live births exceeded 150 in 1902, as compared with 89 in 1922. (Fig. 6) Careful analysis indicates that the decrease was effected largely by the reduction of deaths from so-called preventable causes. While the infant death rate for what are classified as preventable causes fell from slightly above 125 per 1,000 live births in 1906, to less than 50 in 1922, the rate for other causes showed variations from year to year but only a relatively slight decrease during the twenty-year period. The major causes to which the infant mortality in 1922 was attributed, are indicated in Fig. 7.

The Onondaga County Tuberculosis and Public Health Association took an important and active part in the demonstration by co-operating with the Health Department in developing and carrying out a program of popular health education and in organizing occasional neighborhood clinics for tuberculosis. In the field of health educa-

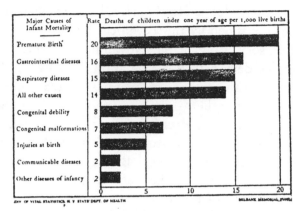

Fig. 7. Major causes of infant mortality in Syracuse, 1922

tion, a large number of health talks was given before local organizations in the city and county under the auspices of this association.

In addition to the preliminary studies which were made for the projects for the control of tuberculosis, the control of communicable disease, the promotion of health education and the improvement of school hygiene, four special surveys were conducted in Syracuse during the year. A study in child health was made by Dr. Walter H. Brown, a study in the control of venereal diseases by Dr. Haven Emerson and Dr. Walter M. Brunet, a study of morbidity statistics by Dr. M. A. Burgess, and a study in industrial hygiene by Dr. Wade Wright. The recommendations embodied in the reports of these investigations will serve as a basis for formulating programs of the future work of the Syracuse demonstration.

The Metropolitan Health Demonstration

At its meeting on November 19, 1923, the Board of Directors of the Milbank Memorial Fund approved in principle the plans for a New York City Demonstration which had been outlined by the Technical Board and sanctioned by the Advisory Council on November fifteenth.* Organization of the demonstration was authorized by the Directors, provided satisfactory co-operative arrangements could be worked out between the several local public and private agencies. This decision followed the careful consideration by the Directors of studies which had been prepared, at the request of the Technical Board, by the New York Association for Improving the Condition of the Poor and which are presented in Chapter V.

The objectives of the New York City Demonstration have been stated by the Technical Board, as follows:

1. To apply to a given area known facts about the prevention of disease.

2. To interest the population of the district in the improvement of its own health.

3. To develop by careful analysis and research, methods of public health administration that are practical and useful in a city of the first class.

4. To supplement existing health agencies, both public and private, to such an extent as to make their facilities reasonably adequate to meet the needs of the population. This implies a health program for the chosen district that, if successful, may be applicable to the whole city and to other urban areas.

5. To integrate the work of the demonstration so thoroughly with the Health Department and other agencies that the gains of the demonstration will be conserved after the demonstration itself is completed.

*Milbank Memorial Fund Quarterly Bulletin, January, 1924, pp. 39-41.

Certain administrative principles for conducting the demonstration have likewise been indicated by the Technical Board. These are briefly summarized, as follows:

1. The demonstration is to be organized on the assumption that the official responsibility for health work in this district, as in all others of the City, rests with the Health Department. The demonstration then must very properly function as a supplement and aid to the Health Department, and all the activities of the demonstration should be carried on in accordance with the Public Health Laws, the provisions of the Sanitary Code and the rules and regulations of the Department of Health.

2. An effort should be made to interest the population in the improvement of its own health rather than to superimpose on it a paternalistic program.

3. The demonstration should undertake to supplement existing agencies insofar as they are not at the moment able to finance a complete program, developing and temporarily conducting health activities under its own direction only as this seems clearly necessary.

4. It is understood that appropriations to both public and private agencies will be in addition to the amount they are already spending, and that such contributions will not permit these agencies to decrease their present expenditures, the appropriations being made in such case only because the resources of the agencies are such as to prevent them from providing an adequate service from their own funds.

5. The Milbank Memorial Fund will look forward to the gradual withdrawal of its financial support from demonstration projects and to the gradual assumption of the financial responsibility therefor by the public and private agencies of the community.

The initial steps in the organization of the proposed New York City Health Demonstration have been completed, the development of the requisite co-operative relationships is proceeding satisfactorily and the program of activities to be undertaken is receiving the careful consideration of those upon whom responsibility for its realization will rest.

Organization and Supervision

The Advisory Council was created by resolution of the Board of Directors of the Milbank Memorial Fund on May 22, 1922. The personnel of this body is listed elsewhere in this volume. During the year, 1923, individual members of the Council made many valuable suggestions regarding the organization and supervision of the New York Health Demonstrations, in their many phases. The Council's sub-committees on bovine tuberculosis, on nutrition, and on statistical procedure have played an important part in shaping the programs and work of the demonstrations. The second annual meeting of the Advisory Council, held in November, 1923, and which was largely devoted to a discussion of the significance of these undertakings, has been reported upon in some length in previous paragraphs.

The Technical Board, which is responsible for the development of the programs of the demonstrations, held monthly meetings during the year for the consideration of problems which arose in connection with the several projects. Its members keep in intimate touch with the work in the areas, making recommendations to the Board of Directors of the Fund as to the ways and means of expediting the demonstrations, and supervising the distribution of functions and funds in accordance with action taken by the Directors. Dr. Donald B. Armstrong, the Secretary of the Technical Board, resigned on December twentieth to become Assistant Secretary of The Metropolitan Life Insurance Company, and Dr. Bernard L. Wyatt, formerly Associate Director of the Rockefeller Commission for the Prevention of Tuberculosis in France, was appointed as his successor.

In June, 1923, the Board of Directors of the Milbank Memorial Fund lost one of its most able and eminent advisors, Dr. Hermann M. Biggs, late Commissioner of Health of the State of New York and a member of both the Advisory Council and the Technical Board. From their beginning, Dr. Biggs was one of the most forceful exponents of the New York Health Demonstrations, contributing much out of his great knowledge, his experience and his vision to the formulation of the policies under which they were inaugurated.* By Dr. Biggs' death, the officers and friends of the Fund who are forwarding these demonstrations have been deprived of a loyal friend and valued counsel. It is hoped that the undertakings will be a factor in the promulgation of that phrase, with which his name is inseparably linked—

> "*Public health is purchasable. Within natural limitations, any community can determine its own death rate.*"

In accordance with its general policy of not duplicating existing agencies, the Board of Directors, on the recommendation of the Technical Board, designated the State Charities Aid Association (New York), in May, 1922, as the organizing and supervisory agency for the demonstrations in Cattaraugus County and in the City of Syracuse. Its plan provided further that the actual operating agencies responsible for the development of the demonstrations activities in these districts should be the local authorities and agencies operating in the health field,† namely, the local public health authorities, the educational authorities charged by law with duties in relation to the health of school children, and the local tuberculosis and public health associations which are the local branches of the State Charities Aid

*pp. 66-75.   †pp. 108-109.

Association State Committee on Tuberculosis and Public Health.

The local health authorities, under the public health law, are subject to the supervision of the State Department of Health and report to that Department. This applies equally to the work done by the local health authorities as a part of the health demonstrations and to the work which such authorities were already carrying on. In addition to the ordinary supervision and assistance which the State Health Department gives to local State health authorities, the Department has taken a very special interest in the New York Health Demonstrations, and the Commissioner and heads of divisions of the State Health Department have advised and assisted in many important ways, including, at times, the detailing of personnel for temporary services.

Similarly, the State Department of Education, through its Division on School Health, supervises, advises and assists the local educational authorities in the demonstration areas in their school health work, although the State Education Department is less well equipped with supervisory and advisory personnel, and its relations to the demonstrations have been less intimate and continuous than those with the State Department of Health.

The State Charities Aid Association Committee on Tuberculosis and Public Health supervises and assists its local associations in the demonstration in the same manner and degree that it supervises and assists its local committees and agencies elsewhere in the State.

In addition to this relationship, the State Charities Aid Association, as the agency through which the Milbank Memorial Fund deals with local operating agencies in the demonstration areas, carries on the following activities, among others:

1. It advises with the local operating agencies in the selection of subjects for special study, leading to the formulation of definite projects to be undertaken as parts of the demonstrations. It advises in the selection and employment of experts when necessary and is the channel through which the co-operation and assistance of national health agencies are secured in the making of such studies and programs.

2. It assists the local operating agencies, upon request, in securing qualified personnel for the demonstrations when such personnel is not found locally.

3. It assists the local operating agencies in formulating in terms of budgets by six-month periods the proposed activities, mutually agreed upon as the result of studies of the character above indicated. It prepares the plan and form of these budgets, considers the budgetary proposals of the different local operating agencies as a total for each locality, and carries into effect plans for securing administrative and financial co-operation by local public authorities and voluntary agencies in financing, as well as administering the demonstrations.

4. It devises and carries on the accounting and finances of the demonstrations, receiving all funds appropriated for the demonstrations by the Milbank Memorial Fund; outlining the plan of authorization and incurring of expenditures and the approval of bills; establishing an accounting system, which will afford, from time to time, proper data as to the cost of each kind of activity; and plans and submits monthly, semi-annual, and annual financial statements to the Technical Board and to the Board of Directors of the Fund.

5. It receives from each of the local operating agencies periodical reports of progress in the development of the demonstration program.

6. It seeks the co-operation of the various national health agencies in promoting the features of the demonstrations in the fields of their respective interests.

7. In general, it exercises primary responsibility for seeing that the recommendations of the Technical

Board and the decisions of the Board of Directors of
the Milbank Memorial Fund, in regard to objectives,
policies, methods, and funds, are actually carried into
effect; that all the authorities and agencies, local,
state and national, which should be consulted, are
actually consulted, and their advice and suggestions
co-ordinated; that co-operation is actually secured
from all authorities and agencies, whose co-operation
and participation should be secured; that adequate
information as to progress and developments is secured from time to time, and important questions of
policy, finance, or administration, which are likely
to arise, are foreseen, defined, and prepared for
submission to the Technical Board.

II

GRANTS OF
THE MILBANK MEMORIAL FUND

AS has been elsewhere indicated, a large portion of the income of the Milbank Memorial Fund has been set aside for the development of the New York Health Demonstrations. During 1923, $137,618.48 was utilized in forwarding these projects. Although the Fund continued during the year to contribute to the support of many of the social agencies which it had assisted in the past, it was forced to decline most of the new applications presented and some requests for renewal of appropriations because of the necessity for holding in reserve sufficient funds to finance its Health Demonstrations. The organizations to which it did contribute have made it possible to give financial assistance in many fields, including public health, health education, child health and child welfare, special health research, social welfare, general education, the co-ordination of social effort, probation work and relief.

The largest single beneficiary during the year was the New York Association for Improving the Condition of the Poor. To this Association was contributed $74,017.44, of which $54,017.44 was for the purpose of furthering the work of the Department of Social Welfare and $20,000 for continuing the Home Hospital demonstration.

THE NEW YORK ASSOCIATION FOR IMPROVING THE CONDITION OF THE POOR

The Department of Social Welfare

The year marked the first decade of activity of the Association's Department of Social Welfare. Made possible by an initial grant from Mrs. Anderson, on March 5, 1913, and by her pledge of annual support during a ten-year period, this Department has enabled the A. I. C. P. to undertake preventive and constructive work for the welfare of the community as a whole, apart from its service to particular families. Its measures have been concerned chiefly with sanitation and hygiene, public health and disease prevention, food problems and child welfare.

Its program has included many pioneer community undertakings. Among these are its activities in the Mulberry Health Center, which is supported jointly by the Laura Spelman Rockefeller Memorial and the Milbank Memorial Fund. Here the Association is endeavoring to develop a constructive health service for a population of 30,000 people, resident in a congested district of the Borough of Manhattan. Recent results accomplished there, particularly in the field of dental hygiene, have stimulated interest in the Center's program in various parts of New York City.

By research and administrative experiment, the Association has effected more and better luncheon facilities in the public schools in the City, service which is now maintained by public support; and has assisted in developing medical, surgical, dental and nursing examinations and care for school children. A significant contribution has also been made in improving the City's public baths, comfort stations and sanitary drinking fountains. Through the operation of the Milbank Memorial Baths and, more recently, the model wet wash laundry, the A. I. C. P. has demonstrated the feasibility of maintaining high standards in the public bath system, and has shown that a thoroughly sanitary community laundry for tenement families can be operated at a reasonable cost.

Special studies of the house fly made by the A. I. C. P. have been of value in helping in the reduction of diarrheal diseases among children. They showed that almost twice as many attacks of diarrhea resulted where flies were numerous as occurred when the pests were a negligible factor, thus clearly establishing the fact of the direct correlation between a high case rate and death rate from infant diarrhea and exposure of children and food to flies.

As a part of the study, much effort was spent, in cooperation with the Department of Health of the City of New York, in the formulation of new measures of fly control, particularly in livery stables in the city. Experiments were made to evolve practical methods of treating stable manure to prevent fly breeding.

Partly because of the more effective control of the insect brought about locally through the Association's three years of intensive activity in its campaign against the house fly, these carriers of disease have been greatly reduced in number in the Greater City. The results of these investigations have been published in pamphlet form and distributed widely.* They provide a scientific basis for the further development of campaigns against flies which are being waged throughout the country.

Because of the achievements of the Department of Social Welfare in the development of preventive social measures, the Milbank Memorial Fund has pledged a continuance of its support of this work. The future program of the Department will emphasize preventive health and social welfare service, particularly for the conservation of the health and welfare of the child. At the same time, the A. I. C. P. plans to continue its interest in the many measures for the improvement of living conditions in the community, which the maintenance of this Department has enabled it to develop during the past decade.

*Flies and Diarrheal Disease, a Joint Study by the Bureau of Public Health and Hygiene of the A. I. C. P. and the Bureau of Child Hygiene of the Department of Health, A. I. C. P., New York, (Publication No. 91), 1915.

The Home Hospital

The Fund also continues its financial assistance in maintaining the Association's Home Hospital, where, as is stated elsewhere,* the practicability of family care of many cases of tuberculosis has been successfully demonstrated. Home Hospital care is humane in that it keeps many families together for whom ordinarily there would be no alternative but the breaking up of the home and sending one or both parents to a sanatorium and the children to institutions. Moreover, ten years' experience in the Home Hospital has shown the effectiveness and economy of such care in dealing with tuberculosis in needy families.

Recently a study was made by John C. Gebhart, Director of the Department of Social Welfare, of the effectiveness of Home Hospital treatment as compared with sanatorium treatment. As a result of his findings, Mr. Gebhart observes that although in no sense intended as a substitute for sanatoria, the Home Hospital, judged by medical results, has proven to be quite as effective as the best sanatoria in the country in arresting and improving tuberculous patients during residence.†

During its decade of operation, no new cases of tuberculosis, either of children or of adults, have developed while a family was in the Home Hospital. This remarkable record, the A. I. C. P. attributes largely to its educational work with resident families. In this environment where there were adequate physical needs, there has been carried out a course of medical treatment and supervision modeled after that of the best sanatoria. But there has also been daily, painstaking educational work on the part of nurses to stress

*p. 80.
†Gebhart, John C., "Tuberculosis, a Family Problem," the story of the Home Hospital of the A. I. C. P., pp. 11–18, A. I. C. P., New York, 1924.

the importance of fresh air, sunlight and wholesome food habits; to emphasize precautions regarding such matters as sleeping arrangements, the use of common towels, glasses and dishes; and to establish right habits of living. In this respect the home-institution is very effective in building up the resistance of well members of families in which there is tuberculosis, thus safeguarding the health of all by preventing the spread of infection.

The policy of the Association in administering the Home Hospital has not been merely to discharge a given tuberculous patient as "quiescent" or "improved." By dealing with the patient as a member of a family, with the family, not the individual patient-member, as the unit, the Board of Managers of the A. I. C. P. believed that there would result the establishment of a standard of living and habits of personal hygiene which would follow the family long after its discharge from the hospital.

In order to test the permanent effect of Home Hospital treatment, the after-history of 306 patients discharged during the first ten years of the institution's history was followed up, and the results compared with similar records from four sanatoria. This study showed that the results secured at the Home Hospital compare favorably with those secured at these sanatoria. A special inquiry showed that practically 60 per cent of the 262 discharged adult tuberculous patients who were interviewed, were at the time able to assume full responsibility toward their families. "Despite the social, educational and economic handicaps which first brought the families to the attention of the A. I. C. P.," observes Mr. Gebhart, "patients discharged from the Home Hospital apparently live longer and are economically more productive than those discharged from other sanatoria."

The survey also indicated that for certain patients who

because of their family relationships were most in need of its specialized care, the relative cost to the community of providing treatment in the Home Hospital "is no more than other plans which are less effective and certainly less humane." Where, for example, "the patient is a widow with three dependent children, the cost of Home Hospital care would be about $4.76 a day, while to place her in a sanatorium and the children in institutions, usually the only alternative, would involve a daily cost of at least $4.21, a difference of only 13 per cent."

The New York State Ventilation Commission

During 1923, the report of the New York State Commission on Ventilation was made public. It will be recalled that this Commission, the personnel of which was suggested by the A. I. C. P. and the studies of which were financed by the Milbank Memorial Fund, was appointed by Governor Sulzer in 1913 to conduct an inquiry into the means of ventilating schools and other public buildings. The volume which is entitled, "Ventilation," embodies twenty-seven chapters, presented in two parts.* An impression of the field covered by the Commission's report is given in the following general outline of its contents:

PART I

A STUDY OF THE PHYSIOLOGICAL SIGNIFICANCE OF THE VARIOUS FACTORS IN VENTILATION, WITH SPECIAL REFERENCE TO THE EFFECTS OF AIR CONDITIONS ON HEALTH, COMFORT AND EFFICIENCY

    I. Historical Development of Knowledge in Regard to the Physiological Influences of Ventilation

    II. General Plan of the Experiments Conducted by the Commission

    III. Physiological Methods Used in the Investigations of the Commission

    IV. Methods of Studying the Psychological Effects of Various Air Conditions

    V. The Effects of Atmospheric Conditions on the Body Temperature

*"Ventilation: The Report of the New York State Commission on Ventilation."— E. P. Dutton & Company, New York, 1923.

VI. The Effects of Atmospheric Conditions on the Circulatory System of the Body

VII. Observations on the Relation of Atmospheric Conditions to Certain Phenomena of Respiration and Metabolism

VIII. The Influence of Chemically Vitiated Air upon Certain Physiological Reactions, upon Human Appetite and upon the Growth of Animals

IX. The Effect of Atmospheric Conditions on the Performance of Physical Work

X. The Influence of Various Air Conditions upon Mental Work

XI. The Effect of Atmospheric Dryness on Nervousness and Neuro-Muscular Achievement

XII. The Effect of Variations in Atmospheric Temperature and Humidity upon the Condition of the Upper Respiratory Tract

XIII. The Influence of Certain Atmospheric Conditions upon Immunity against Infection

XIV. Some Fundamental Physical Factors Affecting the Loss of Heat from a Warm, Moist Surface

XV. General Conclusions in Regard to the Effect of Various Atmospheric Conditions upon Health, Comfort and Efficiency

PART II

A STUDY OF THE PRACTICAL RESULTS ACHIEVED BY THE USE OF VARIOUS METHODS OF SCHOOLROOM VENTILATION

XVI. Historical Development of the Practical Art of Ventilation

XVII. General Plan and Scope of the Field Investigations Undertaken by the Commission, with a Description of the Experimental Plant at School 51

XVIII. A Study of the Relation of Window Ventilation to School Attendance in Certain Selected Schools of Springfield, Mass.

XIX. A Comparative Study of Five Different Methods of Schoolroom Ventilation

XX. A Study of the Results Obtained by Window Ventilation in a Series of Schoolrooms During the Winter of 1915-1916

XXI. A Comparative Study of Window Ventilation and Fan Ventilation in the Winter of 1916-1917

XXII. Comparative Study of the Sensations of Comfort Experienced in Window-Ventilated and Fan-Ventilated Rooms

XXIII. The Prevalence of Respiratory Diseases Among Children in Schoolrooms Ventilated by Various Methods

XXIV. Studies on the Distribution of Air Supply Within the Schoolroom

XXV. A Study of the Effect of the Washing and Humidification of Schoolroom Air upon Health, Comfort and Efficiency

XXVI. Studies of Ventilation by the Use of Re-circulated Air and its Effect upon Health, Comfort and Efficiency

XXVII. General Conclusions in Regard to the Results Produced by Various Methods of Schoolroom Ventilation

In the foreword to the volume, Albert G. Milbank outlines in part the significance of these studies. At the time of the appointment of the Commission, says Mr. Milbank, ventilation, with the kindred problems of hygiene and building sanitation, presented novel aspects. The ventilation of schools, theatres, churches, of factories and of offices was notoriously bad. "Elaborate and expensive equipment for forced ventilation had been devised, but experts freely expressed the opinion that hundreds of thousands and perhaps millions of dollars were being wasted annually in the installation of worthless ventilating devices. They were frank in stating that very little was positively known about the subject of ventilation. It was a dark realm of sanitary science and public hygiene. . . . Disinterested ventilating engineers, physiologists, physicians and sanitarians alike agreed that no satisfactory system of ventilation had been devised."

A Commission of recognized experts* was organized "to undertake the research work and experimentation required to be done before the body of facts could be assembled and recommendations made in accord with which ventilation practice could be based on scientific principles instead of guesswork."

"Each of the members of the Commission, in his own field, has utilized the results of these experiments, and has passed on his experiences in scientific articles which have been read to national and international scientific organizations and published from time to time in scientific periodicals. It is believed that the full report, finding its way to the libraries of colleges and universities, of architects and engineers, of school superintendents and school boards, as well as the public libraries of this and other countries, will constitute a permanent contribution to this branch of science, and will result in general improvement of health and hygiene conditions, particularly among the school children of the land."

*The members of the New York State Commission on Ventilation were: Dr. C. E. A. Winslow, Chairman, Professor of Public Health at the Yale Medical School; Dr. Frederic S. Lee, Dalton Professor of Physiology at the College of Physicians and Surgeons; Dr. James Alexander Miller, Professor of Clinical Medicine at the College of Physicians and Surgeons; Dr. Earl B. Phelps, Professor of Chemistry at the United States Hygienic Laboratory; Dr. Edward Lee Thorndike, Professor of Educational Psychology at Teachers College, Columbia University; and Mr. Dwight D. Kimball, of the firm of R. D. Kimball & Company.

The general conclusions of the Commission regarding schoolroom ventilation were "That either window ventilation or plenum fan ventilation (if the plant be properly designed and operated) yields generally satisfactory results from the standpoint of the air conditions in the average schoolroom . . . and that it is possible to maintain by either of these procedures air conditions in the schoolroom that would be considered satisfactory by all the ordinary physical tests and conditions which are reasonably comfortable and satisfactory to the occupants."*

The volume, which contains 606 pages of text with 134 illustrations, 219 tables and much valuable supplementary data, ends with the assertion that "the avoidance of overheating is the primary essential in all systems of ventilation. Air change, direction of flow, and all other factors are secondary. The most important article of ventilating equipment is the thermometer; and however simple or however complex an apparatus may be installed for air conditioning, a constant and intelligent vigilance in regard to operation and overheating is the price of health and comfort."

GRANTS TO OTHER AGENCIES

Public Health

Including that for the New York Health Demonstrations, the Fund's grants during 1923 for public health work amounted to $215,618.48. Of this amount, $40,000 was appropriated to the Judson Health Center which, by the maintenance of clinics and demonstration day nurseries and by educational work in the interests of community health, ministers to the needs of a congested neighborhood of New York City, inhabited by over 45,000 persons of foreign

*"Ventilation," p. 527.

birth, where health and living conditions are inadequate and where previous to the Center's establishment in 1921 little intensive health work had been attempted. One of the features of the Center is a well-equipped nursery for the treatment and care of poorly nourished and rachitic children.

The Fund's support of the general work of the State Charities Aid Association was continued, and assistance thus given in the maintenance of its activities for the improvement of the administration of charitable institutions, the care of destitute children, the conservation of mental health, and the promotion of efforts to improve public health. The Association during the year led a successful state-wide campaign to enlist public support for a $50,000,000 bond issue for state hospitals and other institutions.

Other beneficiaries in the field of public health include the National Tuberculosis Association, the Public Health Committee of the New York Academy of Medicine, and the Bowling Green Neighborhood Association. A contribution was made to the former to assist in improving its plans for the sale of Christmas seals, from which it and its member state and local organizations derive substantial support in carrying out a nation-wide program for the prevention and control of tuberculosis. The Bowling Green Neighborhood Association operates a health and social center in the neighborhood of Wall Street, inhabited by a large number of newly arrived immigrants.

Health Education

In giving $12,500 to the National Committee for Mental Hygiene, the Milbank Memorial Fund in 1923 brought the total of its grants for the work of this organization in the conservation of mental health to $152,500. The Committee together with its affiliated state societies and committees

aids and encourages work for the conservation of mental
health and for improvement in the treatment of those
suffering from nervous or mental diseases and mental
deficiency.

In addition to making the Committee's general work more
effective, the Fund's contribution has made possible the
organization and operation of a department of information
and statistics. Material collected and codified by this
department has been placed at the disposal of the Federal
Census Bureau, which the Committee has assisted recently
in making a national study of institutional care and treatment for those suffering from nervous and mental disorders
and mental defect. The uniform statistical schedules
planned by this department are now in use in all but twelve
of the state institutions for mental defectives in the country.
Many of the other hospitals for the mentally diseased and
schools for the feeble-minded are co-operating in the Committee's efforts to have uniform methods of record-keeping
universally adopted. Another important phase of the Committee's work to which the Fund's appropriation in 1923 was
devoted was the preparation and publication of educational
material on mental hygiene, which was distributed to professional and lay groups throughout the country, to schools
and to libraries.

Support of the work of the Council on Health Education
in China was also continued, the Fund's interest in the
activities of the Council dating back to a time before Mrs.
Anderson's death, when at a critical period it was given financial assistance. The Council seeks to interest Chinese citizens in improving their country's public health conditions.
Under the leadership there of Dr. W. W. Peter, an effective
campaign is being conducted by this organization to popular-
ize the health movement in China.

Child Health and Child Welfare

Recently the work of the Child Health Organization of America in raising the health standard of school children and that of the American Child Hygiene Association in encouraging measures for the proper care of mothers before, during and after confinement, and for children from birth through adolescence, was amalgamated in a new organization, the American Child Health Association. The Fund made a grant to assist this Association to develop its program which is national in scope and embraces the former activities of these societies. Other appropriations in the field of child health and child welfare went to the Babies' Dairy Association and to the Jacob A. Riis Neighborhood Settlement, both in the City of New York.

Special Health Research

The Saranac Laboratory of the Trudeau Foundation, which is primarily supported by the Fund, is making a series of inhalation studies which, dealing with one of the fundamental problems of this disease, should make a valuable contribution to existing literature on experimental tuberculosis. In addition to these studies, investigations in progress at the laboratory include inquiries by staff members in the following fields:

```
Experimental Tuberculosis Meningitis..............by Dr. W. B. Soper
Experimental Ultraviolet Light Therapy..........by Dr. Edgar Mayer
Experimental Pleurisy.......................by Dr. E. R. Baldwin
```

The inhalation studies on the "Relation of Mineral Dusts to Tuberculosis" have included researches into the action on pulmonary tissues of the dusts of marble, carborundum and quartz. Dr. Morris Dworski and Dr. Leroy U. Gardner, who made studies of marble, have found that this mineral when imbedded (as it frequently is) in silicious rock produces a dust which, when repeatedly inhaled, lowers the resistance of the tissues to attacks of tubercle-bacilli. Similar tests are being made of the dusts of the other minerals.

Recent studies by Dr. Baldwin and Dr. Gardner dealing with "Reinfection in Tuberculosis" indicate that in addition to efforts usually made to safeguard the young from infection, more attention should be paid to protecting both young and old from disease.

The Fund was able in 1923 to assist several special undertakings in the field of general education, although its interest in, and support of, the New York Health Demonstrations have necessitated a degree of retrenchment in the aid formerly given to a number of commendable enterprises. A contribution was made to the Foreign Language Information Service which utilizes popular educational media "to interpret America to the alien and the alien to America;" for the Goldman Band Concerts which during the summer completed its sixth season of outdoor public concerts in the City of New York; to Hampton Normal and Agricultural Institute, one of the country's leading educational institutions for the training of Negro and Indian youth; to the Metropolitan Baptist Board of Promotion and to the World Association of Daily Vacation Bible Schools.

Co-ordination of Social Effort

Financial assistance was extended to the National Conference of Social Work, which in 1923 completed a half-century of leadership in social progress in the United States and Canada. The Fund's appropriation went towards defraying the expenses of organizing and conducting the fiftieth anniversary meeting of the Conference, which was a notable event in the history of social work in America.

The American Country Life Association, which is devoted

to the improvement of rural conditions in the United States, received the support of the Fund during the year, as did also the National Health Council, which was organized three years ago and which marked the first successful attempt to initiate practical co-ordination of the chief national voluntary health agencies of the country. Substantial progress has been made since the formation of the Council, and today the fourteen organizations which compose it are working in closer relationship and greater harmony than might have been predicted earlier. The Milbank Memorial Fund had the benefit of the services of Dr. Donald B. Armstrong, the Secretary of the National Health Council, in developing its health demonstrations program.

Probation Work

Under a pledge extending over a period of years, a grant was made to the National Probation Association. The Association, which was established in 1907, seeks to promote social and effective treatment and prevention of delinquency throughout America, working for the extension of effective probation organization and for co-operation between judges, probation officers, and all concerned in social court work. It also conducts surveys and carries on local campaigns to secure legislation and improved probation work.

Relief

While the philanthropic effort of the Milbank Memorial Fund has since its origin been chiefly preventive, in special instances contributions have been made to agencies engaged in emergency relief work of one kind and another. During 1923, for example, the Fund made an appropriation to the Institute for Crippled and Disabled Men. This voluntary New York City organization aims to discover and provide suitable means to enable men and boys of work age, with a physical disability impairing the use of their limbs, to earn their living and to promote general interest in the problem of the rehabilitation of the disabled. A contribution was made also to the Japanese Relief Fund of the American Red Cross for alleviating the suffering caused by the earthquake catastrophe in Japan.

MILBANK MEMORIAL FUND
FINANCIAL STATEMENT
DECEMBER 31, 1923

Assets:

Investments, Principal Funds	$9,033,280.59
Investments, Special Reserve Fund	148,968.75
Investments, Unexpended Appropriations Account	361,260.23
Cash	153,429.34
Total	$9,696,938.91

Funds and Income:

Principal Fund	$9,050,589.42
Special Reserve Fund	150,000.00
Unexpended Appropriations Account	492,027.89
Balance of Income	4,321.60
Total	$9,696,938.91

INCOME AND EXPENDITURES
During the Year Ended December 31, 1923

Income:

Balance on hand, January 1st.	$166,222.43
Received during the year ended December 31st	543,908.36
Total	$710,130.79

Expenses:

Administration		$29,395.38
Grants Paid:		
Health Demonstrations	$137,618.48	
Other Appropriations	196,767.44	
		334,385.92

Transfers:

To Special Reserve Fund		$25,000.00	
To Unexpended Appropriations Account	$347,783.84		
Less expended during 1923	30,755.95		
		$317,027.89*	
			342,027.89
*Undisbursed Income			4,321.60
Total			$710,130.79

Unpaid Grants and Pledges

Unpaid balances of appropriations made in 1923 and prior years.		$492,027.89
Grants and pledges which become effective in 1924 and following years:		
1924	$465,750.00	
1925	426,750.00	
1926	420,750.00	
		1,313,250.00
Total		$1,805,277.89

*Applicable to Unpaid Grants and Pledges.

SUMMARY OF GRANTS MADE BY THE MILBANK MEMORIAL FUND DURING THE YEAR ENDED DECEMBER 31, 1923

FIELDS OF ACTIVITY	GRANTS
Public Health, including New York Health Demonstrations	$215,618.48
Health Education	15,500.00
Child Health and Child Welfare	6,500.00
Special Health Research	5,000.00
Social Welfare	54,017.44
General Education	13,750.00
Co-ordination of Social Effort	9,000.00
Probation Work	4,000.00
Relief	11,000.00
Total	$334,385.92

GRANTS MADE BY THE MILBANK MEMORIAL FUND TO SOCIAL AGENCIES DURING YEAR ENDED DECEMBER 31, 1923

FIELDS OF ACTIVITY OF RECIPIENT ORGANIZATIONS	GRANTS

Public Health

Bowling Green Neighborhood Association	$1,000.00
Judson Health Center	40,000.00
New York Health Demonstrations of the Milbank Memorial Fund	137,618.48
National Tuberculosis Association	5,000.00
New York Academy of Medicine	2,000.00
New York Association for Improving the Condition of the Poor	20,000.00
State Charities Aid Association	10,000.00
Total	$215,618.48

Health Education

Council on Health Education in China	3,000.00
National Committee for Mental Hygiene	12,500.00
Total	$15,500.00

Child Health and Child Welfare

American Child Health Association..................	$5,000.00
Babies Dairy Association.........................	500.00
Jacob A. Riis Neighborhood Settlement............	1,000.00
Total....................................	$6,500.00

Special Health Research

Trudeau Sanatorium............................	5,000.00
Total....................................	$5,000.00

Social Welfare

New York Association for Improving the Condition of the Poor.....................................	54,017.44
Total....................................	$54,017.44

General Education

Goldman Band Concerts.........................	$3,000.00
Foreign Language Information Service..............	2,500.00
Hampton Normal and Agricultural Institute........	250.00
Metropolitan Baptist Board of Promotion..........	5,000.00
World Association of Daily Vacation Bible Schools....	3,000.00
Total....................................	$13,750.00

Co-ordination of Social Effort

American Country Life Association.................	$2,500.00
National Conference of Social Work................	5,000.00
National Health Council.........................	1,500.00
Total....................................	$9,000.00

Probation Work

National Probation Association....................	4,000.00
Total....................................	4,000.00

Relief

American Red Cross—Japanese Relief Fund.........	10,000.00
Institute for Crippled and Disabled Men............	1,000.00
Total....................................	11,000.00

Grand Total...............................	$334,385.92

PART II

THE NEW YORK HEALTH DEMONSTRATIONS
Their Origin, Scope and Methods

III

THE PURPOSE OF
THE NEW YORK HEALTH DEMONSTRATIONS

IV

THE DEMONSTRATIONS PROGRAM

V

SELECTING THE DEMONSTRATION DISTRICTS

271

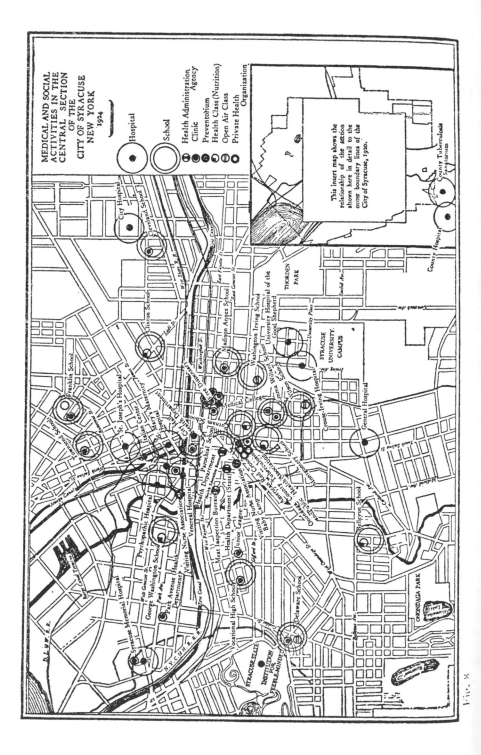

MEDICAL AND SOCIAL
ACTIVITIES IN THE
CENTRAL SECTION
OF THE
CITY OF SYRACUSE
NEW YORK
1924

Hospital

School

Health Administration,
Agency
Clinic
Preventorium
Health Class (Nutrition)
Open Air Class
Private Health
Organization

This insert map shows the relationship of the section shown here in detail to the outer boundary lines of the City of Syracuse, 1920.

III

THE PURPOSE OF THE NEW YORK HEALTH DEMONSTRATIONS

THE chief project now enlisting the interest and support of the Milbank Memorial Fund, is the New York Health Demonstrations. This enterprise grew out of an inquiry made in 1921 by John A. Kingsbury, Secretary of the Fund, with the advice and assistance of Homer Folks, the Secretary of the State Charities Aid Association, Bailey B. Burritt, General Director of the New York Association for Improving the Condition of the Poor, and Dr. Donald B. Armstrong, Executive Officer of the Community Health and Tuberculosis Demonstration at Framingham, Massachusetts.

Consultations with leading health and social workers and an analysis of the activities of the Fund's beneficiaries and of those of allied agencies in the health and social field, resulted in recommendations, subsequently endorsed by the Board of Directors, that the Fund's resources be consolidated to a greater degree than hitherto in a distinctive disease prevention and health promotion program. The results of the Home Hospital Tuberculosis Demonstration of the New York A. I. C. P.* contributed to this conclusion. Even more contributory, perhaps, were the results of the Framingham Health and Tuberculosis Demonstration, as were also the accomplishments of the more adequately financed health and tuberculosis activities in New York State and elsewhere.

To make its demonstrations applicable to communities of different types and thus useful later throughout the

*Milbank Memorial Fund Annual Report, 1922, pp. 44–47.

country, the Milbank Memorial Fund planned to select as localities for the carrying out of such a program: (1) a rural county of 50,000 to 75,000 population, (2) a city of about 100,000 and (3) a metropolitan district of about 200,000. The Board of Directors realized that the selection of these demonstration localities, and of the agencies through which it would operate, as well as the maturing of the plan, would involve further specialized inquiry.

To this end, they adopted a recommendation for the establishment of a Technical Board to render expert assistance in developing a demonstrations program. So that the plan might have the benefit of a wider collaboration and the perspective of greater collective experience, an Advisory Council of experts in the health field was later appointed, its membership to include the personnel of the Technical Board.

In co-operation with the New York State Department of Health, the State Charities Aid Association, the New York Association for Improving the Condition of the Poor and other agencies, the Fund's Technical Board and the Advisory Council spent several months in studying the counties and cities in New York State available respectively for the rural county and the two city demonstrations. Applications from many localities were considered. Because the Milbank Memorial Fund hopes to demonstrate the social possibilities of an intensive health régime not only to the section chosen for demonstration purposes but to communities everywhere, a careful survey of health and social conditions and activities was undertaken in all of the available communities.

These studies resulted in the recommendation of the three localities in New York State where demonstrations are either now under way, or planned. Cattaraugus County was chosen for the rural unit; and Syracuse, for the urban center. The Bellevue-Yorkville district in the Borough of Manhattan of the City of New York was recommended for the metropolitan demonstration, provided satisfactory co-operative arrangements can be made with public and private health agencies operating there.

With the co-operation of interested public and private agencies and with the advice of its Technical Board and its Advisory Council, during a period of at least five years, the Milbank Memorial Fund will endeavor by the application of known facts about disease prevention and health promotion—

1. To develop programs which will illustrate the most effective ways and means of advancing disease prevention and health conservation in the three demonstration areas, each of which represents an important type of the political and administrative units into which this country is divided.

2. To determine if the favorable results obtained in the control of tuberculosis, the reduction of morbidity and mortality rates from other preventable diseases and the promotion of health in smaller population units can be demonstrated on larger and more varied groups.

3. To determine the extent to which tuberculosis and other leading causes of illness and death can further be controlled; and to measure the relative utility of special activities for the control of such diseases.

4. To determine the unit cost of the various health projects undertaken and the per capita cost of adequate general health work, and whether after a preliminary period of financial co-operation with the existing local health officials and agencies, it is feasible for a normal community to assume and permanently maintain adequate machinery for disease prevention and health conservation.

The plan was first publicly announced on May 4, 1922, at the opening session of the eighteenth annual meeting of the National Tuberculosis Association in Washington, by the Secretary of the Fund. A more detailed statement of the undertaking was put before a representative audience of volunteer and professional social workers at the celebration of the Fiftieth Anniversary of the State Charities Aid Association in New York City on May 12, 1922. It was made clear at this time that the demonstrations were not to set up additional operating machinery, but that the Fund anticipated the accomplishment of its aims through established agencies. On May twenty-second, announcement was made that the New York State Charities Aid Association was to be the chief operating agency for the rural and urban demonstrations.

Past Progress in the Control of Disease

At one of the first meetings of the Advisory Council, the late Dr. Hermann M. Biggs, then Commissioner of Health of New York State, reviewed certain records of progress in the public health movement during recent decades which, in part, indicate that the Fund's demonstration plan is soundly conceived and offers hope of success in its general purpose. His speech is paraphrased here at some length.

Dr. Biggs pointed out that public health work in New York City, for example, may be said to have begun in 1892 with the establishment by the New York City Health Department of a public health laboratory. Shortly before this, in 1889, the Department had introduced in a very limited way its first educational campaign against tuberculosis. In 1887, the death rate from this disease in Manhattan and the Bronx was just under 358 per 100,000. (These Boroughs are taken because this period was before the consolidation of the Greater City, and because data from them are available to date.) The accompanying chart (Fig. 9) shows that from that time the rate has steadily and rapidly fallen.

While many health measures, including improved diag-

nosis and better case and death reporting, contributed to
the marked reduction in deaths from tuberculosis, the increase in hospital facilities for the care of sufferers from the

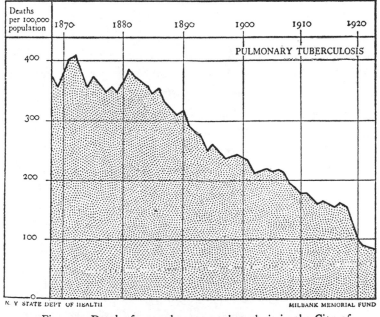

Fig. 9.   Deaths from pulmonary tuberculosis in the City of
New York, per 100,000 population, 1868–1923
Based on combined returns of former cities of Brooklyn and New York
before 1898, and of Greater New York thereafter

disease no doubt played an important part in effecting this
result.   Judging from data collected by Dr. Donald B.
Armstrong in connection with the Framingham, Massachusetts, demonstration, it may be assumed that for every death
from pulmonary tuberculosis there are nine active cases and
approximately the same number of arrested cases of this
disease.   With the adequate hospitalization of cases, the
foci of infection otherwise scattered throughout the city are
decreased at a steady and rapid rate.
Up to 1895 there were less than three hundred beds in

New York City hospitals designated especially for tuberculous patients. Sufferers from tuberculosis were being placed in the general wards. At Bellevue Hospital, for example, thirty-five to forty per cent of the beds in the medical ward were always filled with advanced cases of this disease. As a result of a campaign begun about this time for setting aside beds for patients suffering from pulmonary tuberculosis, the reception of cases in the general wards of general hospitals was absolutely prohibited.

Since this time, the facilities for the hospitalization of cases greatly increased. A census begun by the City Health Department in January, 1907, shows that at that time there were 3,300 patients with pulmonary tuberculosis who had been sent outside of the city for treatment or who were being treated in general public or private hospitals and sanatoria in the city. (Fig. 10) This number gradually increased from year to year until in 1916 there were on the first of January over 9,000 patients with pulmonary tuberculosis being treated outside of the city or in public or private hospital or sanatoria beds in the city. Then the number of patients began to decrease. At the same time, the total of beds available for New York City cases in public and private institutions increased to something over 5,000. The occupied beds began to decrease in 1917 until on the first of January, 1922, there were more than 1,500 vacant beds in the city.

The very rapid reduction in the death rate in late years, to which this increased hospitalization has contributed, is shown by the fact that although the population of the Boroughs of Manhattan and the Bronx has more than doubled since 1887, the actual number of deaths from pulmonary tuberculosis has greatly decreased.

In former days, the death rate from tuberculosis was much higher in the cities than in the country; it was twice

as high in New York City as in the rural districts of the
state. For many years there has been a steady decrease in
the death rate from pulmonary tuberculosis in New York

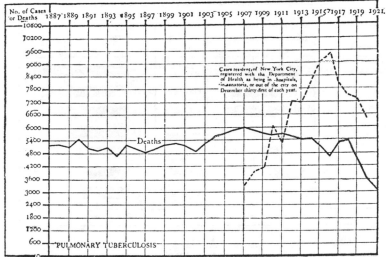

Fig. 10. Number of deaths from tuberculosis in the Boroughs of
Manhattan and the Bronx, City of New York, by years, 1887–1921

Number of cases resident of the City of New York, registered with the
Department of Health as being in hospitals, in sanatoria, or out of the city on
December thirty-first of each year is shown for the period, 1907–1920, inclusive

State outside of New York City. But the present death
rate from this disease in the rural districts is higher
than in any important city of the state. In 1921, for example, the rate in the rural districts was about 110 per
100,000 population as compared with eighty-eight for the
whole state, approximately the same rate for New York
City and about sixty-five for the cities of the state outside
of New York City. At present, the rural rate is thirty-five
per cent above the rate for the cities of the state, excluding
New York City. The reason for this is obvious. It is because, among other things, there has been much more intensive work for the prevention of tuberculosis in the cities.

Dr. Biggs went on to say that at the same time, there has been a noticeable decrease in the general death rate in the United States. This was, in part, a result of the gen-

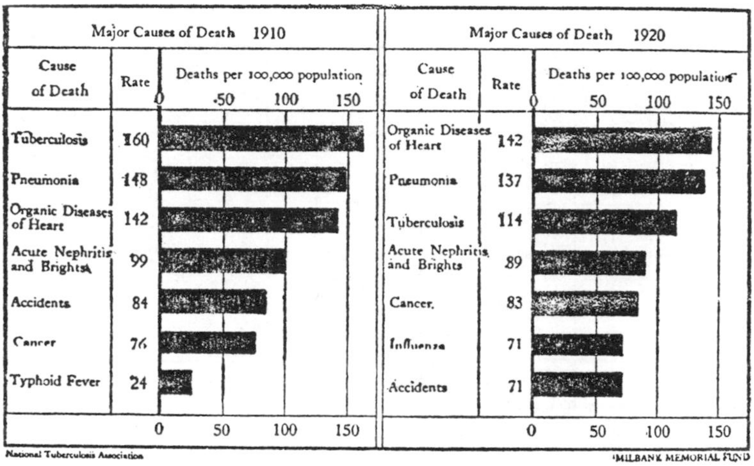

Major Causes of Death 1910			Major Causes of Death 1920		
Cause of Death	Rate	Deaths per 100,000 population 0 50 100 150	Cause of Death	Rate	Deaths per 100,000 population 0 50 100 150
Tuberculosis	160		Organic Diseases of Heart	142	
Pneumonia	148		Pneumonia	137	
Organic Diseases of Heart	142		Tuberculosis	114	
Acute Nephritis and Bright's	99		Acute Nephritis and Bright's	89	
Accidents	84		Cancer	83	
Cancer	76		Influenza	71	
Typhoid Fever	24		Accidents	71	
		0 50 100 150			0 50 100 150

National Tuberculosis Association   MILBANK MEMORIAL FUND

Fig. 11. Major causes of death in the United States (registration area), per 100,000 population, 1910 and 1920

eral educational campaign for the improvement of public health. Improved living conditions, increased wages, the increase in intelligence, possibly the decrease in alcoholism, and many other factors no doubt contributed. (Fig. 11) There have been several distinct lines of work on which public health activities have been centered in these years —these being subjects concerning which specific information was available and to which, therefore, preventive measures could be directed intelligently.

Having reviewed the progress made in the control of tuberculosis, the speaker drew attention to the recent marked decrease in the death rate from typhoid fever. He introduced a chart (Fig. 12) showing that deaths from this disease in New York State (exclusive of New York City) had decreased from thirty-two per 100,000 in 1900, to less than four per 100,000 in 1921. This represents a decrease in the death rate from typhoid fever to one-eighth of what it formerly was. Although the conditions of infection are quite

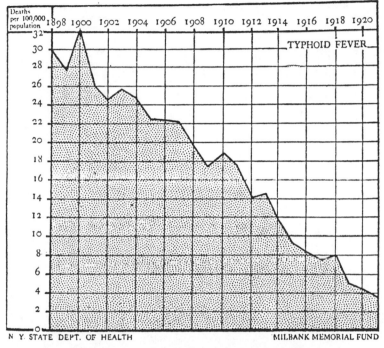

Fig. 12. Deaths from typhoid fever in New York State, exclusive of the City of New York, per 100,000 population, 1898–1921

different, the decrease that has been true of typhoid fever should be true also of tuberculosis, according to Dr. Biggs.

Though work in the prevention of infant mortality does not date back as far as the anti-tuberculosis campaign, Dr. Biggs referred to the significant results which have been accomplished in this field. In 1904, the infant death rate in New York State, including New York City, was 151 per 1,000 live births, while in 1920 it was 86 per 1,000 live births. The death rate from diphtheria, to which the

281

authorities have directed much attention, has been reduced to less than one-sixth of the former rate.

In 1887, tuberculosis, infant mortality, typhoid fever and

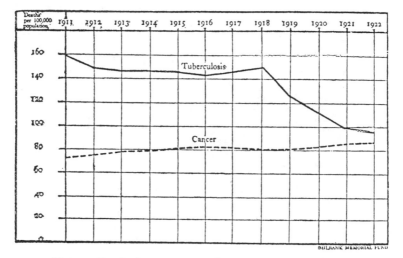

Fig. 13. Deaths from cancer and from tuberculosis in the United States (registration area), per 100,000 population, 1911–1922

diphtheria produced a death rate equivalent to more than two-thirds of the total death rate from all causes in 1921. But comparison of these results with those obtained with diseases where treatment has been handicapped by lack of knowledge, shows quite a different outcome.

There are as yet no adequate methods of preventing cancer. While the death rate from tuberculosis has been decreasing in the United States in the past decade, the corresponding rates from cancer have been slowly increasing. (Fig. 13) The death rate from cancer in the State of New York, excluding New York City, has increased from sixty-six per 100,000 population in 1900 to 109, in 1920. (Fig. 14) Dr. Biggs pointed out that cancer and other diseases, which belong to the degenerative sicknesses of the

middle and advanced periods of life, have a distinct bearing
on the problems of the New York Health Demonstrations
of the Milbank Memorial Fund—stating that in his opinion

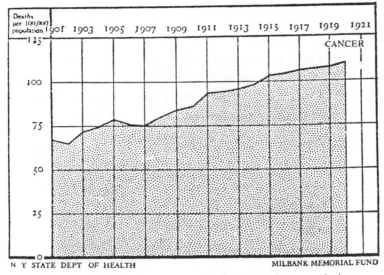

Fig. 14. Deaths from cancer in New York State, exclusive
of the City of New York, per 100,000 population, 1901–1920

it is in a decrease of the death rates from these causes that
great advances are to be made in the future.

With the exception of the enormous increase caused by
the influenza epidemic in 1918, deaths from the acute
respiratory diseases as distinguished from pulmonary tuberculosis show little change. (Fig. 15)   During the epidemic,
the death rate from these causes increased from an average
of about 160 to 600 per 100,000.

During the last three decades in New York State and in
New York City, the death rate from scarlet fever has fallen
rapidly. In the state, it has decreased from about twenty-
two per 100,000 in 1887 to about seven per 100,000 in 1921.
Because there are epidemic years of scarlet fever, there are

times when deaths from the disease will fall to a very low point, only to greatly increase again in spite of any preventive methods which medical men have thus far been able to put into effect.*

In formulating the plans for the New York Health Demonstrations of the Milbank Memorial Fund, it was noted that in the past anti-tuberculosis work has been a most effective factor in promoting general public health and in reducing the general death rates, and that it has been bound up with the whole public health campaign. For example, one of the first measures adopted at Framingham, where effort has been directed chiefly against tuberculosis, was to conduct a general medical examination of as many of the whole population as possible—a procedure which many medical men have long advocated, but largely without results. With periodic examinations, begun early in life, Dr. Biggs said that he had no doubt but that the rising curve for heart and kidney diseases, and for cancer (by bringing about an early diagnosis) could be reversed. Moreover, he said that there is no doubt but that by the practice of known health measures, ten or fifteen years can be added to the average life of the individual. "Years ago," said Dr. Biggs in closing his talk, "we learned from our experience with diseases about which we knew, that with proper machinery we could reduce the death rates with certainty. If we put the proper machinery into effect, there is no question whatsoever in my mind but that we can be absolutely certain of

*Dr. Biggs' speech was made on March 9, 1922. Since that date much information about scarlet fever has been disclosed. According to recent findings, it is practically certain that the disease is caused by a hemolytic streptococcus and tests have been perfected whereby, as in diphtheria, those who are susceptible may be discovered and then by the injection of toxin given protection, or immunized, against the disease. (Recent progress has also been made against measles and chicken pox, although the organisms causing these diseases have not yet been discovered. It is now possible, nevertheless, to temporarily immunize children against measles and chicken pox by the injection of convalescent serum).

reducing the morbidity rates and the death rate. This is true of every one of these diseases concerning which we have accurate knowledge. If we know the causes of diseases, the

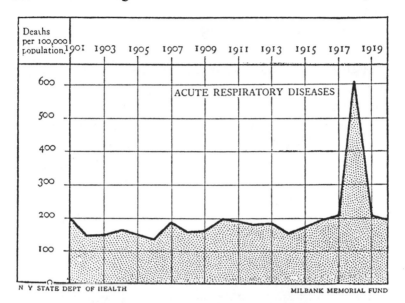

Fig. 15.   Deaths from acute respiratory diseases in New York State, exclusive of the City of New York, per 100,000 population, 1901–1920

means of transmitting them and the methods of treating them, we are able to control them."

The Purpose of the New York Health Demonstrations

In deciding to devote a substantial part of its income to health demonstrations, the Milbank Memorial Fund seeks to determine which diseases more readily yield to concerted attack—to what extent tuberculosis can be further reduced; whether the low infant mortality rate of fifty (per 1,000 born) attained in a few progressive communities can be generally substituted for the rate of 100 or more still prevailing in many parts of the United States; whether diphtheria, for example, can be practically eliminated; what preventive methods are most effective in controlling such diseases as scarlet fever, measles, and chicken pox; what constructive measures are most successful in conserving health; in short, to ascertain what can be accomplished by the intensive application of modern methods to the various problems in the field of public health.

In furthering the demonstrations, the Milbank Memorial Fund is allying itself with a world movement, the aim of which was strikingly expressed at a meeting in Cleveland of the American Public Health Association in October, 1922. At that time, the Committee on Resolutions, consisting of the late Dr. Hermann M. Biggs, Dr. Haven Emerson, former Commissioner of Health of the City of New York, and Dr. Lee K. Frankel, Chairman of the National Health Council, drew up a resolution which said, in part:

> "We, the health workers of our communities, are confident that there is nothing inherently impracticable or extravagant in the proposal we make that many nations may attain such knowledge of the laws of health, appropriate to each age and occupation, to each climate and race, that within the next fifty years as much as twenty years may be added to the expectancy of life which now prevails throughout the United States, and to this goal we dedicate the efforts of our Association."*

This resolution, which was unanimously adopted, directed attention to a century of striking achievements in the science of public health resulting in an accelerated increase in the average length of life. It called attention to the fact that within the past three-quarters of a century the average duration of life has been extended by not less than fifteen years in many of the leading nations of the world, stating

*The American Journal of Public Health, December, 1922, p. 1045.

that the gain in the life span during the last two decades has been greater than during the previous half-century, that while seventy-five years ago one-fourth of all those born in England died before reaching the age of three and one-half years, a decade ago it was not until the age of thirty-three and one-half years that one-fourth died.

As has been said elsewhere, "Elie Metchnikoff reminds us that the significance of life prolongation by disease control, which he made the special object of his studies at the Pasteur Institute, will lie not in adding a few years to old age but in throwing open an expanded maturity for service. It will, he says, make possible an enrichment of the common welfare by the work of developed men and women released from the tasks of earlier years, experienced, yet not constrained by the frailties and inhibitions of age, and thus enabled to give years of mellowed usefulness to mankind.

"The Milbank Memorial Fund exists to utilize its resources in such ways as will assist mankind to enjoy the benefits of health of body and of mind. The demonstrations are undertaken in the conviction that no other method will more surely bring life, not only longer, but more abundant."[*]

[*]Milbank Memorial Fund Annual Report, 1922, p. 38.

IV

THE DEMONSTRATIONS PROGRAM

ECAUSE tuberculosis is yet one of the major causes of death in the United States and because the intensive and extensive health work done in the field of tuberculosis prevention and control has been attended by the improvement of methods and facilities for the prevention of disease and the promotion of public health generally, it was early decided that the Milbank Memorial Fund could with profit formulate its own health demonstrations program in the light of the specialized experience with this disease, and plans for its further regulation. Dr. Biggs has observed that at present tuberculosis is the best "*text*" which a public health program can have. It is the disease which arouses the greatest public interest. Moreover, measures taken in the prevention and control of tuberculosis would be embodied in any public health campaign.

Many factors have contributed to the reduction in mortality from tuberculosis in New York City and in New York State. Improved standards of living have no doubt contributed in large measure to the reduction of mortality from this disease. An effective educational program has been carried on throughout the city and state. Dr. Biggs has referred to the marked increase in hospital facilities. In addition, a large number of clinics has been opened; and there has been a fair degree of nursing supervision of reported cases. Many open air classes have been established in public schools; and large numbers of day camps have been carried on. Then, too, there have been evolved higher standards of relief for families in which there is tuberculosis. With one or two conspicuous exceptions, no one of these factors can be said, however, to have been developed on an adequate scale in any given area; and no one of them is fully developed throughout the whole of the city, nor throughout the whole of the state outside of the city.

The Home Hospital

There is one exception in the Home Hospital, already referred to, which is operated by the New York Association for Improving the Condition of the Poor.* In the belief that it is often not practical or even efficient to treat a tuberculous patient apart from his or her family, this organization equipped one of the Vanderbilt tenements to provide a hospital regimen for families of which one or more members were suffering with this disease. Here both patient and non-patient members of these households receive necessary relief from the Association. The former are under constant medical care and observation, with trained nursing supervision, and the latter are carefully protected from infection. Opened on March 18, 1912, the results accomplished there compare favorably with the best obtained in sanatoria. In 1918, when through gifts of Elizabeth Milbank Anderson the hospital was moved to, and continued in, the Victoria apartments, it was pointed out that 69 per cent of the patients then discharged were well; in 7 per cent the disease was inactive; in only 11 per cent was it still active; and only 7 per cent had died. These results together with those secured there in safeguarding non-patient members of the families from infection and in raising their general vitality, have been highly commended by such authorities as the late Dr. Hermann M. Biggs, Dr. Walter B. James, Dr. James Alexander Miller, Dr. Lawrason Brown, Dr. Edward R. Baldwin and others, who, when through withdrawal of aid from the City of New York it seemed necessary to perma-

*Milbank Memorial Fund Annual Report, 1922, pp. 44-47.

nently discontinue the Home Hospital, urged that it be continued, even if on a smaller scale than hitherto.

The Framingham Demonstration

Another exception is in the demonstration at Framingham, Massachusetts, where over a period of seven years, from 1917 to 1923, inclusive, known methods of tuberculosis prevention and control were applied more extensively than in the Home Hospital and more intensively than hitherto in any other community in the country. Effort was made to discover all existing cases of tuberculosis, whether active or arrested. There were no limitations, arising from lack of funds, in the amount of medical and nursing care, material assistance, or hospital or sanatorium treatment afforded each patient. All persons discovered suffering with tuberculosis received in effect care comparable in thoroughness to that given patients in the Home Hospital.

During the seven-year period, the Framingham Demonstration resulted in the reduction of deaths from tuberculosis by approximately 68 per cent. The significance of this was vastly increased by comparison with results attained in the seven other Massachusetts communities which, because of their comparability to Framingham, were selected as control towns. In these communities the aggregate tuberculosis mortality during the same period decreased only 32 per cent.

Demonstrations in Larger Population Units Needed

There appeared to be no reason why the essential features of the Home Hospital and of the Framingham demonstrations should not be applied to substantially larger units of population with the purpose of demonstrating their feasibility for larger and varied units of population with the definite objective not only of the early and substantial control of tuberculosis, as was achieved in these two instances, but of learning what preventive methods are most effective in controlling disease generally; what constructive measures are most successful in promoting public health; in short, of ascertaining what can be accomplished by intensively applying known measures for disease prevention and health conservation in larger communities and under varying conditions. While in the course of progress in the fields of preventive medicine and hygiene these advances might be made within the next half century, it was thought that by the investment of money and effort in larger population units, relatively comparable to that made available for tuberculosis prevention and control in the Home Hospital and Framingham demonstrations, these improvements might be brought about within a much shorter period of time. This conclusion led to the chief enterprise now enlisting the interest and support of the Milbank Memorial Fund, namely, the New York Health Demonstrations.

The Demonstrations Program

Although the inquiries and discussions which led up to the formulation of the program of the New York Health Demonstrations were perhaps but the logical development of the work in the prevention and control of disease, and particularly of tuberculosis, which, as already pointed out, has been going on in New York State and elsewhere during the past quarter century, the experiences of the Home Hospital and of the Framingham demonstrations were drawn upon in formulating the early tentative drafts of the Milbank plan. Through studies and surveys of the Technical Board and the Advisory Council of the Fund, in co-operation with the New York State Department of Health, the State

Charities Aid Association, the Association for Improving the Condition of the Poor, the New York Tuberculosis Association and various national and local health organizations, access has been had to information about all of the well-known methods of disease prevention and control, and of health promotion.

Its initial demonstrations plans were formulated by the Fund chiefly to have a specific plan at hand to be used as a basis for discussion by its advisors, and to enable its Board of Directors to determine the approximate budgetary requirements for the projects. Fully anticipating that as the program developed the methods for carrying it out would be modified in the light of further study and experience in the demonstration areas chosen, and in the field of public health, the Fund from the first avoided committing itself to a hard and fast plan. Because the success of the demonstration in a given district is dependent upon the enlistment of such community interest, co-operation and participation there that the local authorities and voluntary agencies will, from time to time, take over various features of the program and place them under complete local support and control— that is, because the plan calls for a demonstration *of* the community, not *on* the community, the Fund recognized that it could only generally indicate what activity in the fields of preventive medicine and hygiene might be encompassed in a chosen area within a specified time through local official leadership.

While any general health program will necessarily vary somewhat in its application in the several demonstration communities (as emphasized by certain inevitable differences between, for example, rural Cattaraugus County and metropolitan New York), the fundamental demonstration principles to be applied in all of the areas are the same.

While differences in such factors as population density, difficulty of travel, availability of competent medical assistance, existence of hospitals, clinics, open-air classes and other facilities, the amount of outdoor occupation, on the one hand of extreme poverty, and on the other, of families having assets on which to draw in case of illness—while variations in the present development of the local health, economic and social life of the community and in the general level of the education and intelligence of its population will necessarily modify the details of the procedure when applied practically in a given area—the measures for the control of disease and for the promotion of personal and community health there would remain similar.

It is thought that a program concerned with all of the major problems of public health, wherever projected, will call for intensive efforts in many special fields of work and will include measures for the control of tuberculosis and other communicable diseases; special activities in school hygiene, in maternity, infancy and child hygiene, and in social, mental and industrial hygiene; adequate provision for sanitation and food inspection; and, through attention to the so-called degenerative diseases of adult life, will further the promotion of health conservation and life extension.

The program as here outlined is built upon earlier statements and tentative drafts of proposed activities, which have been modified in the light of experience in initiating and in developing the demonstrations in their early stages in the rural and urban districts. It is intended to give a general picture of the ground to be covered and, while it is subject to the maturing influence of further experience in the demonstration areas, it will be serviceable in directing the trend of the projects.

In developing the program consideration was given to

the assumption that as a result of social and economic factors, there has been in the last few decades a steady decrease in the mortality rates from certain diseases. From available data, particularly about tuberculosis, it seemed reasonable to assume, however, that this decrease has been accelerated by certain direct and indirect influences—by measures aimed specifically against given diseases (as, for example, milk pasteurization, the use of tuberculin in testing dairy herds, and increased institutional facilities for the care of the tuberculous) and at the improvement of general hygienic conditions.

Except for varying differences in the relative urgency of local health problems in the rural, urban and metropolitan areas chosen for demonstration purposes, it is anticipated that the activities of the New York Health Demonstrations will be directed toward comprehensive programs which will include such outstanding factors in the field of preventiv medicine and hygiene as:

> TUBERCULOSIS
> COMMUNICABLE DISEASES
> SCHOOL HYGIENE
> MATERNITY, INFANCY AND CHILD HYGIENE
> SOCIAL HYGIENE
> MENTAL HYGIENE
> INDUSTRIAL HYGIENE
> SANITATION AND FOOD INSPECTION
> HEALTH CONSERVATION AND LIFE EXTENSION

It has been estimated that in all probability $3 per capita per year would be adequate to meet the needs of this "program of health programs," as one writer has called it. It was thought that at any one time during the demonstration period probably not more than $1 per capita per year would be required from special funds, and to meet this need the

Milbank Memorial Fund has set aside $325,000 a year against the time when all of the demonstration units will be in full operation. It is estimated that over a period of five years there may be needed an amount ranging from $1,500,000 to $2,000,000.

It has been noted that one of the important contributions to be made by the New York Health Demonstrations will be to develop in a rural, an urban and a metropolitan community types of administrative procedure whereby results may be most readily and effectively achieved, as well as to make available the experience gained in three typical communities at one time in the different aspects of the public health problem. Because all features of a well-rounded health program require initiation and promotion simultaneously, the order in which the various factors are listed is arbitrary and not indicative of the relative importance of any specific project.

Tuberculosis

Because, as has been previously pointed out, an effective tuberculosis campaign will improve the general health conditions in a community, in planning the New York Health Demonstrations, it was anticipated that the first study in a given demonstration area would be that of the tuberculosis problem, and the first effort toward organization would involve the development of existing local activities in that particular field. Moreover, because there has been more community experience in the prevention and control of tuberculosis, the demonstrations advisors were able to outline plans here in more detail.

While on the one hand, experience has shown that effective tuberculosis work usually stimulates the development of measures to advance the public health, on the other, it has been found that a general health program does not necessarily lead to special activities for the prevention and control of tuberculosis. In a given demonstration district, whether rural, urban or metropolitan, a comprehensive tuberculosis program would involve such special considerations as the following:

1. An intensive case finding campaign to secure adequate medical examination for all cases of tuberculosis, all contacts, and groups of persons particularly susceptible to the disease.

   An essential first step in any campaign is to get as many as possible of the people living in the demonstration area to submit to a medical examination for the purpose of discovering:

   a. All persons suffering from conditions of disease or diminished vitality which might readily lead to the development of tuberculosis.

   b. All active cases of tuberculosis.

   c. All arrested cases of tuberculosis.

   d. All persons suffering from other diseases (such as malnutrition, focal infections, cardiac diseases, Bright's disease, venereal disease and cancer—either in an incipient or a well-developed stage) which are susceptible to some degree of control by public health procedures.

   e. All persons living under such conditions as are likely seriously to diminish their resistance and as are likely thereby to result in infection and the development of tuberculosis or other diseases.

2. An expert consultation service in tuberculosis clinics, in the homes, in schools, and in industrial and other centers.

3. Provision for adequate medical and nursing care through dispensary service; and for home medical care for the tuberculous poor, including visiting, nursing and consultation service to the tuberculous who are patients of private physicians.

   Sufficient supervision of tuberculous patients in their homes and elsewhere by qualified public health nurses —to insure the carrying out of physicians' instructions and recommendations, particularly in regard to the health habits of patients and of the members of their households.

4. Measures, including post-graduate training for physicians and nurses and popular health education for the population as a whole, in order to improve the general knowledge about the prevention of infection and breakdown from active disease; as well as for instruction in the care of the tuberculous.

5. Follow-up service for the promotion of medical examinations and the continuation of medical care for patients having tuberculosis; and for instruction to families of the tuberculous in the methods of preventing the spread of the disease.

   This would involve the periodic medical examination of all persons having active or arrested tuberculosis, of all contacts, of all persons likely to develop tuberculosis, and of all persons in whom some diseased condition or diseased tendency was discovered (to ascertain what forms of treatment, care, or relief are suited to the individual; to learn the developments of any diseased condition or tendency, and to minimize the possibility of infection).

6. Measures to stimulate the use of available sanatoria and hospital facilities and to promote the establishment of sufficient hospitalization for the tuberculous if, and as, the necessity arises.

   A measure which has been especially valuable in the treatment of tuberculosis in New York City has been the Home Hospital, already referred to. This provides for the hospitalization of a selected number of such families as cannot be adequately provided for without bringing them under constant medical and nursing oversight both by day and night.

   Experience at the Home Hospital indicates that the type of building is not so essential as to preclude the possibility of finding sufficient buildings for this purpose in any city district. And this type of treatment perhaps best adapts itself to needs arising in more congested localities.

   A day-home hospital for the day care of both men and women tuberculous patients selected by physicians and nurses would insure daily medical supervision, as frequent medical examinations as are necessary, complete medical control of the amount of rest and of the amount and kind of exercise and work, adequate food, and freedom from the strain of housekeeping, care of children or other home duties unsuited to the proper care of the patient. In connection with this it would be desirable to have a small emergency ward for the temporary care of any emergency cases.

Similarly, a day-preventorium for children primarily of the pre-school age has been found invaluable in the treatment of tuberculosis, particularly in city districts. This day-preventorium would provide lunch for the children and, in the case of children whose mothers were patients at the day-home hospital, dinner also and possibly breakfast. It would be equipped with kindergarten, with opportunities for directed play, with experts in nutrition and with whatever facilities are needed to supply such special care as the medical examination may indicate. Those admitted to treatment here would include:

a. The children of mothers who are patients in the day-home hospital.

b. The children of mothers who are patients, who though remaining at home need to be relieved of the care of their children during the daytime.

c. Other children residing in households in which there is tuberculosis or who are themselves undernourished and predisposed to tuberculosis and in need of special provision for rest, food and health instruction.

d. A certain number of children of school age for whom, owing to the type of building, it may be found impracticable to provide open air classes at the school which they may be attending. The same program would be provided these classes as for the open air classes.

A small emergency night ward would undoubtedly be needed in connection with the day-preventorium, for children of mothers developing an acute illness, for whom it might not otherwise be possible to provide suitable home care at night.

For children not requiring the more intensified care provided by the day-preventorium, open air classes should be established in the public schools. In instances where it is impossible to provide such care, these children needing treatment could be sent to the day-preventorium.

7. A program of occupational therapy for patients under treatment both in institutions and at home. Special efforts to provide the necessary medical, nursing and social service for tuberculous patients cared for in their homes. Resources for vocational instruction, for placement in employment under suitable conditions and for supervision of arrested cases while employed. (Each of these methods has been worked out for certain groups of patients, but not all of them are often available for any given group of patients).

It will be necessary to effect a co-ordination and development of the work of various agencies to be able to provide for occupation as a means of therapy, and for the training of arrested cases in occupations suited to their probable physical condition; and to discover suitable openings for employment, and an adequate degree of supervision to prevent breakdown through continuance in work which, on account of the patient's physical condition, might prove to be unsuitable.

Relief, including skilled case work, with adequate funds to enable each family in which there is a case of tuberculosis to live at such standards as to housing, food, clothing and otherwise as will afford maximum opportunities for care and improvement of the patient and reduce to a minimum any danger of infection of others. This probably need not be more expensive than the relief now given by an organization like the New York A. I. C. P. for allowance to families under its care, in cases in which there is tuberculosis. This includes the working out of standard budgets, calculating the proper income of the family from other sources, and making up the deficit. Such relief supervision would, of course, involve the employment of a sufficient number of trained visiting housekeepers and dietitians and nurses to maintain the best relief standards for the families under care and to fully comply with such medical instructions in regard to rest, food and exercise as are given from time to time.

The organization for carrying out this program would require the following:

1. An expert advisory and administrative service for the general direction of the tuberculosis program, for the co-ordination of various measures and facilities for the control of the disease, and for the evaluation of the results.

2. A consultation and diagnostic service in clinics, in schools, physicians' offices, in homes, factories, etc., including adequate facilities for laboratory examinations of sputum and X-ray examination of the chest, would be furnished primarily by the director of a bureau of tuberculosis.

3. A regular series of tuberculosis clinics at district stations with consultation for cases sent by private physicians; and with dispensary and home service for the tuberculous poor. This service could be in charge of an assistant to the director of a bureau of tuberculosis and of other physicians trained in tuberculosis work, whose services might be obtained from time to time.

4. A public health nursing service from each district station with home visiting for cases requiring it, educational measures for the family and a complete follow-up service for patients, contacts and suspects.

5. A service for instruction to physicians, nurses and health workers carried on chiefly through the demonstrations authorities; and general popular health education in the prevention and control of tuberculosis.

6. A laboratory service furnished without additional cost by the county laboratory.

7. Relief. In New York State existing legislation provides for the indigent sick and efforts should be made to insure the adequate relief in the care of the tuberculous who are in need.

8. A service for occupational therapy and rehabilitation in existing tuberculosis hospitals and sanatoria and in the homes, as a therapeutic agent and a source of economic assistance to indigent patients.

Communicable Diseases

By intensive efforts carried out in a community over a period of years, it should be possible to reduce materially both the morbidity and mortality rates for communicable diseases.

Through Schick testing and immunization and by the earlier and more extensive use of antitoxin, it should be possible to practically eradicate diphtheria. Similarly, through better control of contacts and possibly through the application of newer methods of serum treatment, occurrences of scarlet fever, measles and chicken pox should be greatly diminished. By the prevention of exposure in infancy and the consequent postponement of the disease until a later and more favorable period of life, and also by the use of convalescent serum for infants and children who are particularly susceptible to this disease, the death rate from measles should be reduced. It is assumed that by general vaccination, smallpox, which at present is of rare occurrence, may be practically eliminated. While it is difficult to control the occurrence of whooping cough, chicken pox and German measles, mortality and complications from these diseases may be favorably influenced by education in the proper methods of home treatment, and after care. The essentials of a reasonably adequate communicable disease program, therefore, would include the following:

1. Adequate and prompt reporting to the constituted local and state health authorities.

2. Diagnostic consultation service, including verification of the diagnosis of the major communicable diseases.

3. Laboratory diagnostic service.

4. Isolation and systematic investigation of reported cases.

5. The study of minor outbreaks with prompt measures to prevent epidemics, including vaccination and immunization of contacts, special investigations, isolation, quarantine, etc.

6. Adequate terminal cleansing under the direction of local health officers, assisted by public health nurses.

7. Free supply of vaccines, sera, etc., with assistance to local health officers in their administration.

8. Hospitalization. There should be available in the demonstration areas enough beds to accommodate the

patients, who, because they are afflicted with communicable diseases, require special hospital segregation and treatment. Where such facilities are not available, a pavilion for patients suffering from communicable diseases might possibly be established in connection with an existing hospital.

9. Health education in the prevention of infection, emphasizing the dangers to life of communicable diseases, such as measles and whooping cough, especially if contracted during infancy.

School Hygiene

A very important phase of public health work is that connected with the public schools. Where adequate preventive and protective measures are not taken, the school may be a potent center for the dissemination of communicable diseases throughout the community. On the other hand, here is provided a rare opportunity for the detection of infectious diseases in their early stages, for the discovery and correction of physical defects, and for the instruction of future citizens about essential standards of personal and community health and hygiene. An adequate program in school hygiene would include the following:

1. Routine medical examination of all school children. These examinations should be made in accordance with the uniform system for the collection of such records which exist in the city, county or state where the demonstration is being conducted. Due consideration should be given to existing legislation relative to the frequency and adequacy of such examinations. This routine should provide data concerning nutrition, cardiac and pulmonary conditions, vision, hearing, tonsilar infections and enlargements, and general physical defects.

2. Special examinations from time to time of children selected by teachers and nurses as apparently sick and requiring physical examinations or medical care.

3. Regular and systematic inspection of school children by nurses, with general supervision by a district school nurse.

4. Home visiting by nurses for follow-up service of children showing physical defects.

5. Dental prophylactic service for children in all schools.

6. Expert diagnosis and medical care for certain groups of pupils, such as crippled children and tuberculosis suspects. This could be arranged, in part at least, through consultation clinics. It would also be desirable to have special funds available for treatment of children unable to secure medical care in other ways.

Maternity, Infancy and Child Hygiene

The raising of the standards of the health of children is one of the most important objectives of any community health program. The large number of still-births and of deaths among children of pre-school age, is indicative of the importance of concentration upon the health hazards which confront children of pre-natal, infant and pre-school age. Any comprehensive health demonstration project would, therefore, include a program of maternity, infancy and child hygiene, in which the following provisions would be made:

1. Examination and advisory services for expectant mothers by specialists, including consultation service in the homes.

2. Examination and advisory service for infants and pre-school children, including well baby clinics, classes for mothers and consultation service.

3. A visiting nursing service for the instruction of mothers in their homes; for assistance to physicians at time of delivery; and emergency service in cases of illness among infants and young children.

4. The assistance to expectant mothers in the preparation of supplies to be used at time of delivery (loan baskets) and in securing hospitalization when necessary, including visiting nursing in the homes, dental hygiene, etc.

5. A broad educational campaign, including post-graduate courses for physicians and nurses; educational classes for mothers and young women; and general educational

measures for the prevention of disease. A campaign for breast-feeding and for clean milk supply for children artificially fed and for pre-school children.

Such a program in a given demonstration area may require the following organization:

1. A specialist experienced in the diseases of infancy and in obstetrics for consultations and general direction of the service.

2. A series of regular pre-natal clinics available to all expectant mothers in the demonstration district.

3. A health service for infants and young children, consisting of child health clinics held at regular intervals.

4. Nursing service should be provided at the clinics and nurses should be available for home visiting of expectant mothers and infants. Clubs of "Mother's Helpers" should be organized so that home help for mothers at the time of confinement may be available.

5. A child health educational publicity service should be maintained.

6. Dental service for expectant mothers and pre-school children should be provided and the correction of dental and other defects in children of pre-school age should be carried out during the spring and summer months so that they may enter school free from these handicaps.

Social Hygiene

No general health demonstration is complete which does not include a social hygiene program, including plans for the advancement of sound sex education, for combating prostitution and sex delinquency and for waging an intensive campaign against the venereal diseases. The problems which are presented may be attacked along four lines: educational, recreational, legal and medical.

In planning a program of venereal disease control, it is necessary to bear in mind that the vast majority of patients are ambulatory treatment cases and that "early detection followed by efficient intensive treatment is vitally important not only for the welfare of the patient but for the protection of the public through terminating or shortening the infectious period of the case."

Social hygiene activities should include the establishment of clinics, the provision of adequate laboratory diagnostic service, the development of case finding methods and follow-up supervision and the inauguration of an educational campaign which would emphasize the public health aspects of venereal disease control. Legislation providing for the detention of irresponsible persons who are infected, should be taken advantage of when, and if, necessary.

The utilization of local physicians for the clinics is believed to be highly desirable. The familiarization of local practitioners with the manifestations of venereal disease (especially syphilis of the viscera and nervous system) is of the utmost importance. Frequent medical meetings should be held for the discussion of such problems as pre-natal syphilis, cardiac complications, etc. Emphasis should be placed upon the follow-up work of the nurses, and efforts made to discover contacts and place them under treatment.

Mental Hygiene

Work for the conservation of mental health should be included in the demonstration plan. The larger part of a mental hygiene program would have to do with children of pre-school and school age and the major work entailed would naturally be carried on by those dealing with the health of such children.

The outstanding activities to be undertaken in a comprehensive mental hygiene program should provide for the prevention, detection and treatment of nervous disturbances and mental divergences. The early diagnosis of mental divergences from the normal (either in the nature of deficiency or disturbance) in children of pre-school and school age, is of great importance. The establishment of specialty classes for mentally deficient children; the discovery of conduct divergences and delinquent trends and their treatment, both from a medical and sociological standpoint (including home visitation and supervision and conference with the parents of children apparently deficient); provision for the early commitment to training schools of mentally defective children for whom special class instruction and home supervision are inadequate; co-operation with the juvenile courts; and a well considered educational campaign which would deal with the causes of mental divergences and the means of promoting mental health—are outstanding activities to be undertaken. Occupational therapy must be visualized as an integral part of any complete mental hygiene program. The factor of home as well as custodial care should be kept prominently in mind and attention should be paid to both the amount and the character of the follow-up work by the medical, nursing and social service personnel.

In the initial survey of the demonstration area an effort should be made to discover the psychopathic and neurotic child as well as the defective, insane, etc., and the co-operation of all existing agencies, both state and national, should be solicited not only for suggestions relative to the details of the program but also for assistance in attaining the objectives.

Industrial Hygiene

The active participation of industrial and commercial establishments in promoting the health and welfare of their employees is an important factor in a well-rounded health program. As a result of the demonstration activities in

Framingham, the health work in the industries there has assumed large proportions and has made an important contribution to the results which have been secured. Similarly, in all of the demonstration areas here considered, the support and co-operation of employers of large numbers of workers should be secured.

As a matter of principle, it is generally recognized that industrial health services should be organized and developed by industrial (or mercantile) establishments themselves, rather than by, or through, any outside agency.

The function of the demonstration authorities should perhaps be to co-operate with industrial establishments by providing technical assistance for surveys dealing with factory hygiene, by stimulating the development of such industrial health work as periodic medical examinations, and first aid, and by giving such publicity as may be indicated to the importance of the conservation of the health of industrial workers. Advisory services in industrial therapy and rehabilitation should also be made available.

Sanitation and Food Inspection

In a comprehensive health program there should be adequate provision for the promotion of general sanitation, including the prevention of diseases carried by food and milk. The latter would include such measures as the pasteurization of milk from non-tested cattle, the promotion of tuberculin testing and the control of bovine tuberculosis, etc. This work (which will, of course, bear directly upon the problems confronted in the programs indicated for the control and prevention of communicable disease, and especially of tuberculosis) should include:

1. A service for general sanitation, including advisory service for proper sewage disposal on farms and isolated dwellings.

2. A program for the purpose of insuring the maintenance of a pure water supply throughout the demonstration areas.

3. Regular inspections to insure the maintenance of a pure water supply in hotels, restaurants and public buildings.

4. A service for the purpose of insuring a safe milk supply, including regular and systematic inspection of dairies, testing of the herds and the chemical and bacteriological examination of the milk.

5. A service to provide that food intended for the public is prepared and handled under reasonable sanitary precautions, including the enforcement of regulations requiring the adequate cleansing of dishes and utensils in public eating places.

6. A general service for the improvement of sanitation, including the abatement of nuisances, the sanitary disposal of garbage and refuse, the inspection of public buildings, advisory services for fly and mosquito control, and inspection of labor camps.

7. A general publicity campaign.

Health Conservation and Life Extension

Dr. Biggs has referred to the importance in the New York Health Demonstrations of concentration upon the diseases of adult life, stating that "it is in a decrease of the death rates from these causes that great advances are to be made in the future."*

From the standpoint of mortality, the most important diseases of adult life are included under the group of respiratory diseases, including pneumonia and bronchitis, heart disease, Bright's disease, arterio-sclerosis and certain chronic diseases such as diabetes and rheumatism. While it is stated by some that Bright's disease and arterio-sclerosis, for example, can be prevented only with difficulty, if at all,

*pp. 72-73.

there can be no doubt that under proper medical care and with reasonable attention to hygiene, the mortality from such diseases as Bright's disease and apoplexy may be substantially retarded and the period of life and usefulness correspondingly prolonged.

A program for the prevention of such diseases or for their amelioration, excluding such specific diseases as tuberculosis and venereal diseases, should include the following:

1. A systematic campaign for periodic medical examinations.

2. General health education by means of newspapers, lectures, films, and exhibits. Health education and general information on nutrition and specific information to groups or individuals on the value of proper food.

3. The provision of an effective laboratory service for practising physicians. Laboratory service to include blood examinations for various types of leukemia and anæmia, blood examinations for nitrogenous and sugar content, etc.

4. The provision for a visiting nursing service for adults.

5. The provision of post-graduate courses for physicians. Courses dealing especially with the diagnosis and treatment of such special diseases as Bright's disease, cardiovascular diseases, and diabetes.

6. The encouragement of the establishment of opportunities in clinics and in homes throughout the district, for medical care of the poor, preferably through the assumption of the responsibility for this service by the local health authorities or by voluntary agencies.

7. The establishment of consultation clinics for adult diseases held in district health stations at regular intervals, combined with a consultation service in homes and in physicians' offices.

8. Instruction to individuals and to classes in personal hygiene and in the home care of the sick.

9. Medical Social Service. Such social adjustments as may be found necessary from a health standpoint should be effected in individual cases through the services of experienced social workers. Social service should supplement the medical and nursing service in families where such conditions as poverty and gross neglect of children are considered to be health factors.

10. Occupational Therapy as a means of physical restoration or vocational rehabilitation should be employed in cardiac cases, etc.

General Operations

The organization of the specific activities previously outlined is obviously dependent upon facilities and personnel for administration purposes. Moreover, a comprehensive health program should include the following general services:

1. A bureau of records, reports and vital statistics, responsible for compiling and presenting current mortality and morbidity records and other data of importance in health administration.

2. A general diagnostic laboratory equipped for special bacteriological and chemical examinations.

3. Health Instruction. A general educational campaign in the interest of health conservation and disease prevention should be carried out on a community-wide basis. Probably no phase of the program is of greater importance than that concerned with the instruction of teachers in the teaching of health. Practical methods for the use of teachers, principals and superintendents should be initiated; competent supervision provided; and studies of home and school conditions and of health practices made, so that adequately controlled records of results may ultimately be available. The methods and material required in teaching health to pupils of different ages and the relationship of physical training to health habits should be clearly set forth. Children should be taught how to play and special adjuncts to health education, such as the Modern Health Crusade, Keep-Well Corners and Health Clubs should be included in the program.

4. Nutrition Activities. Special attention should be paid
   to the food habits and diet standards. In addition to
   the instruction of teachers and school nurses in the
   principles of nutrition, a general educational campaign
   to promote the adoption of food habits, based upon
   scientifically determined standards of nutrition, should
   be undertaken.

Demonstrations Extension Program

The New York Health Demonstrations are primarily
educational undertakings. It has been pointed out, on the
one hand, that a vital criterion of their success will depend
upon the extent to which the types of routine services established in the selected demonstration districts continue upon
the termination of the demonstration period and are made
a part of the permanent practice of the community. On the
other hand, their success will depend equally on the extent
to which there may be fostered wider application by adjacent and remote communities of the methods and practices
here developed.

The proposed program should make the demonstration
districts fertile fields for the discovery of additional information about disease prevention and control and about
health administration in general, and should throw new
light upon the social factors involved in such community
undertakings as well as upon the reaction of community
groups to the measures introduced. Fully realizing that the
success of the plan in a given demonstration locality will
depend not only upon its continuance there as long as there
is need for it, but on the degree to which its findings are
used by communities universally, the Milbank Memorial
Fund purposes continuously to study and appraise the results
of the undertaking as a basis for making available through
state and national channels such of its data as would seem
useful to other communities in forwarding their own health

administration, or valuable in increasing the general health knowledge of the public.

It has been pointed out, moreover, that the demonstrations will present an excellent opportunity to offer extension training and field work to physicians, health officers, medical students, nurses and social workers. It was anticipated that institutions giving instruction in public health work, in public health nursing and in social work, might find certain phases of the demonstration activity valuable as field work for students.

Moreover, the facilities for training offered by the project should attract the participation and understanding of the medical profession within the areas selected. To accomplish these results, the demonstrations as a whole will endeavor to establish definite affiliations with recognized institutions for the training of physicians, sanitarians, public health nurses, social workers and nutrition workers.

"About the most difficult thing with which the world has to contend," said Dr. Livingston Farrand at a recent meeting of the Advisory Council of the Milbank Memorial Fund, "is the lack of application of knowledge which is in possession of the experts."* He points out that our enormous advance in scientific knowledge of every kind has been the great characteristic of the last fifty years, and that there is no field in which this is more strikingly evident than in the fields of medicine and of medical science.

"When we view the technical advances that have been made since the days of Pasteur," he says, "when we see, as we do, what would result if these discoveries were fully applied, and when we recognize that practically the only obstacle in the way of that application is recognition on the part of the public of those facts and of the possibilities of

*Milbank Memorial Fund Quarterly Bulletin, January, 1924, p. 30.

their application—then we begin to see why demonstrations of this kind were recommended, after sober consideration by the best counsel obtainable, as being the most promising way of attaining results in human welfare to which a trust, like the Milbank Memorial Fund, could be devoted."

THE NEW YORK HEALTH DEMONSTRATIONS
SUPERVISORY AND OPERATING AGENCIES

STATE CHARITIES AID ASSOCIATION
State Committee on Tuberculosis and Public Health

(Designated by the Milbank Memorial Fund on May 22, 1922, as the Organizing and Supervisory Agency for the New York Health Demonstrations in Syracuse and in Cattaraugus County.)

Officers and Executive Committee

GEORGE F. CANFIELD, *Chairman*, New York.

CHARLES STOVER, M.D., *1st Vice-Chairman*, Amsterdam

HORACE LoGRASSO, M.D., *2nd Vice-Chairman*, Buffalo

HOMER FOLKS, Yonkers

ISAAC ADLER, Rochester

LEE K. FRANKEL, Ph.D., New York

CHARLES GIBSON, Albany

JOHN A. KINGSBURY, Yonkers

MATTHIAS NICOLL, JR., M.D., Albany

WILLARD W. SEYMOUR, Syracuse

MISS LILLA C. WHEELER, Portville

LINSLY R. WILLIAMS, M.D., New York

Executive Staff

HOMER FOLKS, *Secretary*

A. C. BURNHAM, M.D., *Assistant in Preventive Medicine*

GEORGE J. NELBACH, *Executive Secretary*

BERNARD L. WYATT, M.D., *Consultant on Health Demonstrations*

MISS JESSAMINE S. WHITNEY, *Statistical Consultant*

LOCAL OPERATING AGENCIES
CATTARAUGUS COUNTY DEMONSTRATION
County Board of Health

JOHN WALRATH, *President*, Salamanca

WILLIAM C. BUSHNELL, Little Valley

WILLIAM A. DUSENBURY, Olean

MYRON E. FISHER, M.D., Delevan

M. L. HILLMAN, M.D., Little Valley

J. W. WATSON, New Albion

MISS LILLA C. WHEELER, Portville

* * *

LEVERETT D. BRISTOL, M.D., *County Health Officer*

STEPHEN A. DOUGLASS, M.D., *Tuberculosis Consultant*

J. P. GAREN, M.D., *Director of County Laboratory*

County School Health Service

C. A. GREENLEAF, M.D., *Director*

County Tuberculosis and Public Health Association

C. A. GREENLEAF, M.D., *President*

JOHN ARMSTRONG, *Executive Secretary*

SYRACUSE DEMONSTRATION
Syracuse Health Department

THOMAS P. FARMER, M.D., *Commissioner*

GEORGE C. RUHLAND, M.D., *Deputy Commissioner*

GEORGE M. RETAN, M. D., *Director*, Bureau of Child Hygiene

A. CLEMENT SILVERMAN, M.D., *Director*, Bureau of Communicable Diseases

H. BURTON DOUST, M.D., *Director*, Bureau of Tuberculosis

O. W. H. MITCHELL, M. D., *Director*, Bureau of Health Education

H. N. JONES, M.D., *Director*, Bureau of Laboratories

Health Service, Department of Public Instruction

MRS. EDWARD L. ROBERTSON, *President*, Board of Education

PERCY M. HUGHES, *Superintendent of Schools*

JOSEPH C. PALMER, M.D., *Director*, School Health Service

Tuberculosis and Public Health Association

WILLARD W. SEYMOUR, *President*

ARTHUR W. TOWNE, *General Director*

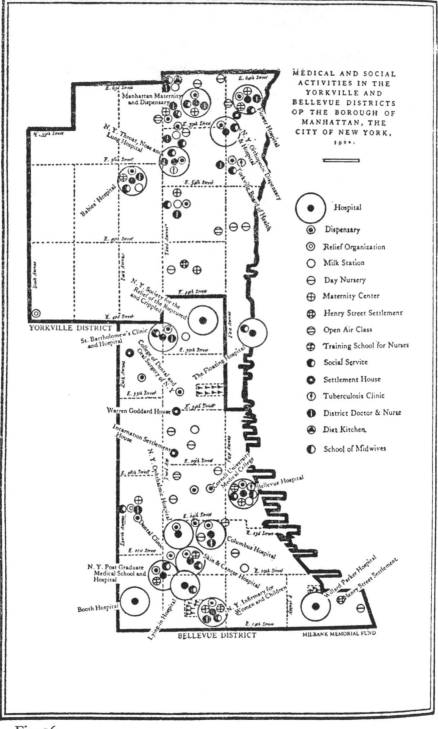

MEDICAL AND SOCIAL
ACTIVITIES IN THE
YORKVILLE AND
BELLEVUE DISTRICTS
OF THE BOROUGH OF
MANHATTAN, THE
CITY OF NEW YORK,
1920.

- ⊙ Hospital
- ⊙ Dispensary
- ◎ Relief Organization
- ○ Milk Station
- ⊖ Day Nursery
- ⊕ Maternity Center
- ⊕ Henry Street Settlement
- ⊖ Open Air Class
- ⊕ Training School for Nurses
- ◐ Social Service
- ● Settlement House
- ⊕ Tuberculosis Clinic
- ◑ District Doctor & Nurse
- ◑ Diet Kitchen
- ◑ School of Midwives

MILBANK MEMORIAL FUND

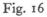

Fig. 16

316

SELECTING THE DEMONSTRATION DISTRICTS

THE program of the Milbank Memorial Fund for a series of community health demonstrations in New York State is unique, not only in the magnitude of the areas and populations covered, and in its application to health problems generally, but also in its plan to utilize existing organizations without the setting up of additional operating machinery. Through its Technical Board and Advisory Council, and their sub-committees, the Fund has had the aid of the best counsel obtainable in formulating its program, in determining the procedure to be followed in the selection of demonstration districts and in the development of the various activities already outlined, the results of which, in terms of reduced morbidity and mortality from preventable diseases, may be measured in the course of time.

It was early recognized by the Fund and its advisors that the State Charities Aid Association (New York), through its Committee on Tuberculosis and Public Health, should be designated as the chief organizing and supervisory agency for the rural and urban demonstrations, this Association having organized a state-wide series of local associations dealing with tuberculosis and public health, and being the only state-wide agency in this field, i. e., New York State outside of New York City. In the metropolitan district a similar though somewhat modified relationship in the investigative phases of the work, was established with the New York Association for Improving the Condition of the Poor.

Through the channels of these agencies, and with the co-operation and assistance of national, state and other city groups, including the National Tuberculosis Association, the New York State Department of Health, the Department of Health of the City of New York and the New York Tuberculosis Association, the Technical Board and the Advisory Council of the Fund spent several months in studying the counties and cities in the state that were most suitable for the rural county and the two city demonstrations. Applications from many localities were considered.

In outlining the more important considerations involved in the selection of the demonstration areas, the Technical Board had the advice of a group of statisticians especially called together for this purpose.* Specific methods were endorsed for the tabulation of facts, including data on population, its distribution as to race, general mortality, birth rates, infant and child mortality, and tuberculosis morbidity and mortality. The actual assembling of these data was under the direction of Dr. Otto R. Eichel, Chief of the Division of Statistics in the State Department of Health, and Miss Jessamine S. Whitney, Statistician for the National Tuberculosis Association.

At the same time, under the direction of Dr. Donald B. Armstrong, Secretary of the Technical Board, and George J. Nelbach, Secretary of the Committee on Tuberculosis and Public Health of the State Charities Aid Association, a careful survey of the economic and social factors in the communities under consideration was undertaken.

Recognizing the importance of having the legally constituted authorities and voluntary agencies in the chosen districts assume their share of the administrative and

*The statisticians who assisted in the preparation of the schedules used in the collection of data in connection with the demonstrations include Prof. Walter F. Willcox, of Cornell University, Consulting Statistician of the State Department of Health, and Dr. Louis I. Dublin, Statistician of the Metropolitan Life Insurance Company, both of whom are members of the Advisory Council; Prof. Robert E. Chaddock, of Columbia University; Dr. Otto R. Eichel, Director of the Bureau of Vital Statistics of the State Department of Health; Godias J. Drolet, Statistician of the New York Tuberculosis Association; and Miss Jessamine S. Whitney, Statistician of the National Tuberculosis Association.

financial responsibilities as rapidly as the desirability and feasibility of such action on their part may be demonstrated, it was early realized that the following would be essential requirements of the demonstration areas:

1. Local desire for the demonstration and local assurance of co-operation, harmony and co-ordination of effort.

2. Local responsibility for participation in, and leadership of, the demonstration—especially on the part of public authorities.

3. Local assumption, in the beginning or as early thereafter as possible, of financial and operating responsibility for newly initiated or freshly developed activities of proven merit.

These requirements naturally assumed on the part of the Fund and its organizing and supervisory agencies as intimate a relationship with the public health, school, relief and other authorities of the areas concerned, as is compatible with the full accomplishment of the purposes of the undertaking. It was in mind also that there would be:

1. Co-operation with all local voluntary health and relief agencies within the districts.

2. Co-operation with all other health and relief agencies doing work in the district but with headquarters elsewhere and covering larger areas. In numerous instances, it might be best to enable such agencies to increase their work in the district selected rather than to build up separate activities.

3. Co-operation with the State Health Department, especially in the rural and urban demonstrations.

4. The setting up of as little new machinery in the community as possible, working rather through existing organizations and local co-ordinated units.

5. A democratic educational effort to interest residents of the community in the improvement of their own health, rather than to superimpose on them a paternalistic system.

Selecting the Rural Demonstration District

Preliminary consideration of information about counties in New York State suitable for demonstration purposes reduced the number eligible for final deliberation to four. These were Cattaraugus, Dutchess, Jefferson and Saratoga counties.* In order to bring before the Technical Board data pertinent to the selection of one of these counties, statistical and sociological surveys were made of each. Tables and schedules presenting the findings of these studies are available at the offices of the Milbank Memorial Fund, 49 Wall Street, New York, and copies will be sent upon request therefor from anyone interested in this phase of the demonstrations.

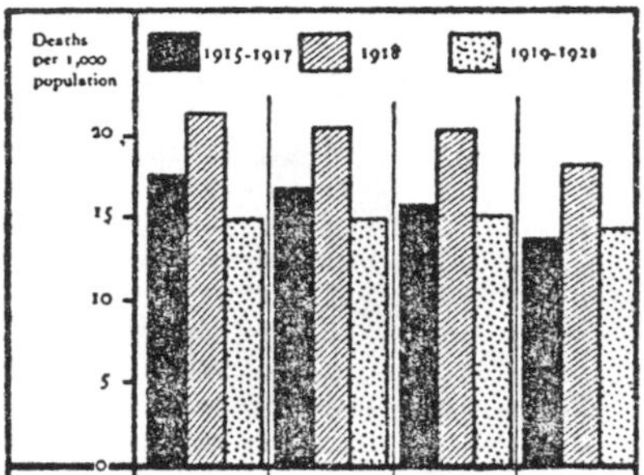

Deaths per 1,000 population	1915-1917	1918	1919-1921		
County	Dutchess	Saratoga	Jefferson	Cattaraugus	
1915-1917	17.6	16.7	15.7	12.7	
1918	21.2	20.5	21.3	18.3	
1919-1921	14.8	14.8	15.1	14.2	

Fig. 17. Deaths from all causes in the four New York State counties considered as areas for the rural health demonstration, per 1,000 population, during the periods, 1915–1917 (inclusive), 1918, and 1919–1921 (inclusive)

The death rates for 1918 are presented separately because during that year they were abnormally high

In the main, these present the following facts about each of these counties (and similar data are available about each of the five cities seriously considered as possible urban demonstration units):

*Other counties were eliminated for various reasons. Some were insufficiently rural in make-up; some had had abnormal mortality rates in the past; in others the local provision of facilities for health work was below the average; in others the constituency of the population was not typical; and for many causes others were excluded from more than preliminary consideration.

1. Percentage of increase or decrease in total population, 1915–1920.

2. Density of population, 1920.

3. Sex and age distribution of population, including groups under 7; 7 to 13; 14–17; 18–44; and 45 and over, 1920.

4. Foreign born population, number and per cent in 1910 and 1920, and distribution by country of birth in 1920.

5. Births and birth rates per 1,000 females between the ages of 18 and 44, average for four years, 1918–1921.

6. General mortality rate by years, 1900–1921, inclusive. (Fig. 17)

7. Infant mortality rates and death rates, per 1,000 population among children under 10 years of age, by years, 1915–1921, inclusive. (Fig. 18)

8. Deaths and death rates from pulmonary and non-pulmonary tuberculosis by years, 1900–1921, inclusive. (Fig. 19)

9. Tuberculosis cases reported by separate years, 1919–1921.

10. Tuberculosis cases reported according to stage of disease, type of disease and promptness in reporting, 1921.

11. Classification by sex and age, of tuberculosis cases and deaths, all forms, reported in 1921.

12. Per capita expenditures for health, education, charities and correction and for cost of government.

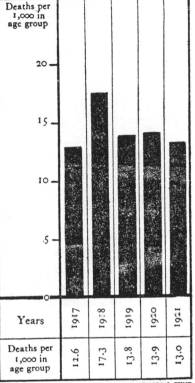

MILBANK MEMORIAL FUND

Fig. 18. Deaths from all causes, of children under ten years of age (per 1,000 children in this age group), in Cattaraugus County, 1917–1921

Years	1917	1918	1919	1920	1921
Deaths per 1,000 in age group	12.6	17.3	13.8	13.9	13.0

13. Tuberculous patients receiving dispensary treatment, showing number of treatments and the number of home visits by nurses.

14. Health stations and clinics and variety of health activities existing in the counties, 1921.

15. Data of economic interest, such as that showing the percentage of the population employed, and the number of factories, 1921.

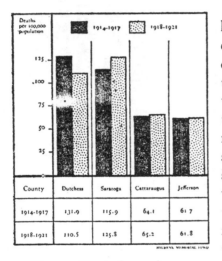

Fig. 19. Deaths from pulmonary tuberculosis in the four New York State counties considered as areas for the rural health demonstration, per 100,000 population,*during the four-year periods, 1914–1917 and 1918–1921

*Exclusive of inmates of state institutions

With this information at hand, it was possible to compare the advantages and disadvantages presented by the several counties and to view each community from the point of view of its relative fitness as a demonstration area. It was desired to select a community with generally representative health, social and economic conditions; with a tuberculosis mortality rate that was fairly average; that already possessed the basic machinery necessary for a comprehensive health promotion program; and that had already made substantial progress in setting up and in conducting a community health program.

Because of its qualifications in these particulars—because its environmental make-up at once presented conditions typical of very sparsely settled rural communities and of semi-rural localities in New York State and in the United

322

States—and because there was emphatic assurance from legally constituted authorities and from voluntary agencies there of the desire and the ability to meet the local obligations of co-operation and participation necessary for the success of the rural demonstration—at a meeting on October 30, 1922, the Executive Committee of the State Charities Aid Association recommended Cattaraugus County for selection. Following the confirmation of this endorsement by the Technical Board on November second, and its approval by the Advisory Council on November sixteenth, the choice of Cattaraugus County as the rural demonstration area was made on November 20, 1922, by the Board of Directors of the Milbank Memorial Fund.

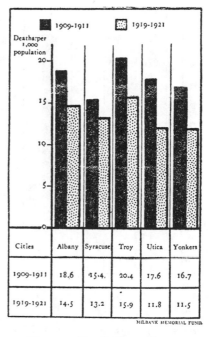

	1909-1911				1919-1921

Cities	Albany	Syracuse	Troy	Utica	Yonkers
1909-1911	18.6	15.4	20.4	17.6	16.7
1919-1921	14.5	13.2	15.9	11.8	11.5

MILBANK MEMORIAL FUND.

Fig. 20. Deaths from all causes in the five New York State cities considered as areas for the urban health demonstration, per 1,000 population, during the three-year periods, 1909–1911 and 1919–1921

The population has been adjusted to the standard million of England and Wales.

Selecting the Urban Demonstration District

The studies of cities in New York State suitable for possible selection as an urban demonstration area, were similar in most respects to those made in choosing the rural unit. Initial surveys resulted in the tentative selection for further consideration of the more eligible communities, on grounds similar to those which entered into the choice of Cattaraugus County.* The choice narrowed down to five cities, namely: Albany, Syracuse, Troy, Utica and Yonkers. Like those

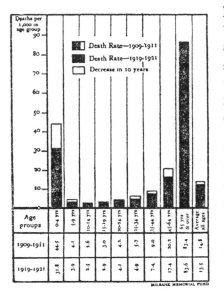

prepared in the case of the counties, the statistical and sociological tables and schedules which were made to advise the Milbank Memorial Fund of the relative qualifications presented by these cities, are available upon request. With the addition of special studies of the standardized death rates of these five cities made by Dr. Otto R. Eichel, Director of the Bureau of Vital Statistics of the New York State Department of Health, the kind of data sought was the same in the case of the cities as it was in the case of the counties. (Figs. 20, 21, and 22)

Fig. 21. Deaths from all causes in Syracuse, per 1,000 population of the age indicated, during the three-year periods, 1909–1911 and 1919–1921

As a result of the study of this material, the considerations and conditions which would enter into the final selection of the urban demonstration area were laid before the health and other municipal authorities and voluntary agencies interested in health in these cities through the local membership association of the State Committee on Tuberculosis and Public Health of the State Charities Aid Association. These were stated in a letter addressed by Homer Folks, Secretary of

*pp. 110-112.

the Association, to the president of the local association, as follows:

1. The demonstration will be carried out through and by local health authorities and voluntary agencies, and these authorities and agencies must be willing to assume the operating responsibilities for carrying out the various features of the local program (with, of course, such counsel and assistance as state-wide authorities and agencies can give).

2. While the particular object of the program will be tuberculosis control, it is believed that this will involve the gradual development of a comprehensive general public health program. The full co-operation of the city is essential to this end. Such general health work would be concerned, as the demonstration progresses, with the following major considerations:

    a. A broad health and anti-tuberculosis educational campaign.

    b. Such specific tuberculosis measures as clinics, home nursing, adequate institutional facilities, open air classes, nutrition classes, adequate relief, consultation service, adequate laboratory facilities, etc.

    c. General health work with the various age groups, including maternity, infancy, pre-school, and child hygiene, mental hygiene, and industrial hygiene.

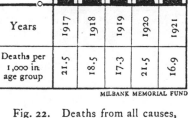

Deaths per 1,000 in age group				
20 —				
15 —				
10 —				
5 —				
0—				
Years	1917	1918	1919	1920	1921
Deaths per 1,000 in age group	21.5	18.5	17.3	21.5	16.9

MILBANK MEMORIAL FUND

Fig. 22. Deaths from all causes, of children under ten years of age (per 1,000 children in this age group) in Syracuse, 1917–1921

 d. General sanitation, including the control of communicable disease, milk and water sanitation, social hygiene, a degree of control of adult life diseases (cancer, heart and kidney conditions, etc.), primarily by means of medical examinations periodically made by the family physicians, etc.

 e. Last, but not least—full co-ordination of the official and voluntary health agencies under responsible local leadership.

3. The Milbank Fund resources will be used to supplement, so far as may seem necessary and desirable, the local health expenditures, public and voluntary, after the approval of each budgetary requirement by the Technical Board of the Fund on the recommendation of the State Charities Aid Association.

4. In considering cities, preference will naturally be given to those most nearly approaching on their own resources the financing of an adequate health program; a further important factor will be the degree of assurance of the city's desire and ability to complete and, after a suitable demonstration period of each activity, to maintain such a program. It is assumed that as the permanent value of each new or experimental phase of work is fully demonstrated, the obligation for its continuance will be locally assumed. A statement from each city, along lines indicated below, about what it will probably be in a position to do, would be welcomed.

It was recognized that it would be impossible for local authorities to make binding definite commitments as to future financial obligations, and that much would have to be left to the convincing educational effects of the various elements of the demonstrations as they develop. It was desired, however, to have as definite and formal a statement as possible by public authorities, voluntary agencies and public spirited citizens that they desired a more complete health program and that they believed that the city authorities and voluntary agencies would be able gradually to assume full responsibility for the continuance of the work as developed successfully during the period of the demonstration. The nature of the evidences of local interest and co-operation desired was indicated as follows:

1. Resolutions of approval and pledges of co-operation from:

    a. The local committee on tuberculosis and public health.

    b. The local medical society.

    c. The local family relief society or kindred organization, if there be one.

    d. The local public health nursing agencies.

    e. Other local organizations having to do with health and social welfare.

    f. The local Chamber of Commerce and other organizations of business men or taxpayers.

    g. Such civic organizations as the Rotary, Kiwanis and Exchange clubs.

2. Endorsement and promise of support from the central federation of labor or kindred organization, and from the owners or managers of important local industrial and mercantile corporations.

3. A formal letter from the Mayor giving assurance from him and his associates on the Board of Estimate and from the Common Council that they approve the undertaking and would favor the gradual assumption by the city of the cost of operating various features of the program of work after their need and value have been demonstrated.

4. A disposition upon the part of the appropriate city authorities to establish a health department under the provisions of Chapter 249, Laws of 1921 (unless this has already been done) in place of the existing Bureau of Health in the Department of Public Safety, with such Health Department directed by a Commissioner of Health with a tenure of office of four years and who shall have the qualifications referred to in the foregoing statute.

5. A willingness upon the part of the appropriate city authorities to work toward the provision of a whole-time health officer for the city, and a disposition to provide a salary for that position sufficient to attract and hold a physician with the requisite qualifications, as defined by law and the Public Health Council.

6. Assurance that such additional hospital accommoda-
   tions as may be needed will be provided, whether from
   municipal, county or private funds.

7. An assurance that the leading newspapers understand
   the proposed demonstration and will give it all reasonable support. The best evidence of such attitude, of
   course, would be editorial approval of the proposed
   demonstration. If, however, a favorable attitude might
   be prejudiced by requesting editorial approval at present, and assurance that the matter has been laid before
   the responsible owners or editors of the leading papers
   and that it receives very cordial approval would be
   sufficient.

Representatives of the cities were invited to present the
qualifications of their respective communities at a joint
meeting of the Executive Committee of the State Charities
Aid Association and the Technical Board of the Milbank Memorial Fund held in New York City on December 28, 1922. The admirable qualifications presented by
the several districts made the choice difficult. But on
the basis of representative conditions, geographic location,
promise of local co-operation and the national significance of
demonstration experience in Syracuse, this city was finally
chosen for recommendation to the Board of Directors of
the Milbank Memorial Fund as the urban demonstration
area. At its meeting on January 5, 1923, the Board confirmed this selection.

Selecting the Metropolitan District

There were many reasons why it was felt that New York
City offered a unique opportunity for the metropolitan
health demonstration. Its problems are typical of those in
many large urban areas, where lives a sizable percentage of
the population of the United States. The rest of the country
is in the habit of looking, more or less, to this city for leadership in different avenues of its life—and because New York

City and New York State have been so often leaders in this field, it looks here, in part, for guidance in its health work. Most of the public health movements that are expressed in voluntary national health organizations have had their origin in and are located in New York City. Then, too, there is here a number of well developed local voluntary organizations, with activities already well coordinated with the work of the public health authorities.*

Careful consideration has been given to the question of where in New York City the demonstration should be held. At the request of the Milbank Memorial Fund, the New York Association for Improving the Condition of the Poor made inquiries into the health facilities of a number of tuberculosis clinic districts in the city to determine which seemed to offer the best opportunities in which to conduct an intensive metropolitan health program. Statistical material regarding these districts was gathered under the immediate supervision of Godias J. Drolet, Statistician of the New York Tuberculosis Association and with the advice of the Statistical Committee of the Milbank Memorial Fund.

Dr. Haven Emerson, in consultation with physicians and authorities on public health administration, recommended the following items, which seemed to be important as determining factors in selecting a population group within the City of New York for the purpose of undertaking the demonstration:

1. Population of approximately 200,000.

2. No such dominance of any special race as to determine racial difference in the tuberculosis and other death rates in the area.

3. No great excess or diminution in the crude death rate, the tuberculosis death rate or the infant mortality rate

*Milbank Memorial Fund Quarterly Bulletin, January, 1924, p. 22.

as compared with the corresponding rates for the Borough or City as a whole.

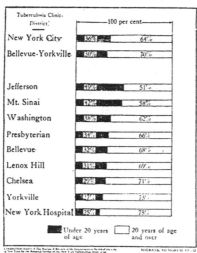

Fig. 23. Percentage of population under and over twenty years of age in the combined Bellevue-Yorkville tuberculosis clinic districts, in other districts, and in the City of New York, 1920

4. The expression by responsible groups of the community in the areas under consideration of eagerness to participate in the proposed demonstration.

5. The absence of any important social or health undertaking which might make it impracticable to draw clear-cut conclusions as to the cost, effect and results properly attributable to the demonstration's method of administrating public health work.

6. Other determining factors as above indicated being equal, preference should be given to a district which has existing educational facilities for training in public health work.

In the first place, the Technical Board of the Fund has determined that the district selected should include a population of approximately 200,000 persons, this because a population of less would not offer an adequate statistical basis for the demonstration. This means that in view of the fact that most of the tuberculosis clinic districts are just over 100,000 in population, consideration has been given to the wisdom of combining two tuberculosis clinic districts in New York City as the demonstration unit. Believing in the importance of selecting a demonstration area whose limits are so far as possible coterminous with areas selected by the Department of Health for their administrative purposes, the Technical Board has assumed from the beginning that the demonstration district should be chosen, having in mind first the sanitary districts, which are the smallest health units in the city, and, second, the tuberculosis clinic districts which are composite of a certain number of sanitary districts of Federal Census tracts. With the Federal Census returns for these several districts and the mortality data obtainable from the records of the Health Department, it is possible to compute for each district the local mortality rates. The study, therefore, included comparative inquiries into the several tuberculosis clinic district areas which seemed most likely to offer satisfactory conditions for the conduct of the demonstration.

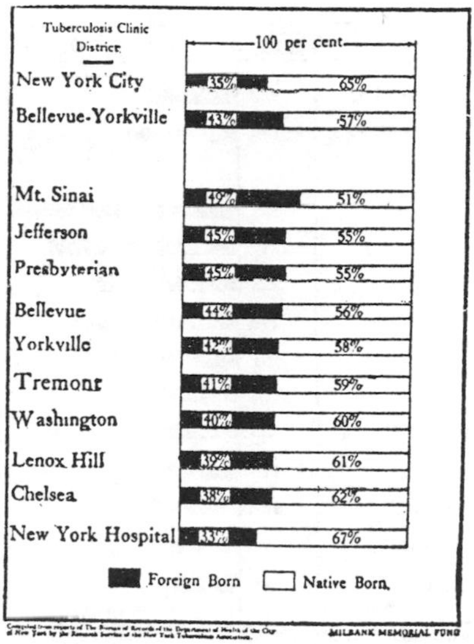

An interesting fact in connection with the popu-

Fig. 24. Percentage of native and foreign born in the combined Bellevue-Yorkville tuberculosis clinic districts, in other districts, and in the City of New York, 1920

lation study is that in practically every district in Manhattan there has been a loss of population during the past ten years. In the Bronx, on the other hand, the districts are growing at an annual rate of almost 10 per cent. The density of the population per acre of those districts studied is largest in the Mt. Sinai tuberculosis clinic district and lowest in the New York Hospital district. Concerning the population in each district, a very important factor to be borne in mind is that because of the general displacement, due to the industrial and business factors, there are two different groups of population utilizing most of the districts

331

at different times of day. The Census gives only the night residential population, and all the vital statistics are based upon this population; but it must be remembered that during the day another group of workers comes into these districts and is exposed and subject, as far as health is concerned, to all the conditions prevailing locally. The additional problems arising from these two populations within a district are, however, typical of a condition now becoming common in the heart of all business centers and large cities. A solution of the dangers to the health both of the residential population and of those at work should prove of interest and value to all concerned with the welfare

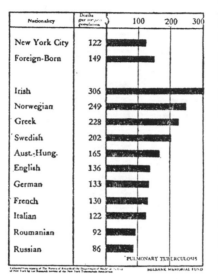

Fig. 25. Deaths from pulmonary tuberculosis among foreign born in the City of New York, per 100,000 population in each respective group, during the four-year period, 1918–1921

of urban populations. With this in mind, information was secured from the State Department of Labor, giving the factory population for most of the tuberculosis clinic district areas. In the Bellevue tuberculosis clinic district the number of persons employed in factories is 24,656, which is the largest number found in any area.

Age Distribution

Studies of the population indicate that certain districts have a very high percentage of children while others have an exceedingly low one. (Fig. 23) For instance, the Jefferson district has more than 48 per cent of its population under 20, which is 15 per cent more than the average for Manhattan, while the New York Hospital district has only 25 per cent of its population under 20. In recommending a district in which the Demonstration should be conducted, the Technical Board of the Milbank Memorial Fund has been mindful of the importance of securing a district in which the age distribution is typical.

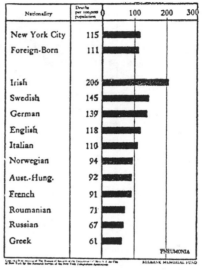

Nationality	Deaths per 100,000 population
New York City	115
Foreign-Born	111
Irish	206
Swedish	145
German	139
English	118
Italian	110
Norwegian	94
Aust.-Hung.	92
French	91
Roumanian	71
Russian	67
Greek	61

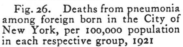

Fig. 26. Deaths from pneumonia among foreign born in the City of New York, per 100,000 population in each respective group, 1921

Foreign Born

The percentage of foreign born in the several districts likewise varies greatly. (Fig. 24) The Mt. Sinai district, which is largely Russian or Jewish, has 49 per cent of its population foreign born, while the lowest percentage of foreign born is found in the New York Hospital district, in which only 33 per cent of the population is foreign born. The percentage of foreign born in Manhattan is 43 per cent and for New York City as a whole, 35 per cent. A comparison of the death rates from pulmonary tuberculosis, pneumonia, cancer, organic heart diseases, and Brights disease among foreign born in New York City is shown in Figs. 25, 26, 27, 28, and 29.

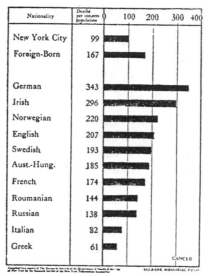

Nationality	Deaths per 100,000 population
New York City	99
Foreign-Born	167
German	343
Irish	296
Norwegian	220
English	207
Swedish	193
Aust.-Hung.	185
French	174
Roumanian	144
Russian	138
Italian	82
Greek	61

Fig. 27. Deaths from cancer among foreign born in the City of New York, per 100,000 population in each respective group, 1921

The largest group among the foreign born in most of the districts in Manhattan is the Italian. This is in spite of the fact that there is a smaller percentage of Italians in the City as a whole than Russians. In the Jefferson tuberculosis district, for instance, 68 per cent of all the foreign born are Italians, which is the highest percentage of any foreign born group in any of the districts. In the Washington district, on the lower west side, 59 per cent of their foreign born population is Italian, while the smallest Italian group is found in the Lenox Hill district, where only slightly more than 4 per cent of all the foreign born is Italian. The largest percentage of foreign born Russians is found in the Tremont district, in the Bronx, and Mt. Sinai district in Manhattan, in which the Russians represent 45 per cent of all the foreign born. The largest percentage of foreign born Irish is found in the New York Hospital tuberculosis district, where 30 per cent of all the foreign born were born in Ireland, while the smallest percentage is found in the Jefferson district, where only 3 per cent of the foreign born are Irish.

General and Infant Mortality

The general and infant mortality rates by tuberculosis clinic districts were made available beginning with the year, 1920 from the vital statistics segregated by sanitary areas classified by the Department of Health, with the assistance of the Red Cross. In 1920 the highest general death rate, 21.2 per 1,000, was in the New York Hospital district. Outside of Lenox Hill, Mt. Sinai, and probably Tremont, the general death rate of all the other districts under consideration exceeded the city's death rate. The birth rate was highest in the Jefferson district and lowest in the Lenox Hill dis-

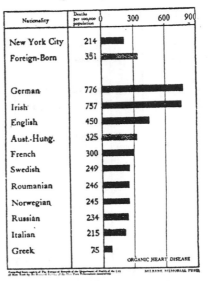

Fig. 28. Deaths from organic heart diseases among foreign born in the City of New York, per 100,000 population in each respective group, 1921

trict. The infant mortality rate was considerably higher in most of the tuberculosis clinic districts studied than for the city as a whole. (Fig. 30) The Bellevue clinic district exceeded the city rate by 56 per cent and the Jefferson district by 45 per cent.

Tuberculosis Mortality

The annual mortality rates from pulmonary tuberculosis for the eight-year period, 1915–1922, inclusive, were secured for each Manhattan district. (Fig. 31) While the pulmonary tuberculosis death rate decreased in New York City 49 per cent during these years, and 45 per cent in Manhattan, the decrease in the several districts studied varied from a decrease of only 26 per cent in the Jefferson district, where the rate has been and is now very low, to 58 per cent in the Chelsea district. The very great differences in tuberculosis mortality in the districts in 1922—183 per 100,000 in the New York Hospital district and 52 in the Tremont district, are accounted for in some degree by various racial groups and by the difference in the age distribution of the several populations. (The annual average death rate from pulmonary tuberculosis in each sanitary area in the Borough of Manhattan for the six-year period, 1915-1920, is shown in Fig. 32.)

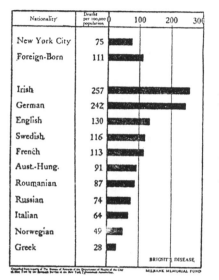

Fig. 29. Deaths from Bright's disease among foreign born in the City of New York, per 100,000 population in each respective group, 1921

Tuberculosis Morbidity

The total number of known living cases of pulmonary tuberculosis registered in New York City on October 1, 1922, was 27,321, giving a morbidity rate of 468 per 100,000. In the Washington district the morbidity rate was 1,277 per 100,000, while it was lowest in Tremont, where the rate was 485. The percentage of known tuberculosis cases under medical care in New York City was 47 per cent. The highest percentage under medical care was in the Presbyterian district where it reached 58 per cent. The largest number hospitalized or in sanatoria was in the Bellevue district, where 31 per cent of all the known cases were in institutions.

Standardized and Specific Death Rates

For the years 1921 and 1922, the pulmonary tuberculosis death rate was standardized in the several districts studied on the basis of an age composition of the population similar to that of New York City as a whole. The effect of the standardization by age has been to raise the rate where a larger number of children is contained in the population and to lower it where the proportion of adults is

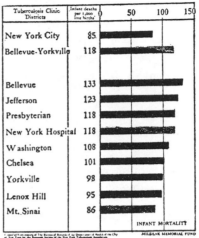

Fig. 30. Deaths of children under one year of age, per 1,000 live births (infant mortality), in the combined Bellevue–Yorkville tuberculosis clinic districts, in other districts, and in the City of New York, 1920

greater. When larger areas are standardized, as in the Borough of Bronx, the crude death rate of 1922 is found to differ by only one point, and in Manhattan by 4 points, where the standardized rate is found to be 102 instead of 106, the crude rate. In the Jefferson district, with its large number of children, the standardized rate is 17 per cent higher than the crude rate. The standardized tuberculosis death rate in each district permits, of course, a more accurate presentation of the tuberculosis situation and also allows a real comparison to be made between the various sections. In the preparation of standardized rates an opportunity occurs to note the specific death rates at certain age groups in each clinic area. The table included as part of this report shows the variation of death rates in each district, in five important age groups of the population for 1922.* The varying rates, especially among children under fifteen, should not be given too much weight as there were few deaths in these groups; but the larger numbers available in the adult sections of the population give greater value to the rates found. In general, in New York City, the tuberculosis mortality rate is higher among people over 45 than those between 20 and 44. The highest death rate among young adults, that is between 15 and 19, is in the Bellevue district, where it was 172 per 100,000 living at that age group in 1922. The lowest in that same group was in Mt. Sinai district, where it was 66 per 100,000.

Tuberculosis by Racial Groups

The death rate in the various nationalities from pulmonary tuberculosis is a crude rate as the details of the age com-

*Standardized death rates from pulmonary tuberculosis in the Bellevue, Yorkville and other tuberculosis clinic districts, in the Borough of Manhattan and in the City of New York, 1921 and 1922. Showing the specific death rates by age groups, 1922.

Tuberculosis Clinic Districts	Standardized Death Rate (a)		Specific Death Rates by Age Groups in 1922 (b)				
	1921	1922	0–5	5–14	15–19	20–44	45
City of New York	89	86	14	8	83	117	137
Borough of Manhattan	106	102	28	14	103	128	163
Bellevue	158	146	19	0	172	172	282
Chelsea	131	127	23	0	138	146	257
Jefferson	129	117	31	18	110	154	176
Lenox Hill	82	88	0	6	147	105	149
Presbyterian	111	111	48	17	99	140	175
Yorkville	92	79	27	7	100	123	67
Mt. Sinai	83	68	24	8	66	85	111
N. Y. Hospital	188	159	0	39	153	202	256
Washington	157	146	10	11	102	202	236

(a) Standardized on basis of an age composition of the population in each district similar to that of New York City as a whole.

(b) Death rate per 100,000 persons living at these particular age groups.

position of the population in each different age group are not available. This probably explains in a measure the higher pulmonary tuberculosis death rate among the foreign born, which was 113 in 1921 against 80 among the native born. During the four-year period, 1918-1921, the tuberculosis death rate was highest among the Chinese, the annual rate for this period being 825 per 100,000. The second is that of the negro population, which was 398 against the city rate of 122. Other rates considerably higher than the city rate are found among the Finns and the Irish. (Fig. 25) Lower rates than the city average prevail especially among those from Russia and Roumania.

Deaths of Transients

Separate information was secured in each district as to the deaths from pulmonary tuberculosis of non-residents of New York City occurring within the different sections. During 1922 in all of New York City, 154 such deaths occurred. These are at present included in the total of 5,035 deaths from pulmonary tuberculosis charged by the Bureau of Records to New York City, as no distribution out of town could be made of these deaths. In Manhattan, where there is no permanent tuberculosis hospital, the proportion of deaths of transients is very small, being only 49 such deaths against a total of 2,412 which occurred in the borough. The largest number of deaths of non-residents from pulmonary tuberculosis in any district was in the Bellevue district, where six such deaths were charged in the total of 175 for the district. The present number of deaths charged against each district includes not only those of residents of the district who died within the district, but also those of district residents occurring in institutions in other parts of the city.

Health Facilities of the Districts

In addition to the study of the vital statistics of the city, a very careful inquiry was made into the health agencies

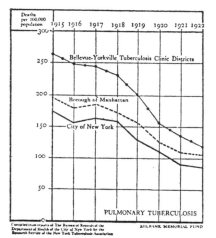

of the Borough of Manhattan, and a careful analysis made of their work in each of the respective districts. In addition to this, the service rendered by local agencies was noted and all of this information placed in the hands of the Technical Board. This study included a careful inquiry into the tuberculosis facilities of the district, the maternity service, the infant hygiene service, pre-school work, school hygiene work and service in such special fields as industrial hygiene, mental hygiene, venereal disease, hospital social service and health education. The extent of the several agencies' work in all of these fields has been carefully surveyed and analyzed. The study of this information, together with the vital statistics, has led the Technical Board of the Milbank Memorial Fund to recommend that the demonstration be held in the Bellevue-Yorkville district, the approximate boundaries of which are between 14th and 64th Streets, and from 4th Avenue to the East River. (Fig. 16)

Fig. 31. Decrease n deaths from pulmonary tuberculosis in the combined Bellevue-Yorkville tuberculosis clinic districts, in the Borough of Manhattan, and in the City of New York, per 100,000 population in each respective region, 1915–1922

Following are some of the reasons why the selection of

this combination of tuberculosis districts over any others seemed wise:

1. The combined Bellevue-Yorkville districts make a satisfactory unit population.

2. The percentage of the foreign born in the Bellevue-Yorkville district is but slightly more than that of the whole city and there is no predominant racial group there.

3. The density of the population is about the same as in the Borough of Manhattan.

4. The clinic facilities are fairly adequate. It is believed that a smaller expenditure of funds will be needed for clinic work in this area than in any of the other areas.

5. The age distribution in the Bellevue-Yorkville district is practically the same as for Manhattan.

6. The birth rate is practically the same as the rate for Manhattan and for the greater city.

7. There is a larger percentage of pre-natal and maternity cases under competent medical and nursing supervision in this area than in any other area.

8. The general nursing facilities of this area, while inadequate, are relatively as well developed as in other areas, with the exception of two sanitary areas in the Jefferson district.

9. Hospital social service is as well developed in the Bellevue-Yorkville district as in any of the other districts.

10. Facilities for dealing with tuberculosis are relatively well developed in the Bellevue-Yorkville district.

11. The social service and public health agencies in the Bellevue-Yorkville district are accustomed to working together effectively, so that the Trustees of the Fund would be assured of the co-operation of the health and social agencies.

12. The Milbank Memorial Bath Building, erected in 1904 at a cost of $150,000, and presented to the A. I. C. P. by Mrs. Elizabeth Milbank Anderson, is no longer used as a bath building. It is possible that this building— a fireproof, substantial, well lighted and well ventilated structure, might be made available by the A. I. C. P. as headquarters for the demonstration.

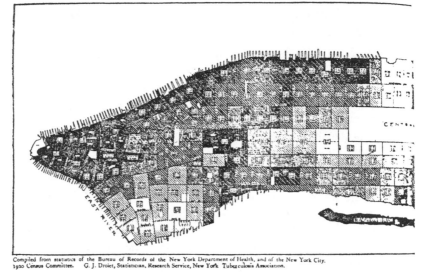

Compiled from statistics of the Bureau of Records of the New York Department of Health, and of the New York City.
1920 Census Committee. G. J. Drolet, Statistician, Research Service, New York Tuberculosis Association.

Fig. 32. Deaths from pulmonary tuberculosis in the B
of Manhattan of the City of New York. Annual

Methods of Procedure in Organizing the Demonstrations

It was anticipated that to secure effective results in the promotion of a comprehensive health program in each of the areas chosen and at the same time to make of as much value as possible the correlated experience of all three demonstrations, uniform methods of general procedure would need to be carried out in each district by the local operating authorities in co-operation with the supervisory operating agency appointed by the Milbank Memorial Fund, upon the recommendation of its Technical Board and Advisory Council. Such measures as the following were considered essential:

1. A local survey of the prevalence and distribution of disease, of the community's general health needs, and of the available facilities for meeting those needs.
2. The perfection by the community of its own organization to meet the opportunities and requirements of the

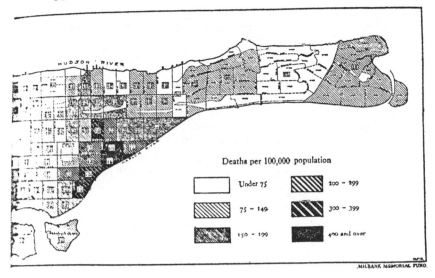

Deaths per 100,000 population

	Under 75		200 - 299
	75 - 149		300 - 399
	150 - 199		400 and over

.MILBANK MEMORIAL FUND.

ᵈᵉᵃᵗʰ rate, per 100,000 population in each sanitary area for the six-year period, 1915-1920

demonstration, to place non-experimental phases of its work on a permanent basis, and to supplement agreements arrived at previous to its selection as a demonstration area. It was thought that this would involve:

a. The development of an adequate official health organization which could be supplemented or modified as the demonstration progressed.

b. The initiation of steps to co-ordinate the voluntary and official health work of the community, enlisting the integrated co-operation and aid of all groups, including those working in the medical, nursing, educational, industrial and religious fields; and the organization of necessary local committees.

3. The setting up of effective machinery interrelating the demonstration unit, the operating agencies and the Fund—arranging for records, reports, the handling of finances, etc.

4. The securing of qualified personnel.

5. The establishment of necessary co-operative relations with state and national agencies, official and voluntary.

6. The acquainting of the people in the community with the motives, methods and practical objectives of the demonstration.

7. The selection of "control" communities. These would be counties or cities having similar health problems, the health improvement of which would be measured yearly along with that of the demonstration county, to discover whether the increase in health activities and facilities in the demonstration resulted in greater health improvement than that shown in the "control" areas.

8. The formulation of indices by which an attempt will be made to measure, year by year, results of, and progress in, the demonstration.

The survey would include a detailed study of the health conditions and health hazards in the community and of the facilities available for adequate treatment, supplementing the statistical and sociological data secured before the community was selected as a demonstration area. Such information will serve as a basis for determining the methods of procedure necessary to the successful development of the demonstration. It will be advisable perhaps to start with the activities more obviously needed and begin operations in certain fields of work before the survey has been entirely completed. A community analysis would include:

1. The appraisal of the health machinery of the community, supplementing information acquired previously and building on such preliminary steps as may already have been taken. This would include:

   a. The study of official equipment, of voluntary activities, and of their interrelations; of public appropriations and private expenditures for health; of the adequacy and character of existing personnel; of the character of existing health organization and services, such as perhaps the districting of the community, etc. It would also include a careful analysis of the provision made by the community for specific health services, including those for special age groups, and those to deal with specific disease problems.

    b. A special study of the local nursing services, the extent to which they are specialized or general in character; their adequacy to the community need; the training required of nurses.

    c. A study of hospital provisions, of out-patient clinics, and the adequacy of measures for contagious disease control.

    d. A study of the laboratory needs of the community.

    e. A study of the local facilities for disseminating information about the public health movement, including those maintained by the voluntary agencies, the school authorities, the Health Department, etc., such as special training courses for nurses, special lecture and clinic courses for physicians, health officers and veterinarians, and bulletins, exhibits, lectures, films and newspaper publicity to reach the public at large.

2. A study of the environment which would include the following major considerations:

    a. Facilities for food control, including the milk supply; the bovine tuberculosis problem; the housing problem; the water supply; a review of existing sanitary legislation; and a survey of general sanitary conditions.

    b. Hygienic equipment of the schools, including the drinking water supply, lighting arrangement, ventilation and toilet facilities.

    c. General working conditions in the community, including factory sanitation and occupational hazards.

3. A study of the general health conditions in the population, and of the efforts made to meet local health problems. This would include specific inquiries along the following lines:

    a. Tuberculosis.—To ascertain the number of tuberculosis cases reported, supplemented by a preliminary intensive case-finding study; to learn the adequacy of institutional provision and of laboratory and X-ray facilities for the treatment of this disease.

    b. Communicable Diseases.—To learn the prevalence of communicable diseases and the adequacy and effectiveness of control measures therefor.

c. School Hygiene.—The extent of contagion and defect (medical and dental), corrective measures instituted, special activities, if any, for diphtheria control, the existence of clinics, how often children are examined, the adequacy of staff (physicians, nurses, dietitians, dental hygienists, dentists, and physical educators), and the completeness and effectiveness of the health educational procedure in the school.

d. Maternity, Infancy and Child Hygiene.—The infant and child morbidity and mortality rates; the extent of hospitalization of maternity cases; the adequacy of provisions for infant hygiene.

e. Social Hygiene.—To learn the prevalence of venereal diseases and the adequacy and effectiveness of control measures therefor.

f. Mental Hygiene.—To ascertain the prevalence of nervous disturbances and mental divergences and the means for their prevention, detection and treatment. The survey should attempt to discover the psychopathic and neurotic child as well as the defective, insane, etc.

g. Industrial Hygiene.—The incidence of occupational and other diseases, the frequency and severity rates for industrial accidents, the conditions of factory hygiene and the scope and adequacy of the facilities for the supervision of the health of the workers.

h. Sanitation and Food Inspection.

i. Health Conservation and Life Extension.

A possible study might be made of general economic conditions, wages, income, family stability, the prevalence of poverty and the adequacy and efficiency of existing relief measures.

APPENDIX

THE original program of the Milbank Memorial Fund placed primary emphasis on tuberculosis and made other public health problems ancillary to it. Subsequently, as a result of further study and consultation with recognized experts, the emphasis was reversed and a general public health program adopted, with tuberculosis as one of its main features.

The original program, as well as the subsequent modifications of it, have been submitted to test and review from varied points of view, and efforts made to forecast the results of a comprehensive public health program adequately supported by effective co-ordination of community forces and resources.

One of the most interesting and suggestive of these forecasts which played an important part in focussing the attention of the Fund's Directors and their advisors upon the possibilities of public health work, was prepared by Dr. Haven Emerson for the New York Association for Improving the Condition of the Poor, through which the Milbank Memorial Fund was conducting its preliminary surveys in New York City. This study dealt with the original tentative program entitled, "The Next Steps in the Control of Tuberculosis," and is here presented because of its historical interest to the Fund and as an interesting contribution to the discussion of the economic aspects of tuberculosis.

347

BRIEF FOR INVESTMENT IN ADEQUATE HOME TREATMENT FOR THE PREVENTION OF TUBERCULOSIS

By Haven Emerson, M. D.

ALTHOUGH it has been a matter of common knowledge to most physicians and to many of the laity that the loss of life, wealth and resources from tuberculosis, both pulmonary and other forms, for many generations has been the greatest drain from disease upon all classes of the population and upon all races of our country, the actual present-day extent of the damage due alone to this preventable and curable disease has not yet been expressed in a brief and convincing manner.

The direct losses of tuberculosis can be described from the point of view of the community most simply in terms of:

1. Deaths attributable to this disease.
2. The estimated shortening of the expectancy of life due to deaths from tuberculosis.
3. Cases of prolonged total disability, or persons suffering for long periods from semi-invalidism from tuberculosis.
4. The loss in wealth due to deaths, sickness and shortened lives.

Status of Death Loss in United States and New York City

Using the population of continental United States as 108,500,000 (estimated exactly to be 108,468,099 on January 1, 1922) and that of the City of New York as 5,850,000 (estimated at 5,841,187 on January 1, 1922) and basing our estimates of deaths, sickness and other losses upon 80 deaths per annum from pulmonary tuberculosis per 100,000 of the population, a rate below any so far recorded for the City or the Nation for a year (89 in 1921), we find that we shall lose in 1922 in continental United States 86,800 lives and in the City of New York, 4,680 lives from pulmonary tuberculosis alone, and at a rate of 10 deaths per annum per 100,000 of the population (17 in New York City in 1920) from other forms of tuberculosis, or 10,850 lives in the Nation and 585 for the City in addition, or a total number of deaths from all forms of tuberculosis of 97,650 for the United States and 5,265 for the City of New York in 1922.

Sickness from Tuberculosis in United States and New York City

Studies of the incidence of tuberculosis in many parts of the United States show that there are quite certainly seven times as many people suffering from the disease at any time as there are

349

deaths from tuberculosis in the population in the given year. In arriving at this figure of seven cases per death per annum we are considering only those who are definitely handicapped, if not totally disabled by the active process of the disease, and who require medical and nursing direction and care.

If all the devices and resources which were used at Framingham, Mass., are used in an average community we may expect to discover as many as 10 cases with demonstrable signs of pulmonary tuberculosis for each death from this form of the disease per annum, but, since the actual experience in New York City with the available means of the public and private agencies has been that not more than seven cases of active disease per death per annum are found, we are using the more conservative number.

Further, instead of charging against the disease the cost of sickness care of all the cases of tuberculosis, many of which will have to suffer little in the way of interference with their work or manner of living, it is considered reasonable to arrive at the number of persons with tuberculosis who will need medical care and direction, and during this period will be unable to work, by multiplying the number of deaths per annum by the factor two and one-third, or the number of years found to be the usual duration of complete disability prior to death of cases of pulmonary tuberculosis. (Sir George Newman uses three years in his statements upon duration of sickness prior to death from tuberculosis.)

There will be found in all probability during 1922 not less than 683,550 people in continental United States and 36,855 in the City of New York suffering from the active stages of tuberculosis and needing almost constant professional direction and many also financial aid.

Financial Cost of Deaths and Sickness

Although the value of life, including consideration of all factors, of age and sex, and of social, economic or racial status of the individual, has never been estimated to the entire satisfaction of economists, and even less to the satisfaction of the family from which a life has been taken, it is possible to arrive at the cost of the annual death loss from tuberculosis by showing what this means in terms of shortened lives. Our annual loss of life from tuberculosis applied to the entire population of all age groups means the shortening of the duration of life of all of the population by not less than two and one-half years. Without rehearsing the evidence upon which the cost of reduction in life expectancy is based, it can be said that $100 is considered by well informed and reliable and conservative statisticians and economists as representing the loss in national wealth due to a loss of a year of time by any individual.

Tuberculosis is cutting two and one-half years or $250 from the life or wealth resources of each person in the United States during the span of his life, or for all of those now living in the continental United States $27,125,000,000, or for all of those now living in the City of New York the sum of $1,462,500,000 during their life-span.

Since present day expectation of life is approximately fifty-two years, we shall be wasting lives in 1922 from tuberculosis deaths in New York City and the United States equivalent to a loss in the wealth of the Nation and the City of $521,634,615 and $28,125,000, respectively, in the year 1922, or $4.81 per capita of the entire population.

Additional Cost of Care of the Tuberculous Sick

In spite of the impracticability of giving accurately all the elements in the cost of care of those suffering from various forms of tuberculosis, we are well within the facts of expense when we use the figures obtained from relief agencies which care for the dependent sick.

The group of the population of the City of New York for whom the cost of care has been calculated is precisely those of the community whose standards of living are such that the cost of their care can be met by a minimum expenditure for housing, nutrition, clothing and professional supervision. The higher the economic and social status of the patient the more expensive is the cost of his care during tuberculosis. Therefore, the estimate now offered is considered to be well within the most conservative limits for the entire population. It now costs in New York City not less than $1,500 a year to give adequate care to a patient in the active stage of tuberculosis; this cost including, as it must, the protection of members of the patient's family against the major risks of exposure to the disease, as well as provision of medical observation for the family to detect and correct promptly any evidence of early development of an active tuberculous process in other members of the household.

There must be added, therefore, to the cost of deaths from

tuberculosis the cost of care of the sick which for the United States and New York City would be $341,775,000 and $18,427,500, respectively, for the year, 1922, or $3.15 per capita of the population.

The combined wastage from tuberculosis in terms of dollars alone in 1922 will be for the continental United States $863,409,615 and for the City of New York $46,552,500, or $7.96 per capita of the population for the year.

If, instead of picturing the aggregate loss in wealth and in cost of services for care of the tuberculous sick as a burden shared equally by all members of the community alike, whether in city or nation, we try to express the losses from the point of view of the handicapped minority of the people who suffer from tuberculosis, not from any personal fault or neglect or misdeed of their own, but largely because the community has not fully safeguarded its young and dependent, its wage earner and its school child, we see the problem in a somewhat more serious and painful perspective. It may be said that an annual per capita loss of $7.96 can be better borne, while the gradual decrease of tuberculosis is being accomplished by the expenditure of a fraction of that amount each year, than can an annual outlay not far from the actual cost of the disease, for the sake of a more rapid elimination of it. But what does this look like from the point of view of the 683,550 in the United States and the 36,855 in New York City, whose losses have been theoretically distributed among all the people? These tuberculous patients will lose in 1922 $1,262 apiece as well as such of the amenities of life as may constitute their particular share of happiness, and one in seven will die, to boot.

Reduction in Tuberculosis

The reduction in all forms of tuberculosis has been notable and progressive in recent times as can be seen from the percentages of fall in the death rates of tuberculosis per 100,000 population in the City of New York and the United States during the past ten years.

	Death rate per 100,000 from Tuberculosis			Per cent of reduction	
	1910	1920	(1921)	1910–20	1910–21
New York City...............	210	126	(103)	40.0%	50.9%
United States (continental).....	160	114		28.7%	
(Reduction in New York City, 1920–21............18.3%)					

Variations in the Death Rate from Tuberculosis among Nations, States and Districts of a City

Whether we look on the death rates from tuberculosis as students of international relations or as analysts of regional variations among the states of the Union, or as interested citizens of our own metropolis, we find wide variations in the death rates from tuberculosis. Several cities* and large parts of the rural population in central and eastern Europe show death rates even in 1920 as high as 400 per 100,000 per annum, while Australia boasts a rate of under 75. Among our cities, where there is a preponderance of colored or Irish population, rates of 250 or over are not uncommon, while in the states of Kansas (1,800,000) and Utah (449,396) and Oregon (783,000) the rates per 100,000 for 1920 were Utah 40.8, Kansas 47.4 and Oregon 86.2. Similarly, within the City of New York there are large units of the population so favored by race, education and economic status that rates of 50 and under prevail among them (96,289) while in others less fortunately situated to resist disease we find 231,780 of our fellow citizens supporting a tuberculosis death rate of over 300 per 100,000 per annum. (Fig. 32)

Reduction of Rates Not a Matter of Chance

That these wide discrepancies in the burden of deaths tolerated by different communities, be they urban, statewide or national, are not accidental but result from controllable factors of environment and human relationships is known to physicians and economists.

That reductions, where they have occurred, are due and in proportion to consistent effort and intelligent direction in the prevention and treatment of the disease is accepted by special students of, and authorities on, tuberculosis.

That there is nothing unreasonable or improbable in the expectation that we can accomplish a reduction of 50 per cent in the incidence and deaths from tuberculosis by applying well-known measures to groups of urban and rural communities is shown by the experience with logical and adequate preventive services demonstrated at Framingham, Mass., during the past five years where as a direct result of combined medical and social attack

*1920 Death rate per 100,000 population from Tuberculosis. Vienna, 405; Warsaw, 338; Budapest, 376; Prague, 324; Paris, 279; Berlin, 177; Amsterdam, 156; Florence, 298; Koln, 179.

upon tuberculosis in a population of 17,000 the death rate has been reduced from a rate of 121 to one of 40 per 100,000, a reduction of 67 per cent.

The Cost of Preventive Service

Experience with the treatment, prevention, cure and education of the tuberculous even under the difficult conditions, as to race and economic status, which prevail among the crowded and partly dependent tenement house dwellers of this City, demonstrates the practicability of accomplishing very great reductions in the development of the disease and postponement of deaths from the disease such as have already been attained at Framingham, Mass. at a total cost to the community of $2.40 per capita per annum.

Costs and Savings in the Reduction of Tuberculosis

Admitting for the sake of discussion the correctness of the estimates of losses which are likely to be suffered from tuberculosis by the Nation and by the City of New York in 1922; namely, $863,409,615 and $46,552,500, respectively, a reduction in the death rate of 50 per cent with an equivalent and simultaneous reduction in the sickness from tuberculosis would mean a saving of $431,704,808 for the Nation and $23,276,250 for the City in the year 1926. Theoretically this can be accomplished at an expenditure of $3.00 per capita for five years, or for the two population groups $17,550,000 per annum for the City and $325,500,000 for the Nation.

It is not within the limits of exact facts to picture the reduction from year to year during the five-year period but if we believe we can accomplish a reduction of 50 per cent in the fifth year we must have faith and confidence that during the five years and prior to the completion of the service there will have been exhibited substantial reductions each year. We can properly consider that each year the cost of service should fall with a steadily diminishing number of people sick with tuberculosis to be cared for and when we start at the sixth year we find ourselves facing not the 1922 situation over again but a community suffering only one-half the losses of 1922 and already losing but $3.98 per capita in 1927 from the disease and a much diminished cost of service, how much less it is impracticable to estimate since one of the most effective means to be counted upon for final reduction of the disease is an annual periodic medical examination of each member of the community and up to the present time the costs of this have not been determined, although it is difficult to see how the cost of a preventive service could be reduced much below $3.00 and still give the protective diagnostic skill which would be needed.

In a broad way, we can reasonably expect increased savings from a decreased expenditure:

Losses in 1922 per capita of population..........................$7.96
Estimated cost of preventive service per capita of population annually
  1922–26, inclusive.. 3.00
Losses in 1926 per capita of population........................... 3.98
Estimated cost of preventive service per capita of population 1927.. 2.75

A Practical Trial within our Reach

Presuming that it would be no matter of great difficulty to obtain a sum adequate to meet the cost for a period of five years to extend a demonstration, which has already been carried to a successful conclusion in Framingham, Mass., to a district within the City of New York or in the populations adjacent to the city which can be properly described as suburban or rural, a study of the elements which might determine the selection of a population group or a district within which to apply such a fund at the rate above suggested has been made.

Presuming that an expenditure of $1,500,000 a year for five years was provided for from public and private sources to apply a consistent and liberal policy for prevention of tuberculosis, according to the best available present-day knowledge, in not more than three groups in New York City and State with a combined population of not over 500,000, we would doubtless show savings in the year, 1926, in terms of deaths postponed, sickness avoided and costs of life reduced in these groups of

225 deaths from tuberculosis postponed; 1,575 cases of sickness from tuberculosis avoided. $1,990,000 spared to the community because of reduced costs of deaths and disease.

Deaths at rate of 90 for tuberculosis, all forms, in population of 500,000 would be 450 a year. A 50 per cent reduction would result in 225 deaths postponed in 1926. Sickness from tuberculosis at rate of 7 active cases per death per annum would be 3,150. A 50 per cent reduction would result in 1,575.

Cost of sickness at rate of two and one-third years of sickness and $1,500 per year for professional care or care and relief would be $1,575,000. A 50 per cent reduction in cost of sickness would be $787,500.

Cost of deaths among 500,000 population at the rate of cost for a city of 5,850,000 would be $2,403,847. A 50 per cent reduction in cost of deaths per 500,000 would be $1,201,928.

There will remain as a burden upon the community of 500,000 people a wastage of $1,989,428 in the sixth year due to tuberculosis, in the reduction of which we should obviously have to expend a smaller sum per capita of population than has been supposed to be needed in the first five years. In other words, the costs of preventive service will fall, though not at an equal rate with the diminution in losses to the community from the disease.

That this measures only certain crude savings is obvious to any one familiar with past experience where any large group of diseases or cause of a large group of deaths as the enteric diseases, the diseases of infancy and the acute infectious fevers have been materially reduced, since in the case of each such material reduction of particular diseases, there has been a notable and persistent reduction in many other causes of sickness and deaths not obviously related to the particular disease reduced.

Furthermore, in dealing with a carrier disease, of which the distribution is due to the great prevalence of carriers of the tubercle bacilli which are commonly discharged in the sputum and over very large periods of time in the lives of many of the unrecognized cases and in a majority of those acutely ill with the disease, a reduction of 50 per cent in the deaths and prior sickness from the disease will result in a greater reduction in the community cost in subsequent years, and an increasing relative savings in lives and cost in proportion to the expenditure of time, effort and money in control and prevention by isolation.

In other words, the savings expressed in terms of dollars in the fifth year of the undertaking represent not an individual or unique saving for one year, but a stage in an increasing and continuous saving to endure at least at the same rate and probably at a greater rate in subsequent years.

In fact, now that the gradually developing evidences of result from the many years of intelligent educational, sanitary, and medical effort in the control of tuberculosis are becoming manifest, it is apparent that this disease can actually be rendered a negligible factor in mortality and morbidity if we push our attack with the liberality called for in the premises.

With the facts in hand, as to the burden in loss of life and wealth which tuberculosis still causes, in spite of the reduction in deaths from the disease in the more favored countries, cities and economic groups; and accepting as sound and practical the methods, by which in Framingham, Mass., a further great reduction in deaths and sickness from this disease has been accomplished; and admitting as reasonable and accurate the estimates of cost, of a repetition of such services in New York City based upon the experience of the A. I. C. P. in its Home Hospital experiment during the past seven years: it is presumed that the logical next step is to invest further in life-saving, with the obvious and calculable result of earning for the population group selected, dividends in amount, whether expressed in human life or wealth, to justify an expenditure at least twice the per capita cost of the best modern municipal public health service.

It is believed that if three population groups of approximately 200,000 each, one in New York City, one in a city of the second class in New York State and one including a smaller city and a large rural or country area in New York State, were so served by the judicious investment of $3.00 per capita for the prevention and treatment of tuberculosis among them in addition to the expenditures now made by these various communities for purposes directly or remotely assisting in the control and care of tuberculosis, as to reduce the death rate per 100,000 per annum in 5 years by 50 per cent, the effect upon the districts selected, upon the nation, and upon the opinion and wealth of the world as a whole would be such as to convince all nations and communities of their obligation to make at least the same effort and probably to oust tuberculosis from its position as the greatest single destroyer of life and property today.

January 17, 1922.

MILBANK MEMORIAL FUND

QUARTERLY BULLETIN

NEW YORK HEALTH DEMONSTRATIONS

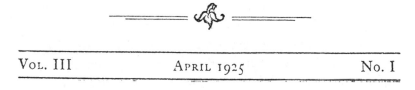

| Vol. III | April 1925 | No. I |

TWO YEARS *of* PUBLIC HEALTH DEMONSTRATION

by John A. Kingsbury, *Secretary*
Milbank Memorial Fund

IN the light of two years' experience in their organization and development, it was possible at a recent meeting of its Technical Board to re-examine the aims and purposes of the three health demonstrations which are at present enlisting the chief interest and support of the Milbank Memorial Fund. Work done in the rural health demonstration in Cattaraugus County and in the urban health demonstration in Syracuse, was reviewed, and an attempt was made to assess the relative importance of the various health activities included in the programs being carried out in these communities. The discussion included an inquiry into the social significance of the major health problems presented in these localities and in the Bellevue-Yorkville district of New York City, as a means of determining anew the degree of emphasis which should be placed on the various projects included in the health demonstration programs. Two days, February twenty-seventh and twenty-eighth, were given over to the discussions.

The Milbank Memorial Fund QUARTERLY BULLETIN is published by the Milbank Memorial Fund, 49 Wall Street, New York.

Although the New York Health Demonstrations are concerned with measures which have been for the most part settled by experiment, the procedure of development has been and will continue to be essentially experimental, with all that implies. It is believed that the health demonstration districts provide fertile fields for the discovery of additional information about disease prevention and control and about health administration in general, and that they should throw new light upon the social factors involved in such community undertakings as well as upon the reaction of community groups to the measures introduced and their willingness to support them. The health demonstrations deal with large population groups, varied in character, living under different environmental conditions. They are concerned with all age groups. There is general participation, every organization, both public and private, and every individual in the demonstration units being included. There is no sharp time limit on the undertakings. They deal with health, not in its narrowest sense, but rather in the broader sense of its social implications. Always pertinent, therefore, is a critical review, such as that made at the recent Technical Board meeting, of the general health demonstrations program, its aims, methods and procedures.

In addition to making an appraisal of the available health and social statistical data, the Technical Board examined the types of organization and health services which had been set up and developed in Cattaraugus County and in Syracuse; the co-ordination which has been effected between existing public and private health agencies; and the measure of success which has been attained in perfecting co-operation between the voluntary health agencies, the private organizations and the public health officials. The Board reviewed the qualifications of the directing personnel and attempted to measure the success they had had in adjusting themselves to the local situations which they had found and to the changes which had arisen. Through a consideration of the sums it was found necessary to include in the budgets, the Board also attempted to determine the amount and importance of the local community participation in the health demonstrations, as measured by their assumption of the costs of the new elements in their community health program.

All of the work of the rural health demonstration in Cattaraugus County, it was reported, has been carried on under the appropriate local authorities and agencies there. The County Board of Health, with an adequately equipped personnel, is operating in an efficient manner. Village and town health officers have participated in the demonstration, and there has been no opposition to the project by either lay or medical groups. The press has been generally favorable to the work. Both public appropriations and volunteer contributions to public health work in the County have greatly increased since the beginning of the demonstration there.

The general death rate and the infant mortality rate were shown to have decreased in the County in 1924, as compared with the average for the previous five years, and with those of the control counties as a whole—Jefferson, Steuben and Washington, all in New York State. The death rate from tuberculosis also shows a slight decrease. For the length of time the rural health demonstration has been under way, its work in the prevention and control of tuberculosis, measured by the number of cases under supervision, the percentage of incipient cases reported, and the increase in the numbers under sanatorium or home care, compares favorably with the results achieved in the Framingham project, which specialized in this disease.

Progress in the urban health demonstration in Syracuse,

New York, has been made wholly through the development of the work of the Department of Health there, together with that of the Bureau of Health Supervision, which is under the supervision of the local Board of Education, and that of existing voluntary agencies, including the Onondaga Health Association. Effort has been directed toward securing effective administrative organization and control of important and developing health services in the City.

Various bureaus of the Health Department have been strengthened, particularly those in charge of tuberculosis work, communicable diseases, medical work in parochial schools and child hygiene. An effective Bureau of Public Health Education has been established, and the Bureau of Records and Reports has been made more potent.

As in Cattaraugus County, public appropriations for health work in Syracuse have materially increased since the demonstration started. There is evidence of full understanding and complete appreciation by the fiscal authorities of the value of the demonstration activities, their benefits to the people of the City, and the propriety with which many of them could become municipal charges.

The general death rate, infant death rate, tuberculosis death rate, and other rates, show a very favorable comparison with the previous five years, and while, as yet, the demonstration activities have not been in operation long enough to trace this decrease to the demonstration, it is probable that in some measure, the improved position of Syracuse in relation to the control cities (Albany, Troy, Utica, Rochester and Yonkers) of the State in this respect is due to the health campaign.

In both the Cattaraugus County and Syracuse projects, there has been gratifying co-operation and generous participation by the New York State Department of Health, the

State Mental Deficiency Commission, and by the State Department of Education. Although at first unofficially organized, the rural school health work in Cattaraugus County has already led to legislation which not only makes official the school hygiene program carried out there, but which makes permissive the establishment of county school hygiene districts throughout New York State.

While the demonstration in the Bellevue-Yorkville district of New York City is still in its initial stages, it is reported that the active co-operation of both public health and voluntary health organizations has been secured and the foundations laid for the successful operation of the proposed program for this demonstration.

The Cattaraugus County Board of Supervisors recently appropriated $10,000 for the construction of an addition to the County tuberculosis sanatorium. The present institution, which has a bed capacity for the treatment of forty patients, has recently undergone repairs and renovation.

Forty patients were admitted to the County Sanitorium during the fiscal year ending in 1923, and eighty-four during the same period in 1924—an increase of 110 per cent.

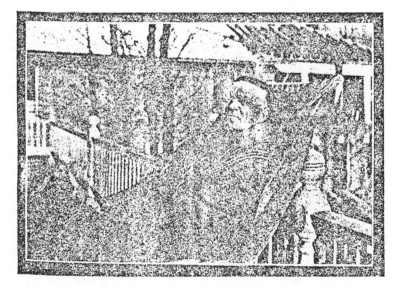

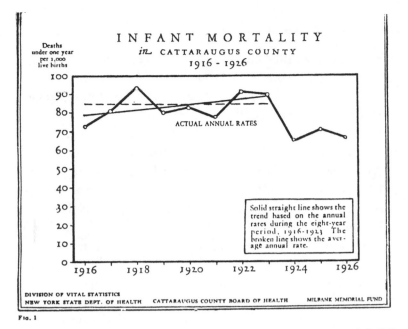

INFANT MORTALITY in CATTARAUGUS COUNTY 1916 - 1926

Deaths under one year per 1,000 live births

ACTUAL ANNUAL RATES

Solid straight line shows the trend based on the annual rates during the eight-year period, 1916-1923. The broken line shows the average annual rate.

DIVISION OF VITAL STATISTICS
NEW YORK STATE DEPT. OF HEALTH   CATTARAUGUS COUNTY BOARD OF HEALTH   MILBANK MEMORIAL FUND

Fig. 1

INFANT MORTALITY IN CATTARAUGUS COUNTY*
by Dorothy Gerard Wiehl
Assistant Statistician, United States Public Health Service

RECENT years have recorded a sudden decline in Cattaraugus County in the mortality of infants under one year of age. During the three years 1924, 1925 and 1926, the infant mortality rates there were lower than in any of the previous eight years, the decline marking a definite departure from an upward trend which had been in progress from 1916 to 1923. Study of the causes to which these infant deaths had been attributed, shows that the three-year decline was due principally to a falling off in the number of deaths from diseases generally designated as preventable, that is, from communicable diseases, from gastro-intestinal diseases and from respiratory diseases. Comparisons have brought out that, during the years 1924 and 1925, the infant mortality

*From the Statistical Office of the Milbank Memorial Fund.

from these preventable causes was higher in each of four other New York counties than it was in Cattaraugus.

That the mortality among children under one year of age in Cattaraugus showed an improvement in the years 1924, 1925 and 1926 over the preceding eight years is obvious from the annual rates* shown in Table 1 and Fig. 1. The rate in each of these years was lower than the rate for any of the previous eight years and it follows that the average rate for the three years was much lower than the average for the eight years.

The significance of this improvement can be judged from (1) comparison with the changes in the annual mortality in the County in previous years to determine whether such a decline might have been expected and (2) comparison with other areas to determine whether or not this decline has been common to other rural sections of the State and nation.

Comparison of Current with Earlier Years

In the first comparison, it is necessary to decide on the basis of eight years' experience in Cattaraugus County what might reasonably have been expected in the next few years if the factors affecting infant mortality in the County had continued unchanged. The shortness of the period and the wide variation in the rates for these eight years make it very difficult to determine any real trend in the mortality in the County. The actual rates plotted in Fig. 1 suggest a tendency for the mortality to increase from 1916 to 1923, and a straight line fitted to the eight points by the method of least squares† has a decided upward slope, as shown in the chart. It is quite evident that the slope of this trend line is influenced greatly by the low rate in 1916, which was offset to some extent by the high rate in 1918, and by the two high rates in 1922 and 1923. In some years the actual rates do not

*Throughout this study, the rates are based on infant deaths and births exclusive of Indians.
†The line was fitted to the eight annual rates by the equation $y = a + bx$.

Table 1. Deaths of children under one year of age, per 1,000 live births (infant mortality) in Cattaraugus County, 1916-1926.*

NUMBER AND RATE	YEAR										
	1916	1917	1918	1919	1920	1921	1922	1923	1924	1925	1926
Death rate per 1,000 live births	73.0	81.6	94.7	80.6	83.4	78.1	91.9	90.2	65.8	71.6	67.0
Number deaths under 1 year	109	115	147	118	129	129	145	130	97	102	95
Number live births	1,493	1,409	1,553	1,464	1,547	1,652	1,578	1,442	1,474	1,425	1,417

*The deaths of Indian children under one year of age and Indian births in Cattaraugus County have been excluded.

fall very close to the straight line, and it is doubtful that this line can be taken as representative of any real trend for the period as a whole. In fact, when the significance of the slope of the line is tested statistically, the slope (b in the equation) is found to be only three and a half times its probable error. It would seem very likely, therefore, that the trend of infant mortality in the County had been upward for this specific period, but it is not possible to determine accurately a defifinite rate of increase.*

Therefore, instead of comparing the infant mortality in 1924, 1925 and 1926 with the high point of 1923, or with an "expected rate" in those years based on a projection of the trend line for the preceding eight years, the more conservative comparison is made between the average rate for the eight years from 1916 to 1923, and the succeeding years. The difference between the average rate for the years 1916-1923, and the average rate for the years 1924-1926 was sixteen per 1,000 births, which is more than five times the probable error of the difference in the rates and undoubtedly indicates a significant change for the better in the infant mortality.

*The deaths under one year of age, but not the births, are available back to 1900. The infant death rates based on the total population of the County for the years 1900-1915 indicate an upward trend for this longer period, though the upward slope is less marked than for the eight years 1916-1923.

Table 2. Deaths of children under one year of age, per 1,000 live births (infant mortality) in Cattaraugus County, in Rural New York State, and in the Rural Birth Registration Area,* 1916-1926.

AREA	DEATHS UNDER ONE YEAR PER 1,000 LIVE BIRTHS										
	1916	1917	1918	1919	1920	1921	1922	1923	1924	1925	1926
Cattaraugus County	73.0	81.6	94.7	80.6	83.4	78.1	91.9	90.2	65.8	71.6	67.0
Rural New York State	83.1	85.4	92.8	76.9	78.2	73.7	74.2	76.9	67.5	66.8	73.1
Rural Birth Registration Area*	96.7	87.8	93.5	82.9	79.4	73.7	72.2	76.1	68.9	71.5	

*Area as of 1917, exclusive of Rhode Island, except for the year 1916.

Comparison of Cattaraugus County with Other Areas*

The second comparison is shown in Figs. 2 and 3 and in Table 2. Here, the trend of the infant mortality rate in Cattaraugus County during the eight-year period, 1916 to 1923, is compared with that in the rural area of New York State and that in the rural birth registration area of the United States, as of 1917.

The actual rates in the rural area of New York and in the rural birth registration area of the country show much less annual variation than Cattaraugus County due to the fact that they are average rates for many areas such as Cattaraugus County, in which the chance fluctuations compensate giving a more *stable* rate. The straight line trends fitted to these rates indicate a definite *downward* course and the slope of the lines in these larger areas is statistically significant. If "expected rates" for these two rural areas were computed by

*The sources of the data used in this study are as follows: the data for Cattaraugus County are taken from two sources—(1) special tabulations for the years 1916 to 1924, inclusive, made for the Milbank Memorial Fund from the records of the Division of Vital Statistics, New York State Department of Health; and (2) tabulation of duplicate death certificates for 1925 and 1926, now in the files of the Cattaraugus County Health Department.

For other counties and for rural New York State, the data up to 1924 are from the annual reports of the Division of Vital Statistics. For the year 1925, a special manuscript table was supplied by the Division of Vital Statistics. For the year 1926 only the gross infant mortality rates were available, and these are provisional figures from the *Annual Supplement* to the *Monthly Vital Statistics Review*.

Statistics for the rural birth registration area of the United States are from the annual reports of the Census Bureau on Birth Statistics and Infant Mortality for the years 1916 to 1924. Figures for 1925 were furnished by the Census Bureau in manuscript, but for 1926 no data were available.

projecting the trend lines for the years following 1923, the rates so obtained would not vary greatly from the actual rates. In other words, the experience in these two large areas indicates a continuation of the same downward trend in 1924 and 1925, which had been in progress for the previous eight years. In Cattaraugus, however, a sharp decline occurred in 1924, and was maintained in 1925 and 1926. Whether this break is measured from an upward trend or from a level it seems to indicate a significant change in the rate.

A comparison of the annual infant mortality in Cattaraugus County with that in four other New York counties is

Fig. 2. Deaths of children under one year of age per 1,000 live births (infant mortality)in Cattaraugus County and in the rural areas of New York State, 1916–1926.

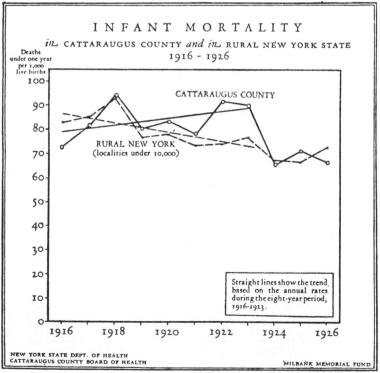

made in Table 3. The mortality in Chautauqua and Jefferson Counties shows a definite downward trend throughout the period, similar to that for rural New York State. The course of the mortality in Steuben and Washington has been very irregular and unlike that in Cattaraugus County or the other two counties. In these counties, the mortality from 1923 to 1926, inclusive, was less favorable than in the preceding years. The general level of the rates in all four counties in the three most recent years is very similar to that in Cattaraugus, but none show the same abrupt improvement.

Important Causes of Infant Mortality in Cattaraugus County

The most important causes of mortality in the first year of life are (1) premature birth, (2) congenital defects and other conditions of early infancy, (3) injury at birth, (4) communicable diseases, (5) gastro-intestinal conditions and (6) respiratory diseases. The first three causes are subdivisions of the broad group of conditions classified by the International List of Causes of Death as "Malformations and Early Infancy." These six causes in nearly every year were responsible for approximately nine-tenths of all the infant deaths in Cattaraugus County. The percentage distribution of the infant deaths according to these important causes is shown in Table

Table 3. Deaths of children under one year of age, per 1,000 live births (infant mortality) in Cattaraugus County and in four other counties in New York State, 1916-1926.

| COUNTY | DEATHS UNDER ONE YEAR PER 1,000 LIVE BIRTHS | | | | | | | | | | |
	1916	1917	1918	1919	1920	1921	1922	1923	1924	1925	1926
Cattaraugus	73.0	81.6	94.7	80.6	83.4	78.1	91.9	90.2	65.8	71.6	67.0
Chautauqua	87.9	89.0	85.3	78.4	75.7	70.6	67.0	74.7	72.2	61.0	56.2
Jefferson	118.3	105.1	107.3	77.4	93.5	90.7	88.0	75.7	75.8	68.3	83.9
Steuben	78.2	81.9	96.4	67.7	65.4	65.7	60.1	94.9	67.6	67.9	83.0
Washington	86.8	107.3	112.3	65.3	75.3	64.1	75.3	87.9	72.0	77.2	86.3

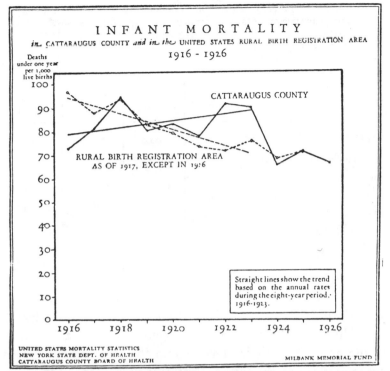

Fig. 3. Deaths of children under one year of age per 1,000 live births (infant mortality) in Cattaraugus County and in the rural birth registration area of the United States as of 1917, except in 1916, 1916–1926.

4, after the annual figures were combined into three periods of years. Since the number of deaths from specific causes in a single year is small and subject to wide fluctuation, the average numbers for several years give a more reliable picture.

Premature birth stands out as the most important cause of·infant death in Cattaraugus County. In each of the three periods it was responsible for from 32 to 36 per cent of the total deaths. Malformations, debility and other congenital conditions caused approximately 18 per cent of the deaths in the periods 1916-1920, and 1921-1923, and 25 per cent in the period 1924-1926. Injury at birth added another 5 to 8 per

Table 4. Percentage distribution of deaths of children under one year of age (infant mortality) by important causes,* in Cattaraugus County, in three periods of years, 1916-1920, 1921-1923, and 1924-1926.

Cause* of Death	Per Cent of Total		
	1916-1920	1921-1923	1924-1926
TOTAL	100.0	100.0	100.0
Communicable diseases (1-16)	5.0	3.5	3.4
Respiratory diseases and pulmonary tuberculosis (97-107, 31, 37a)	14.8	14.4	8.2
Gastro-intestinal diseases (112-113)	14.1	15.3	10.9
Malformations and early infancy (159, 160, 161, 162, 163)	56.2	56.4	69.4
Premature birth (161a)	33.7	31.7	35.7
Injury at birth (161b)	5.2	6.4	8.5
Congenital malformations, debility, and other infancy (159, 160, 162-163)	17.6	18.3	25.2
All other causes	9.9	10.4	8.2

*Numbers in parentheses refer to classifications in the International List, 1920 Revision.

cent to the mortality from the broad group of causes classed as "Malformations and Early Infancy." The total deaths from this general group was 56 per cent of all infant mortality in the first two periods of years and the large amount of 69 per cent in the latest period. Respiratory diseases and gastro-intestinal diseases were each, as a group, of about equal importance and were responsible for approximately 15 per cent of the total deaths during the years 1916-1920 and 1921-1923, but for the period 1924-1926, these groups caused 8 and 11 per cent respectively of the total deaths. Communicable diseases* in most years was not a very important cause of death, the average mortality from this cause for the three periods ranging from 3.5 to 5 per cent of the total.

The trend of the mortality from each group of causes in the County, except communicable diseases, is shown in Fig. 4 in which the annual rates shown in Table 5 have been plotted on a logarithmic ordinate scale. The five lines in this

*This group includes number 1 to 16, inclusive, of the International List, but in Cattaraugus from 1916 to 1926 deaths were reported only from measles, whooping cough, diphtheria and influenza.

Table 5. Deaths of children under one year of age (infant mortality), from important causes,* in Cattaraugus County, 1916-1926.

CAUSE* OF DEATH	DEATHS UNDER ONE YEAR PER 1,000 LIVE BIRTHS										
	1916	1917	1918	1919	1920	1921	1922	1923	1924	1925	1926
All Causes	73.0	81.6	94.7	80.6	83.4	78.1	91.9	90.2	65.8	71.6	67.0
Communicable diseases (1-16)	2.7	0.7	5.8	2.0	10.3	1.8	1.9	5.5	3.4	1.4	2.1
Respiratory diseases (31, 37a, 97-107)	10.7	16.3	18.0	8.9	7.1	10.9	12.7	13.9	4.7	6.3	5.6
Gastro-intestinal diseases (112-113)	12.7	12.8	14.2	11.6	7.1	14.5	13.3	11.8	6.8	8.4	7.1
Malformations and early infancy (159-163)	42.9	41.2	47.6	46.4	53.0	43.0	53.9	49.9	43.4	49.1	49.4
Premature birth (161a)	30.8	27.7	29.0	25.3	25.2	27.2	27.2	27.7	22.4	25.3	25.4
Injury at birth (161b)	2.0	2.8	4.5	4.1	7.8	3.6	6.3	6.9	6.8	4.2	6.4
All other infancy (159, 160, 162-163)	10.0	10.6	14.2	17.1	20.0	12.1	20.3	15.3	14.2	19.6	17.6
All other causes	4.0	10.6	9.0	11.6	5.8	7.9	10.1	9.0	7.5	6.3	2.8

NUMBER OF DEATHS UNDER ONE YEAR											
All Causes	109	115	147	118	129	129	145	130	97	102	95
Communicable diseases (1-16)	4	1	9	3	16	3	3	8	5	2	3
Respiratory diseases (31, 37a, 97-107)	16	23	28	13	11	18	20	20	7	9	8
Gastro-intestinal diseases (112-113)	19	18	22	17	11	24	21	17	10	12	10
Malformations and early infancy (159-163)	64	58	74	68	82	71	85	72	64	70	70
Premature birth (161a)	46	39	45	37	39	45	43	40	33	36	36
Injury at birth (161b)	3	4	7	6	12	6	10	10	10	6	9
All other infancy (159, 160, 162-163)	15	15	22	25	31	20	32	22	21	28	25
All other causes	6	15	14	17	9	13	16	13	11	9	4

*Numbers in parentheses refer to classifications in the International List, 1920 Revision.

figure are strikingly different, and it is quite apparent that the mortality from some causes has increased during the eleven years from 1916 to 1926, while from others it has decreased. Deaths from premature birth show the least fluctuation but the logarithmic line indicates a slight downward trend. Other conditions of early infancy have shown just the opposite trend and the mortality both from injury at birth and from congenital defects had a marked increase during the first five years of the period after which it seems to have remained approximately on a level, although wide fluctuations have occurred in some years.

When the trend of infant mortality from respiratory diseases and from gastro-intestinal conditions is considered a more encouraging outlook is obtained. The course of both groups for Cattaraugus County has been decidedly similar: the mortality from each group was high in 1917 and 1918, followed by a drop to quite a low rate in 1920, after which another high period of three years occurred and was succeeded by a decline in 1924, which lasted three years. With the exception of the low rate in 1920, mortality from gastro-intestinal diseases shows relatively small variations about a level for the years from 1916 to 1923, but that from respiratory diseases shows greater variation. The sharp decline in mortality in the three years 1924 to 1926, which was so marked in the death rate from all causes is found to be common to that from respiratory and gastro-intestinal diseases.

For a comparison of the percentage increase or decrease in the different causes, the average mortality in the last three years of the study has been compared with the average for the preceding three-year period which, in turn, has been compared with the five-year period 1916-1920. The mean rates and the percentage change are shown in Table 6.

The mean infant mortality rate in Cattaraugus County for the three years 1921-1923 was approximately 5 per cent higher than for the five years 1916-1920. Each of the major causes showed some increase, except premature birth, which remained the same, and communicable diseases which showed a decrease.* The increase in infant mortality from respiratory diseases was not significant being only 2 per cent.

*When deaths from influenza are excluded from the communicable disease group the mortality in the two periods is nearly constant, being 2.3 per 1,000 live births in the first period and 2.1 in the second.

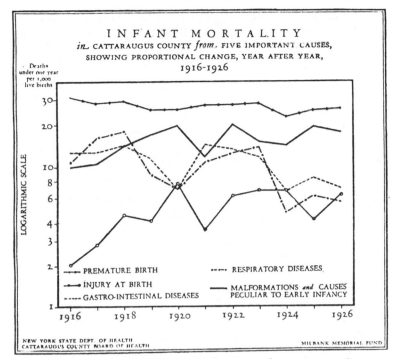

Fig. 4. Deaths of children under one year of age per 1,000 live births (infant mortality) in Cattaraugus County from five important causes, showing proportional change, year after year, 1916–1926.

The increase in the mortality from gastro-intestinal diseases, from malformations and other congenital conditions and from "all other causes" ranged from 10 to 14 per cent. Deaths from injury at birth increased 30 per cent, but this figure is based on a small number of deaths.

The abrupt decline in the three latest years (1924-1926) brought the mean infant mortality from all causes in the County a little more than 20 per cent lower than the mean mortality in the preceding three-year period. It is interesting to note that the decline in the mortality from specific causes bears no relation to the increase that had occurred in the previous years. Thus, deaths from injury at birth showed a

Table 6. Per cent of change in deaths of children under one year of age (infant mortality), from important causes,* in Cattaraugus County, in the three-year periods, 1921-1923 and 1924-1926, over the average rates for a preceding period.

CAUSE* OF DEATH	RATE PER 1,000			PERCENTAGE CHANGE	
	1916-20	1921-23	1924-26	1921-23 OVER 1916-20	1924-26 OVER 1921-23
TOTAL	82.51	86.47	68.12	+ 4.8	−21.2
Communicable diseases (1-16)	4.15	3.00	2.32	−27.7	−22.7
Respiratory diseases (97-107, 31, 37a)	12.19	12.41	5.56	+ 1.8	−55.2
Gastro-intestinal diseases (112-113)	11.65	13.27	7.41	+13.9	−44.2
Malformations and early infancy (159-163)	46.34	48.80	47.27	+ 5.3	− 3.1
Premature birth (161a)	27.59	27.40	24.33	− 0.7	−11.2
Injuries at birth (161b)	4.29	5.57	5.79	+29.8	+ 3.9
Congenital malformations, debility and other infancy (159, 160, 162, 163)	14.47	15.84	17.14	+10.94	+ 8.2
All other causes	8.17	8.99	5.56	+10.0	−38.2

*Numbers in parentheses refer to classifications in the International List, 1920 Revision

further slight increase, and the deaths from malformations, debility and other conditions of early infancy increased 8 per cent. Deaths from premature birth, which had not increased in the former period declined 11 per cent. The most significant decrease was in the deaths from gastro-intestinal and respiratory diseases which declined 44 and 55 per cent.

Of the specific causes considered separately in the above tables and discussion, three are recognized as largely preventable. Deaths from communicable diseases, the respiratory diseases and from gastro-intestinal diseases should be very rare if modern knowledge of sanitation, control of diseases and infant care were utilized to the fullest extent by individual families and health departments. It is, therefore, extremely encouraging to find that the infant deaths from these three groups of causes in Cattaraugus County in the years 1924 to 1926 was 15.3 per 1,000 live births against 28.7 in the preceding three-year period, a decline of 47 per cent in the mortal-

ity rate and a saving of thirteen infant lives out of each one
thousand born alive.

In marked contrast is the very slight decline which has
occurred in the mortality due to congenital defects and conditions at birth. These causes obviously are associated with
heredity and prenatal conditions for the prevention of which
specific activities are not as yet well defined. The mean mortality in the period 1924-1926 from these causes was 47.3 per
1,000 live births against 48.8 in the preceding three-year
period, a decline of only 3 per cent and a saving of only three
infants out of each two thousand born alive. These congenital
and early infancy conditions offer a very difficult and complex problem which is a challenge to any health department.

Important Causes of Infant Mortality in Four Other New York Counties

Only the mean infant mortality from certain important
causes for the first five years was available for counties other
than Cattaraugus. These rates are shown in Table 7. The
annual deaths from 1921 to 1925 were available but these
have been combined into two periods, and the mean rate for
the three years 1921 to 1923, and for two years 1924 to 1925,
are shown in the same table with corresponding rates for
Cattaraugus County. Although these unequal time periods
are not ideal they give a satisfactory basis for several interesting and probably significant comparisons. To set forth
more clearly the relative mortality in the different counties
the ratios of the mortality rates in the several counties from
each cause and in each period to the corresponding rate in
Cattaraugus County are shown in the table.

Considering first the earliest period, we find that the mean
infant mortality in Cattaraugus County from each of these
causes except premature birth was approximately the same
or lower than in the other counties with the exception that

Table 7. Deaths of children under one year of age (infant mortality), from important causes,* in Cattaraugus County, compared with four other counties in New York State in three different time periods from 1916 to 1925.

COUNTY	Deaths Under 1 Year Per 1,000 Live Births			Ratio of Rates in Other Counties to Cattaraugus Rates†		
	1916-1920	1921-1923	1924-1925	1916-1920	1921-1923	1924-1925
Total Under 1 Year						
Cattaraugus	82.8	86.5	68.6	1.00	1.00	1.00
Chautauqua	83.4	70.8	66.7	1.01	.82	.97
Jefferson	100.1	84.9	72.0	1.21	.98	1.05
Steuben	78.1	73.0	67.7	.94	.84	.99
Washington	89.7	75.8	74.5	1.08	.88	1.09
Communicable Diseases (1-16)						
Cattaraugus	4.4	3.0	2.4	1.00	1.00	1.00
Chautauqua	6.7	5.0	2.7	1.52	1.68	1.12
Jefferson	7.7	5.2	2.9	1.75	1.73	1.19
Steuben	6.8	4.1	3.7	1.55	1.37	1.52
Washington	7.1	2.3	3.9	1.61	.78	1.61
Respiratory Diseases (31, 37a, 97-107)						
Cattaraugus	12.2	12.4	5.5	1.00	1.00	1.00
Chautauqua	11.7	9.3	9.1	.96	.75	1.65
Jefferson	13.0	11.0	6.9	1.07	.88	1.24
Steuben	8.7	10.0	7.3	.71	.80	1.33
Washington	16.5	8.6	9.5	1.35	.69	1.71
Gastro-Intestinal Diseases (112-113)						
Cattaraugus	11.7	13.3	7.6	1.00	1.00	1.00
Chautauqua	15.0	9.3	8.1	1.28	.70	1.06
Jefferson	16.0	11.1	7.7	1.37	.84	1.02
Steuben	9.9	10.3	11.6	.85	.78	1.53
Washington	15.3	10.9	12.2	1.31	.82	1.61
Premature Birth (161a)						
Cattaraugus	27.6	27.4	23.8	1.00	1.00	1.00
Chautauqua	20.8	20.9	17.6	.75	.76	.74
Jefferson	25.5	20.6	21.1	.92	.75	.89
Steuben	21.1	18.7	18.9	.76	.68	.79
Washington	23.6	23.3	21 7	.86	.85	.91
Congenital Malformations, Debility and Other Infancy (159-160, 161b, 162-3)						
Cattaraugus	18.8	21.4	22.4	1.00	1.00	1.00
Chautauqua	21.3	20.0	20.3	1.13	.94	.90
Jefferson	24.9	25.3	22.3	1.32	1.18	.99
Steuben	23.6	21.5	20.1	1.26	1.00	.90
Washington	17.7	19.0	20.0	.94	.89	.89
All Other Causes						
Cattaraugus	8.2	9.0	6.9	1.00	1.00	1.00
Chautauqua	7.9	6.3	8.9	.96	.70	1.29
Jefferson	13.0	11.7	11.1	1.59	1.30	1.61
Steuben	8.1	8.4	6.1	.99	.93	.88
Washington	9.4	11.7	7.2	1.15	1.30	1.05

*Numbers in parentheses refer to classifications in the International List, 1920 Revision.

†Ratios are computed on rates to two decimals.

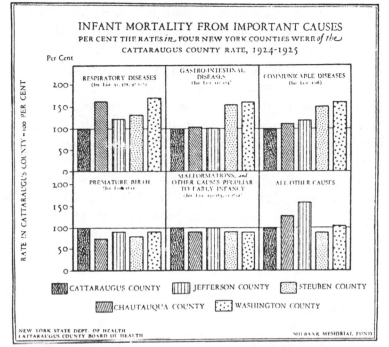

Fig. 5. Deaths from important causes of children under one year of age per 1,000 live births (infant mortality). Per cent the rates in four New York Counties were of the Cattaraugus County rate, 1924–1925.

the mortality from both respiratory and gastro-intestinal diseases was lower in Steuben County than in Cattaraugus. The mortality from premature birth, on the other hand, was 8 to 25 per cent lower in each of the other counties than in Cattaraugus. The excess infant mortality in Chautauqua, Jefferson and Washington Counties as compared with Cattaraugus County was greatest in deaths due to gastro-intestinal diseases and to communicable diseases.

In the period 1921-1923, when the mortality from most causes had increased in Cattaraugus County, the death rate from each cause except communicable diseases was considerably lower in at least two and in some instances all of the other counties of comparison than in Cattaraugus County. The deaths due to respiratory and gastro-intestinal diseases and from premature births were from 12 to 30 per cent lower in each of the other counties than in Cattaraugus.

The relative mortality from the various causes in the two years 1924 and 1925 in the four other counties and in Cattaraugus is shown graphically in Fig. 5. The average mortality from all causes was fairly similar in all these counties, being only 3 per cent and 1 per cent lower in Chautauqua and Steuben respectively than in Cattaraugus, and 5 and 9 per cent higher in Jefferson and Washington Counties. The mortality from specific causes, however, was very different in these counties. Mortality in the four counties due to premature birth was from 9 to 26 per cent lower than in Cattaraugus County. In three of the four counties, the death rate from congenital defects and other conditions of infancy was 10 per cent under that in Cattaraugus. On the other hand, the mortality from each of the three groups of "preventable" diseases was lower in Cattaraugus than in any of the other counties; the greatest difference is shown in the mortality from respiratory diseases.

Conclusion

It is not the purpose of this inquiry to seek to determine how much, if any, of the recent decline in the death rate of Cattaraugus County infants has been due to a recent increase in the County's public health work. Since 1923, the County has been participating in a health demonstration, the chief task of which has been the building up of the services of its County Board of Health and its County School Health Service, both newly established in that year. As a part of this program, specific activities for the protection of the health of infants have been gradually developed. No special bureau for work in infant and maternal hygiene was established until the summer of 1926, but considerable direct work for the protection of infants was carried on by the public health nurses as part of the generalized nursing service, inaugurated in 1923. During the first two years of the operation of this service, the nurses visited only special cases for which care was sought or which were discovered through the various activities of the Board of Health. In October, 1925, however, routine visiting of all new-born infants was started. The comparison made in the accompanying table of the nurses' home visits in successive years is, therefore, indicative of an increase in the growth of the County's work for the conservation of the health of its infants. Mothers' Health Clubs for group study had been organized as early as 1924, but intensive prenatal care was not developed until 1926, when the bureau of maternity, infancy and child hygiene was established under a medical director.

It may be presumed, however, that such activities, accompanied by others included in a general public health program, may have affected the health of the infants in the County. But the fact that a decline in the deaths of infants took place at this time does not establish what factors brought about this decline. And, as I have pointed out, it is not within the province of this study to establish a relationship between any specific conditions or activities in the County and a lowered mortality.

To sum up the more important indications revealed by this analysis, however, the reduction in deaths which occurred in the last three years was almost wholly the result of a decrease in the deaths from communicable diseases, respiratory

Type of Service	Number of Nurses Home Visits*			
	1923	1924	1925	1926
Prenatal and maternity	25(1)	1,208	1,739	1,738
Infant hygiene (under 2 years)	460(2)	1,829	3,800	4,492

(1) Prenatal visits only.
(2) Includes all visits to children of pre-school age.
*Does not include visits made by Olean City nurses.

and gastro-intestinal diseases, the death rate from these preventable causes in the period 1924-1926 being approximately 50 per cent of the rate in the preceding three-year period and well below the rate in the four other counties in the years 1924-1925. Although the death rate from premature birth declined 11 per cent in the three-year period 1924-1926, it exceeded that in the four counties. Furthermore, the mortality from congenital defects and other conditions peculiar to early infancy increased and it also was higher than in three of the four counties. More than two-thirds of all infant deaths in the period 1924-1926 were attributed to the causes classified as "Malformations and Early Infancy." These causes obviously are a very important problem in Cattaraugus with reference to its infant hygiene work. Even though the decline in deaths from the preventable causes continues, it will have an increasingly slight effect on the gross infant mortality and the reduction in the infant mortality will be limited unless the mortality from these early infancy conditions also can be reduced.

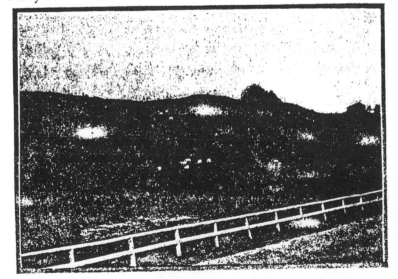

THE DECLINE IN THE TUBERCULOSIS DEATH RATE IN CATTARAUGUS COUNTY

by EDGAR SYDENSTRICKER, *Statistician in the United States Public Health Service and Statistical Consultant to the Milbank Memorial Fund*

꩜

DURING the past five years a public anti-tuberculosis program has been developed in Cattaraugus County, New York, by the Board of Health of that County, that, according to the judgment of competent critics, embodies and practices modern principles and procedures of tuberculosis prevention, relief and cure.

During the same period and in the same area all five annual death rates from tuberculosis have been lower than the rates as predicted from the experience of the previous twenty-two years. For each of the last three years the tuberculosis death rate has been lower than in any year of its previous recorded history which goes back as far as 1900. Furthermore these three successive low rates constitute an event which has not been paralleled in this area since 1900.

To most persons, especially to those who are conversant with the modern anti-tuberculosis program, this decline will appear as a result due in large measure to the development of an efficient public health administration in Cattaraugus County, more particularly of its anti-tuberculosis work. For, the prolongation of the lives of tuberculous individuals, the prevention of new cases, and the arresting of incipient cases, by modern methods of controlling the disease, are well established facts in the experience of those who are intimately engaged in these activities. But to the coldly scientific mind, accustomed to caution and trained in the habit of doubt, any conclusion as to a causal relationship between

383

the two series of events should rest on more complete evidence and should be established by more elaborate methods of appraisal. The situation may be likened to that in which the laboratory research worker finds himself. He may be honestly convinced of the soundness of his hypothesis and of the accuracy of his results but at the same time he realizes that his work must stand the test of scientific scrutiny not only for his own intellectual satisfaction but also in order that it may be established in other critical minds.

In a sense, therefore, the tuberculosis experience of Cattaraugus County, as well as that of any area or population group, may be regarded as an "experiment" in that it requires the application of the principles and the methods of scientific experimentation in measuring results of a specific factor especially when that factor has been deliberately introduced in order to bring about a definite result.*

The measurement of the results of anti-tuberculosis efforts, however, is not an easy task. We are accustomed to attempt it in terms of mortality, although we realize, or ought to realize, that a death rate is a poor index of what we are trying to evaluate. It is a faulty statistic for the reason that it may indicate on the one hand the prevalence of the disease, and on the other hand its fatality. It measures neither the one nor the other accurately. Furthermore, the annual number of deaths is so small in an area the size of Cattaraugus County as to be subject to wide variation from fortuitous circumstances. Again, it is a poor measure because the greatest emphasis in an anti-tuberculosis program is on preventing the disease, and on arresting it in those persons in whom the tubercle has been activated; the tuberculosis death rate can therefore measure only a fraction of the full

*Annual Report, Milbank Memorial Fund, 1926, Part II: The Measurement of the Results of Public Health Work.

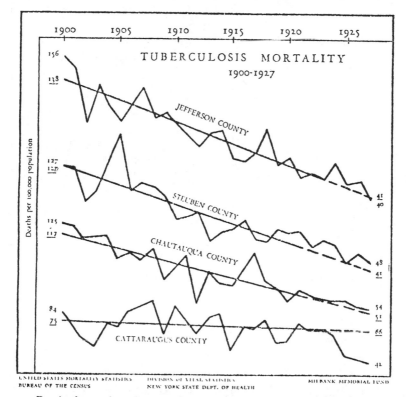

TUBERCULOSIS MORTALITY
1900-1927

Deaths from tuberculosis, all forms, in Cattaraugus County and in three other counties in New York State, per 100,000 population, 1900-1927. The straight lines indicate the trend of the death rate based on the period 1900-1922.

force of the campaign. Moreover, in the measurement of anti-tuberculosis efforts we observe the effects of various preventive and curative activities upon a stream of many continuous cases, each of which has its own course over a period of time. From this point of view the measurement of anti-tuberculosis work in adolescent and adult ages should be by different methods from those by which we measure an effort to prevent a definite event, such as a case of diphtheria or a death from measles. For the anti-tuberculosis campaign is not an effort directed toward a single objective; its objectives

MORTALITY *from* TUBERCULOSIS
in CATTARAUGUS COUNTY
1900-1927

In the following table are given the data upon which the tuberculosis mortality rates for Cattaraugus County for 1900-1927 are based. The deaths of Indians are excluded for the reasons that it is believed that registration of deaths among Indians on the reservation situated in the County has been incomplete and that the Indian population has not been included in the health activities of the County. The Indian population has been deducted in the manner stated in a footnote. Deaths of non-residents in the J. N. Adam Memorial Hospital at Perrysburg, which is primarily an institution for residents of Buffalo, have been excluded, but no other correction for residence of decedents has been made.

YEAR	POPULATION		DEATHS					Death Rate per 100,000
	Total (1)	Exclusive of Indians (2)	Indians (3)	Non-residents (4)	Total Indians and non-residents	Total (5)	Net including Indians and non-residents	
1900	65,645	64,645	3		3	57	54	83.5
1901	65,673	64,673	3		3	49	46	71.1
1902	65,701	64,701	3		3	41	38	58.7
1903	65,729	64,729	3		3	37	34	52.5
1904	65,757	64,757	3		3	50	47	72.6
1905	65,785	64,785	3		3	48	45	69.5
1906	65,813	64,813	3		3	58	55	84.4
1907	65,841	64,841	3		3	61	58	89.4
1908	65,869	64,869	3		3	63	60	92.5
1909	65,897	64,897	3		3	43	40	61.6
1910	66,035	65,035	3		3	61	58	89.2
1911	66,592	65,592	3		3	53	50	76.2
1912	67,148	66,148	3		3	46	43	65.0
1913	67,705	66,705	3	1	4	56	52	77.9
1914	68,262	67,262	3	1	4	59	55	81.8
1915	68,818	67,818	3	2	5	39	34	50.1
1916	69,375	68,375	0	5	5	53	48	70.2
1917	69,932	68,932	3	4	7	54	47	68.2
1918	70,488	69,488	1	3	4	57	53	76.3
1919	71,045	70,045	4	4	8	48	40	57.1
1920	71,546	70,546	4	7	11	52	41	58.1
1921	72,000	71,000	2	4	6	58	52	73.2
1922	72,453	71,453	3	15	18	66	48	67.2
1923	72,907	71,907	3	9	12	61	49	68.1
1924	73,360	72,360	4	14	18	64	46	63.6
1925	73,814	72,814	2	14	16	49	33	45.3
1926	74,267	73,267	5	25	30	62	32	43.7
1927	74,720	73,720	3	25	28	59	31	42.1

(1) Population estimates on following basis: Period 1900-1920, on Federal censuses; 1920-1925, on Federal census of 1920 and State census of 1925.

(2) Assumed deduction of Indian population: 1,000 annually. Census enumeration showed the Indian population to be 1104 in 1900, 1013 in 1910 and 1162 in 1920 (XX Census Volume III: 678).

(3) For period 1900-1915, number of deaths of Indians estimated at 3 annually.

(4) Non-residents dying at the J. N. Adam Memorial Hospital in Perrysburg.

(5) Mortality data from the following sources: Period 1900-1914 from U. S. Mortality Statistics; 1915-1924, from New York State Department of Health; 1925-1927, from Cattaraugus County Department of Health.

Mortality from tuberculosis (all forms) at different ages in Cattaraugus County in 1916-1924 and 1925-1927.

(Indian deaths and non-residents dying at the J. N. Adam Memorial Hospital are excluded.)

AGE	RATE PER 100,000		TOTAL NUMBER OF DEATHS		POPULATION ESTIMATED JULY 1	
	1916-24	1925-27	1916-24	1925-27	1920	1926
All Ages	67.1	43.7	426	96	70546	73267
0— 4	14.5	14.5	9	3	6913	6887
5— 9	15.0	0	9	0	6673	7143
10—19	35.3	12.5	40	5	12577	13342
20—29	129.3	59.0	127	19	10912	10741
30—39	121.1	78.8	110	25	10095	10580
40—49	61.6	66.6	47	18	8478	9005
50—59	65.3	42.1	41	9	6977	7122
60—69	53.4	51.7	23	8	4790	5158
70 & over	67.4	81.1	19	8	3131	3290
Unknown			1	1		

are several, each calling for a different kind of activity. It includes efforts to prevent incipient tuberculosis, to prevent the development of incipient cases into more serious stages; to arrest active cases, and to relieve cases in very advanced stages, and so far as possible to prolong their lives also. Obviously any single measure is inadequate for evaluating precisely the complete results of so varied a program.

In reviewing the experience thus far of Cattaraugus County, therefore, it is essential to keep in mind that the mortality rate for a period as short as three years, or even as five years, can reflect the results of specifically those anti-tuberculosis activities which affect the prolongation of lives of tuberculous individuals. In other words, the tuberculosis mortality rate in so limited a period can measure, and with a fair degree of definiteness, the effect of public health efforts upon the *fatality* of active cases only, rather than the activities that seek to prevent incipient cases or new "active" cases.

With the limitations set before us by these necessary definitions, it is proper to examine the tuberculosis death rates of Cattaraugus County from at least two points of view:

(a) the statistical significance of the decline in the gross rate, and (b) the nature of the decline as indicated by the changes in the rates among persons of different ages. Other analyses of the mortality record will be made later when further experience is available, and the case and morbidity data are now being studied for the purpose of ascertaining more precisely the results of other kinds of anti-tuberculosis activities.

So far as we know, no marked change in the ordinary conditions that affect the tuberculosis death rate, other than those which were generally prevalent and common to similar communities, has occurred in Cattaraugus County in the five years 1923-1927. Provisionally at least, therefore, we are warranted in assuming that the only factor of major importance, so far as possible effects upon the tuberculosis death rate are concerned, was the development of a modern anti-tuberculosis administration during this period.

Now in judging of the statistical significance of the decline in the tuberculosis death rate in Cattaraugus County in 1925-1927, we have so far attempted to answer three questions: (1) Could any of these low rates have been a variation arising solely from the small numbers involved, since only about 30 deaths have occurred in each of the three years? (2) Do these three rates constitute a unique occurrence judging by past variations in the tuberculosis rates in Cattaraugus County itself? (3) Is the Cattaraugus County experience of the past three years unique in comparison with generally similar areas in the same period.

The data for Cattaraugus County are given in the accompanying table, together with certain explanations as to the sources of the statistics used and certain corrections and eliminations made in order to render the statistics as comparable as possible throughout the period covered.

In applying any one of these tests, it is necessary to ascertain as accurately as possible what the trend of the tuberculosis death rate was in Cattaraugus prior to 1923, as well as in the other counties with which comparisons were made. For Cattaraugus County it was found that the tuberculosis death rate since 1900 had been practically on a level* with annual variations above and below this level which is indicated by the straight line on the accompanying chart. The experience of Cattaraugus was unusual in this respect. For in twelve other counties with whose tuberculosis mortality rates a comparison is made later in this report, the mortality was higher at the beginning of the period and a definite decline is shown since 1900. Why Cattaraugus has had such a favorable rate, we are unable to say until certain inquiries now under way may afford some explanation. But, feeling assured that the mortality record is reasonably accurate, this fact need not concern us here except in a respect which may be stated as follows: The intensive anti-tuberculosis work in Cattaraugus County was undertaken in an area where the death rate from the disease was already relatively low and had been on a low level for some years, and the further reduction of the death rate under such conditions becomes an experiment of unusual interest. Now, if no change in the trend of tuberculosis mortality had occurred subsequent to 1922, we would expect the value of this level to be about 67† per 100,000 in 1925-1927. As a matter of fact, the actual rates (45.3, 43.7 and 42.1) were from 34 to 37 per cent below the expected trend values.

Applying the first test, the probability that rates in three successive years as far below the trend values as the ob-

*A straight line fitted to the rates for 1900-1922 showed that the slope (value of b) was -0.33 ± 0.09 per 100,000 per year.

†66.8$\pm$6.4 for 1926, using .67449 of $\sqrt{\dfrac{pq}{n}}$ where n=estimated population as of July 1, 1926.

served deviations would occur, as a result of fluctuations due to small numbers, is about 4 in a million. So that the decline can not be ascribed to these "chance" fluctuations.

Changes in the mean annual tuberculosis death rate by age groups in Cattaraugus County 1916-1924 over 1925-1927.

Age Group	Actual change in Rate per 100,000	Relative Change Per Cent
Under 5	0	0
5— 9	—15.0	—100
10—19	—22.8	— 64
20—29	—70.3	— 54
30—39	—42.3	— 35
40—49	+ 5.0	+ 8
50—59	—23.1	— 35
60—69	— 1.7	— 3
70 and over	+13.7	+ 20

Applying the second method, the probability that rates in three successive years as far below the trend values as the observed deviations would occur, using the annual deviations in the period 1900-1922 as the basis, is about 1 in 100,000.* In other words, if we can apply the theory of probability to such a problem as this, and assuming the independence of the events considered (and, statistically speaking, they may be so assumed), the occurrence of three rates as low as these for 1925-1927 may be judged as constituting a distinctly unique event.

Applying the third method we have used very roughly as "controls," twelve other counties in New York State, namely, Otsego, Ontario, Delaware, Fulton, Chenango, Columbia, Herkimer, Montgomery, Tompkins, Steuben, Chautauqua and Jefferson. A preliminary selection of these counties was made on the grounds that they were generally comparable with Cattaraugus in that they did not contain any cities with a population of 50,000 or over, had established a county tuberculosis sanitorium during the period of consideration (1900-1927), do not constitute or contain a

*The value of *sigma* of annual deviations from the trend of the rates per 100,000 in 1900-1922 is 11.34.

suburban area, and included no State institutions or large private sanatoria. The annual variations were considered in the same way as those for Cattaraugus County. On the accompanying diagram three of them have been plotted as illustrations (page 43). A preliminary analysis indicates that the rates for 1925, 1926 and 1927 in these twelve counties were either above or not significantly below the expected rate for these years.*

The latter comparison has not been carried to the point of completion by any means. In order that more precise and complete comparisons will be possible, it is expected to refine them and to continue them in ensuing years, to study the comparability, in important respects, of these counties, as well as possibly other areas, with Cattaraugus; and to obtain data on the character and volume of the anti-tuberculosis work in some of the counties generally comparable in other relevant respects with Cattaraugus County.

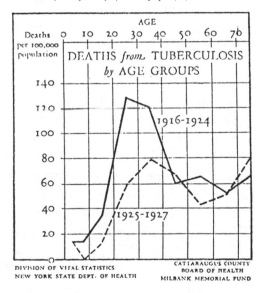

Deaths from tuberculosis, all forms, by age groups in Cattaraugus County, per 100,000 population, in 1916–1924 and 1925–1927.

Of greater significance, in the writer's opinion, than the

*For Tompkins County each of the tuberculosis death rates as recorded for 1924-1927 was below the trend value but the difference in each instance was not statistically significant. Taking the four successive rates together, however, an apparently significant change is indicated.

results of purely statistical tests, such as the first two employed in the foregoing paragraphs, is the fact that the decrease in the Cattaraugus County tuberculosis death rate has taken place in the younger ages. This fact is clearly indicated by the accompanying table and diagram which compare the mean annual rates for 1916-1924 with those for 1925-1927 at different ages. The actual changes in the rates, as well as the relative changes, were as shown in the accompanying table.

The rate among children under 5 years of age shows no change, but it was already low in comparison with other areas,* the largest number of deaths in any year during the period 1916-1927 having been 3. The decreases in the succeeding age periods up to 40 years were considerable and were consistent. This is in contrast to the absence of such changes in the older age periods (40 years and over). If we make a division of the ages in three groups—under 5 years, 5 to 40 years, and 40 years and over—which is roughly characteristic of the ways the disease manifests itself in different periods of life, the decline in the tuberculosis rate in 1925-1927 was confined to the ages of later childhood, adolescence, and young adults, the decrease amounting to about 50 per cent of the mean rate for the previous nine years, and being in itself statistically significant.†

*For example: the 1924 rate among white persons under 5 years of age in the registration states of 1920 was 38 per 100,000; the 1925 rate among all persons under 5 years of age in New York State (exclusive of New York City) was 40 per 100,000.
†Since the downward trend of tuberculosis mortality for all ages in the period 1916-1922 was of negligible importance, and since no definite trend was indicated for the rates at any age, the comparison made above seems justifiable. The difference in the mean rates for the ages 5-39 years is 8 times its probable error, as shown below:

| Age Group | Mean Annual Rate per 100,000 | | |
	1916-1924	1925-1927	Difference
0 – 4	14.5	14.5	0.0
5 –39	78.9 ±3.1	39.1 ±3.8	39.8 ±4.9
40+	61.8 ±3.7	58.3 ±6.0	3.5 ±7.0

It may be stated that most of the differences in the mean rates for the more refined age groups in the ages 5-39 are also statistically significant when judged according to their ratios to their probable errors, and that the age distributions of the deaths in the two periods (using the quinquennial and decennial divisions) are significantly different when the Chi Square test is applied.

The Duke Endowment

An Address on

The Duke Endowment

ITS ORIGIN, NATURE AND PURPOSES

BY

William R. Perkins

DELIVERED BEFORE

The Sphex Club

AT LYNCHBURG, VIRGINIA

OCTOBER 11, 1929

WITH AN APPENDIX CONTAINING THE INDENTURE
ESTABLISHING THE DUKE ENDOWMENT AND THE
PROVISIONS OF THE WILL AND OF A TRUST
OF JAMES B. DUKE SUPPLEMENTING
THE ENDOWMENT

PUBLISHED BY
THE DUKE ENDOWMENT
POWER BUILDING
CHARLOTTE, N. C.

Mr. Chairman, and Members and Guests of The Sphex Club:

I have very real pleasure in being with you on this occasion. The privilege of appearing before such a gathering is an honor most highly esteemed, I assure you. And then Lynchburg is home. Here are the familiar scenes of years gone by. Here I received the impetus to whatever of achievement I may lay claim. And here, God willing, still linger many of the friendly faces that are nearest and dearest. Of all the beautiful pictures that hang on memory's wall, the ones of the old Hill City, they seem to me best of all.

My subject is The Duke Endowment, its origin, nature and purposes, which I have been told, and can well understand, is of interest to you. It is one of the outstanding philanthropies of all time. It is of our Southland. It is for our Southland. While located in the Carolinas where the Dukes were born and the Duke Power System operates, undoubtedly its influence will permeate and its activities will benefit elsewhere, as through the great educational institution it is constructing at Durham on your border. And if the income prove more than sufficient within the Carolinas the trustees, in their discretion, may use the excess for hospitalization beyond their confines, giving preference to adjoining States, in which category, of course, comes Virginia.

All that exists or happens is the expression of a personality. Such is the case with business and pleasure,

397

our good deeds and our bad, our homes and habits, and
even the clothes we wear; for the apparel oft proclaims
the man. This world of ours is the expression of a great
personality. I know that on this subject some assert in-
sufficient knowledge to form a belief and others enter an
ignorant denial; but to me the marvel of creation has always meant the existence of a Superior Being, and I be-
hold in the act which is my theme this evening a product
of this Superior Being working through the hearts and
consciences of mankind.

The Duke Endowment was an expression of the personality of James Buchanan Duke, though it presented a
side of him which then seemed little known to the public.
I well recall the surprise voiced by the Press in its announcement. As a matter of fact, this was one of the
highest compliments ever paid the quiet, unpretentious
way in which Mr. Duke carried forward his plans. Yet
I confess to quite a feeling of resentment at the time because I knew this lack of understanding had its source in
the persistent ways in which he had been depicted as a
malefactor of great wealth by those who sought to secure
their own preferment by his detraction.

There should have been no surprise. Mr. Duke came
of a family of benefactors. His father, Washington Duke,
and his brother, Benjamin N. Duke, were both notable in
this respect. The aggregate of their donations was imposing. Mr. Duke himself had been generous in his gifts
and his intimate friends were well aware that he contemplated, to use their oft repeated phrase, "big things
for God and humanity". Mr. Duke's mind was busy

with the subject as far back as when I became his personal counsel and for over ten years there lay in the drawer of my desk a draft of the document which eventually embodied The Duke Endowment.

You wonder at this elapse of time. The answer is the unique basis of the Endowment, which distinguishes it radically from other large philanthropies. The Press notice stated simply that Mr. Duke had given $40,000,000 to charity. The Indenture described the donation as so many shares of stock. What Mr. Duke really contributed in major part was control and operation of a business.

Many years ago, while in the midst of his tobacco merchandising, Mr. Duke had his attention called to a hydro-electric development on the Catawba River in South Carolina. An investigation was followed by an investment. And thus there began what, for him, was the real business fascination of his life, culminating in the acquisition and development of the great Saguenay River in the Province of Quebec, Canada and giving rise, contrary to popular belief, to much the larger portion of his fortune.

Mr. Duke was a builder. He loved to create and establish. This quality was preeminent in his make-up and found full scope for its exercise in harnessing the great natural resource—water power—and turning it to the service of mankind. He threw himself wholeheartedly into this field of endeavor. He erected dams and power plants and transmission lines. By participation in financing and otherwise, he encouraged the location of industries on these lines. He even projected an electric railway, parts of which he constructed and would have completed the whole but for the World War and its aftermath. The result was that the portions of North and South Carolina, in which these activities centred, became a synonym of progress and prosperity. The Duke Power System took its place in the front rank of public utilities, with plants producing millions of kilowatt hours of electrical energy which it distributed over miles of transmission lines to thousands of customers, including many towns and cities. And there was borne in upon Mr. Duke the great thought which lies at the very foundation of his Endowment—why not let his philanthropy take the form of giving this power system to the communities it served in a manner whereby through it they could finance their own charities by simply doing business in the usual and ordinary way.

I shall never forget the delight with which Mr. Duke in the utmost confidence unfolded the idea to me. He felt it met the test of real assistance. It helped others to help themselves. And he illustrated by saying it was easy enough to give a fellow food or shelter or raiment or money, but the best of all gifts was a job. He asked me to embody the plan in a draft of indenture, which I did, and he went about its performance with the enthusiasm of a boy, refusing to accept from the Companies even the expenses of his services, much less any compensation, though much stock was in the hands of the public.

Hence the ten years which I mentioned; for Mr. Duke was unwilling to turn over the properties until he regarded them as complete for the purpose. And what a ten years! There was the war, with its stress and havoc and deluge of blood and tears, when all our resources and energies were bent to the one essential, victory. During the war there came the greatest flood ever known in the Carolinas. The Catawba River, where most of the Duke plants are, rose some fifteen feet higher than any previous record and washed away every bridge from the mountains to the sea. So dams had to be carefully reinforced and a large impounding reservoir built high up on the water shed to provide amply against such future occurrences. Again, the war left wages and other costs so high that the rates obtaining for electric current were found materially inadequate. So proceedings had to be instituted which, after a bitter fight, secured a comparable increase. And it was only when all these things had been accomplished that Mr. Duke regarded the situation ripe for dedicating the properties to his magnanimous conception.

Of course, meanwhile the conception had grown immensely in amount and scope. Such was always the case with what Mr. Duke undertook. The $40,000,000 value put into the Endowment at its inauguration embraced largely more than stock in the Duke Power System. One-fifth of each year's net income he required to be accumulated until thereby another $40,000,000 was added to the principal of the Endowment. And his Will probably added as much more. For it bequeathed the Endowment $10,000,000 by Item VIII and by Item XI, as amended by the codicil, two-thirds of his residuary estate, subject only to an annuity to his widow.

But through it all runs the basic thought on which the philanthropy is bottomed and the Indenture expressly and broadly so states. Thus in his declarations for the guidance of the trustees Mr. Duke says:

> "For many years I have been engaged in the development of water powers in certain sections of the States of North Carolina and South Carolina. In my study of this subject I have observed how such utilization of a natural resource, which otherwise would run in waste to the sea and not remain and increase as a forest, both gives impetus to industrial life and provides a safe and enduring investment for capital. My ambition is that the revenues of such developments shall administer to the social welfare, as the operation of such developments is administering to the economic welfare, of the communities which they serve."

And with these views in mind he not only recommended the securities of the Duke Power System as "the prime investment for the funds of this trust", but required such funds to be invested by loans to, or acquiring the securities of, the Duke Power System "if and to the extent that such a loan or such securities are available upon terms and conditions satisfactory to said trustees"; otherwise investments could be only in first-class Federal, State or Municipal Bonds. He not only advised the trustees not to "change any such investment except in response to the most urgent and extraordinary necessity", but he stipulated that such securities could not be disposed of, in whole or part, "except upon and by the affirmative vote of the total authorized number of trustees at a meeting called for the purpose, the minutes of which shall state the reasons for and the terms of such sale''. And he requested the trustees ''to see to it that at all times these Companies be managed and operated by the men best qualified for such a service''.

I feel justified, therefore, in stressing this striking characteristic of the Endowment which I believe to be unique. I have supreme faith in its efficacy because I have just that faith in the common sense and loving kindness of the people on whose shoulders has fallen this mantle of beneficence. When they understand the conception they will appreciate and fulfill it. And if they do not, the trustees by unanimous action have a way out so that the Endowment will not thereby be jeopardized.

Another feature of the Endowment worth dwelling upon is its duration. This subject was brought again to the fore in an article by Mr. Julius Rosenwald which appeared in the Atlantic Monthly for May 1929 and has since been distributed in pamphlet form. Mr. Rosenwald makes vehement opposition to perpetual endowments and, suiting his action to his word, has required that every dollar of his donations, both principal and income, be expended within twenty-five years of his death.

I have read the article with much interest. Its controlling thought is that perpetual endowr ⸱s unduly tie up capital and outlive their usefulnes: And, within proper limits, there is merit in the view. For, undoubtedly, as Bobby Burns well said, ''the best laid schemes o' mice and men gang aft agley''. But I do not believe the subject admits of the broad generalizations and strictures which Mr. Rosenwald indulges nor that his illustrations of outlived usefulness are the kind upon which to base a universal rule of conduct. Rather do I think the determining factors to be the nature of the object desired and its attendant circumstances, as objects differ greatly in their endurance and requirements.

For instance, I cannot see any parallel to the great causes of health and education in the cases cited by Mr. Rosenwald of funds established for ''worthy and distressed travelers and emigrants passing through St. Louis to settle for a home in the West''; to furnish ''a baked potato at each meal for each young woman at Bryn Mawr''; to provide for Boston ''fortifications, bridges, acqueducts, public buildings, baths, pavements or whatever may make living in the town more convenient for its people and render it more agreeable to strangers''; to pipe water from Wissihicken Creek for the City of Philadelphia or to make Snug Harbor in Brooklyn ''a haven for superannuated sailors''. Those examples are the extremes, the freaks, of history, though some were by men both eminent and wise. One has but to consider the probable fate of Harvard, Yale, Princeton, Johns Hopkins, Leland Stanford, had each of their benefactors been of Mr. Rosenwald's mind.

The same thing is true of Mr. Rosenwald's ungracious comment on Mr. Hershey's noble provision for orphans, that ''orphan asylums began to disappear about the time the old-fashioned wall telephone went out''. I suspect

Mr. Hershey was much better informed concerning orphanages than Mr. Rosenwald. For ten percent of the net income of the Duke Endowment is given to institutions in the Carolinas which, as a charity, take care of white and colored whole or half orphans. And so far we have found no diminution in such institutions or their need for funds.

Besides, Mr. Rosenwald's view runs counter to the great incentives of life and athwart the prevailing traits of humanity. Men prefer to write in brass, not water, to leave their footprints in rock rather than upon the shifting sand. They are unwilling, unless necessity compels, to trust their cherished ambitions to something so precarious as posthumous charity, not that coming generations will prove uncharitable, but that they may have other plans of their own.

Mr. Duke could not envisage the fruition of the University he was founding or the Hospitalization he was inaugurating except through substantial permanence in his provision for them. He therefore expressly provided that the Endowment should endure forever under the management of a self-perpetuating board of fifteen trustees who could expend none of the principal except the $17,000,000 for erecting and equipping Duke University. At the same time he gave the trustees such ample discretion about income as safely to accommodate his philanthropy to the changes time may work. If any beneficiary ceases to exist the income allotted it may be used for any other object of the Endowment. As respects any year and any object except Duke University the trustees may withhold the income allotted and use it either for "any such like charitable religious or educational purpose" within the Carolinas or for "any such like charitable hospital purpose which shall be selected therefor by the affirmative vote of three-fourths of the then trustees" at a meeting called for the purpose; and without such vote the trustees may use in any State the income allotted to Hospitalization, in excess of that needed in the Carolinas, giving preference to those States adjoining the Carolinas. Even as to Duke University if, in the judgment of the trustees, it "incur expense or liability beyond provision already in sight to meet same" or "be not operated in a manner calculated to achieve the results intended" they may withhold the whole or any part of the income allotted that institution and use it for any other object of the trust.

You thus see that the trustees have the widest discretion for use of income within the Carolinas and outside those States may use the whole income of the Endowment to extend aid to hospitalization, according to Mr. Duke's plan, unto the four corners of the earth.

The objects of the Endowment may be conveniently classified as religion, hospitalization and education, of which the provision for orphans has already been mentioned.

To appreciate the provisions for religion one must realize that Mr. Duke was a Methodist of the rural district type and such had been his father and his grandfather before him. And a first-rate type it was and is.

The Circuit Rider had entered deep into the warp and woof of their lives, as into the lives of many others. Mr. Duke often remarked: "My old daddy always said that if he amounted to anything in life it was due to the Methodist circuit riders", to which he invariably added: "If I amount to anything in this world I owe it to my daddy and the Methodist Church." And may I add that I do not believe any son ever cared more for a father? As the years sped it ripened into a veneration beautiful to contemplate, of which I might give you numerous incidents. I could but marvel at the man Washington Duke must have been, thus to have impressed and influenced for good the life of his great descendant. It made me realize the possibilities, the responsibilities, of fatherhood as nothing else and always brought an intense yearning that my life, each father's life, might deserve and receive such a blessing.

You will not be surprised, therefore, to know that the Endowment's provisions for religion took the form of allotting six percent of the distributable net income to assist in building Methodist Churches in the sparsely settled rural districts of North Carolina and four percent of such net income to assist in maintaining and operating Methodist Churches in those districts. In addition, two percent of such net income was allotted for the care and maintenance of needy and deserving superannuated preachers and widows and orphans of deceased preachers who shall have served in a Methodist Conference in North Carolina, a provision which perpetuated a gift Mr. Duke had been making yearly for some while through Trinity College by way of supplement to the Conference fund for the same purpose. Up to July 1, 1929 the Endowment had paid in round figures $66,250 to superannuated preachers and their families, $93,000 for operating rural churches and $148,000 for building rural churches, this amount being about ⅛ of the total for such building.

Hospitalization appealed strongly to Mr. Duke because he considered the cause splendid and the need very great. He therefore provided much more liberally for it than for any other purpose. The Indenture allotted to it thirty-two percent of the distributable net income arising from its principal and accretions. Mr. Duke's Will, in giving two-thirds of his residuary estate to the Endowment, specified that ninety percent of the net income therefrom should be used for hospitalization under the terms of the Indenture. And it is the only object for which the trustees may use net income beyond the confines of the Carolinas, in the manner and to the extent I have already indicated.

This aid to hospitalization took two forms, helping people to get needed hospital attention and helping to secure hospitals adequate to such needs.

To the former Mr. Duke gave precedence because he regarded it more immediately pressing and less likely to be met sufficiently. His provision for it was a direction to the trustees to pay to each and every hospital in the Carolinas, whether for white or colored, not operating for private gain, such sum (not exceeding $1) per free bed per day for each and every day such bed may have been occupied during the period covered by such payment free of charge by patients unable to pay as the amount available for the purpose will pay on a pro rata basis.

This form of assistance is based on what is almost axiomatic, that if you take care of the charity patients the hospital will take care of itself. It was adopted only after thorough study and in accordance with the best modern thought. Hospitals must serve the people. They should not, can not, turn suffering humanity away. But most of the cases come from those who are unable to bear the expense and pay patients may not be charged sufficient to carry fully this extra burden. It is just here, where the shoe pinches, that Mr. Duke's plan supplements in an amount which an elaborate analysis of hospital costs and experiences indicated would be proper, namely, not exceeding $1 per free bed per day. In reality he has to this extent endowed hospitals in proportion to the charity work they do. And it constitutes a great forward stride in enabling hospitals to realize their true mission.

The second form of help in hospitalization consists in securing adequate hospitals by assisting in the erection of those not operated for private gain. And to this Mr. Duke has dedicated the surplus of the funds allotted to hospitalization left after making the free bed payments. While thus subordinated, this second form should not be minimized, for the two forms of assistance are, in fact, coordinate.

The practice of modern medicine is dependent upon and therefore centres around the hospital. This is a well-known fact and the reason is plain. The great progress in the sciences and surgery, as well as in mechanics, has made hospital facilities indispensable in both diagnosis and treatment. But hospitals, for the most part, are yet located in cities and large towns. And the result is a vast disproportionateness between our urban and rural populations as respects the amount, nature and caliber of the medical facilities open to them.

Mr. Duke saw and appreciated this inequality and sought its relief. His conception was a network of hospitals so located and constructed that they and their attendant staffs would be adequate and accessible to all who might need. And as the climax, the capstone, of this system of hospitals his Will bequeathed $10,000,000 to the Duke Endowment, of which $4,000,000 was to be used in building and equipping at Duke University a Medical School, Hospital and Nurses' Home, and the net income of the whole turned over to Duke University for their operation.

The trustees have earnestly set themselves to the task of fulfilling this program for hospitalization. They have been fortunate in securing for direction of this work the services of Dr. W. S. Rankin, a splendid, capable man of fine experience whose enthusiasm knows no bounds. Real progress is being made, though co-operation in full measure in building and equipping hospitals will come slowly because only education brings a true realization of this need. To July 1, 1929 in round figures the free day bed payments have aggregated about $1,-500,000 and the expenditures and commitments for building and equipping hospitals about $1,125,000, exclusive of the Hospital and Medical School at Duke University. The construction of the latter is well on the road to completion. They are expected to be open by September 1930. Their head will be Dr. W. C. Davison, formerly Assistant Dean of Johns Hopkins, another really splendid and capable man. He has been giving his close personal attention to the construction and assures us that in location, structure and appointments they will compare favorably with the best now existing.

The magnitude of this program for hospitalization can not be overstated. One is simply overwhelmed by the contemplation of its sweep through the years, nay ages, to come. It is not too much to say that it will prove a veritable tree of life whose leaves are for the healing of the nations.

While the Endowment allots five percent of the net distributable income to Davidson College, a Presbyterian institution located at Davidson, N. C., a like amount to Furman University, a Baptist institution located at Greenville, S. C. and four percent of such net income to the Johnson C. Smith University, an institution for colored people located at Charlotte, N. C., and these are appreciable gifts, Mr. Duke's real provision for education is Duke University.

In 1838 the Methodists and Quakers joined in establishing a school in Randolph County, N. C., which they appropriately called "Union Institute". Later it was incorporated as "Normal College" and the Governor of the State became chairman and other State officials became members of the Board of Trustees. This mingling of state with school soon ended, and the institution was turned over to the North Carolina Methodist Conference, by which it was renamed "Trinity College".

Mainly through the efforts of Mr. Washington Duke, in the early nineties Trinity College was moved to Durham, N. C. in order to secure better facilities and a larger outlook. To accomplish this he pledged for buildings $85,000, which he later increased to $180,000. And thereafter he gave for endowment amounts totalling $300,000. Part of this latter was on condition that young women should be given all the privileges granted to young men as students there, the condition was accepted and thereby Trinity College became, and Duke University will be, a co-ordinate school of education for young men and young women.

Following in the footsteps of his father, Mr. James B. Duke, when the Endowment was established, had contributed to Trinity College some $100,000 for buildings, $158,500 for expenses, and approximately $3,000,000 for endowment, besides uniting with his brother, Mr. Benjamin N. Duke, in adding 27½ acres to the old campus and $800,000 to endowment. Mr. Benjamin N. Duke, besides his participation I have mentioned, had contributed around $100,000 to endowment, some $250,000 for expenses and over $300,000 for building purposes. And other members of the Duke family had made further contributions, notably Mr. Angier B. Duke, who gave $30,000 for expenses, joined with his sister, Mrs. Mary Duke Biddle, in contributing $25,000 to the erection of the

Alumni Memorial Gymnasium and by his will bequeathed $250,000 to endowment.

You thus realize that at the time of the creation of the Endowment Duke generosity had played a most prominent part in locating, building and maintaining Trinity College at Durham and augmenting its endowment funds. And you see how entirely natural and fitting it was that Mr. Duke should think in terms of Trinity College in planning his philanthropy for education. Accordingly, he provided that by taking the name "Duke University", Trinity College might be the Duke University contemplated by the Endowment so long as it retained that name and was not operated for private gain, subject, however, to discretionary power in the Endowment trustees to withhold the whole or any part of the income allotted the University should it incur expense or liability beyond provision in sight to take care of same or, in their judgment, be not "operated in a manner calculated to achieve the results intended" for education through Duke University under the Endowment.

In some quarters it has been suggested that in this power to withhold might lie seeds of future conflict and embarrassment. But no such apprehension exists among those who bear the responsibility. Rather do they think it an element of strength, preventing the ill-considered and making for stability like the checks and balances of our National Government. The response from Trinity College was immediate and complete. It welcomed this call to greater usefulness. The name was promptly changed from "Trinity College" to "Duke University".

And in good faith and perfect harmony its trustees and officials and those of the Endowment are co-laboring, and in the years to come will continue so doing, to fulfill the purposes of the Endowment as to Duke University, all parties well understanding that this was not simply a change of name or acquisition of funds for building or maintenance, but a dedication of Trinity College to achieving these intended educational results.

What are these purposes, these intended results? They embrace both construction and operation.

The construction program, as outlined for the Endowment, consisted in expanding and extending Duke University, acquiring and improving lands and erecting, remodeling and equipping buildings for that purpose, to the end that Duke University might include Trinity College as its undergraduate department for men, a school of religious training, a school for training teachers, a school of chemistry, a law school, a coordinate college for women, a graduate school of arts and sciences, a medical school and an engineering school. For it the Endowment allotted $6,000,000, Mr. Duke gave an additional $2,000,000, and by his Will he bequeathed $11,000,000 more, making a grand total of $19,000,000. It was to be carried out by the Endowment trustees. And this they are now doing in two steps or stages.

The first step was enlarging the existing Trinity College into what will be the Co-ordinate College for Women of Duke University. Here the plans required the removal of three buildings and the addition of eleven build-

ings, constructed of red Baltimore brick, trimmed with
Vermont marble, in the Georgian style of architecture.
And this unit has now been completed and is in use. Its
main buildings are grouped about a quadrilateral, at one
end of which is the entrance while the other end is closed
by the Auditorium with its spacious dome, which consti-
tutes the dominant feature of the ensemble. And the
whole comprises a campus of 108½ acres, located on
Main Street in the western part of Durham, enclosed by
a fine stone wall and beautifully planted; the auditorium
seating 1,400 people, a union building with offices and
dining and service rooms, as a centre of student activities, a capacious library, three science buildings, three
other classroom buildings, an apartment building containing 18 suites for faculty members, 10 dormitories
arranged to house over 1,200 students, besides several
residences, a heating plant, and other buildings; also an
athletic field provided with grandstand, bleachers and
cinder runningtracks, and a finely appointed gymnasium
with splendid bathing pool.

The second step was the creation of a new unit, the
College for Men and Graduate and Professional Schools
of Duke University. This is now well on the road to completion, with the hope of opening in September 1930.
For it there has been acquired a campus of some 5,000
acres lying about a mile to the southwest of the old
campus and connected with it by an avenue which passes
under Main Street and the railroad. Here roads are
being laid out, the grounds planted and construction is
proceeding. The architecture is Gothic and the material
native stone from a nearby quarry with tile roofs and

trimmings of Indiana limestone. Again the main buildings are grouped about a quadrilateral. The dominant feature, as you approach the grounds, will be a chapel with imposing spire rising upwards of 200 feet. To your right, as you face the chapel, will be the school of religion, the library, the law school, the chemistry building, the medical school and hospital, the botany and zoology building and the physics and science building; while to your left will be the auditorium seating 1,500 people, the union, again with offices and dining and serving rooms, as a centre of student activities, and three groups of dormitories arranged to house 1,500 students. Farther still to the left are the gymnasium with swimming pool, the athletic fields and the stadium, or horseshoe bowl, seating 35,000 people, recently opened, as you no doubt saw in the papers, with a game between Duke and the University of Pittsburgh. There is also the heating plant and laundry. Plans are now being made to erect some appropriate houses for officials and faculty members. And eventually there will be tennis courts, golf links and probably a lake sufficient for aquatic sports.

I realize, of course, that what I have said gives you the merest thumbnail sketch of the physical features of Duke University. But neither time nor talent avail for more. Come and see for yourself. The trip is well worth while and a cordial invitation is extended. Though other institutions have finer individual buildings and a larger aggregate accumulated over the years, this is the greatest piece of scholastic construction ever consummated at a single time. And we feel confident that in arrangement, structure, ornamentation and appointment it will be an outstanding accomplishment.

The operation of Duke University is in the hands of its trustees, officials and faculty. For it the Endowment allotted thirty-two percent of the distributable net income arising from its principal and accretions. And the Will gives all the net income arising from the $10,000,000 and ten percent of the net income arising from the portion of the residuary estate which it bequeathed to the Endowment, less the $11,000,000 it directed to be spent for building and subject, of course, to the power of withholding I have mentioned.

In respect of the operation of Duke University Mr. Duke declared for the guidance of his trustees:

"I have selected Duke University as one of the principal objects of this trust because I recognize that education, when conducted along sane and practical, as opposed to dogmatic and theoretical, lines, is, next to religion, the greatest civilizing influence. I request that this institution secure for its officers, trustees and faculty men of such outstanding character, ability and vision as will insure its attaining and maintaining a place of real leadership in the educational world, and that great care and discrimination be exercised in admitting as students only those whose previous record shows a character, determination and application evincing a wholesome and real ambition for life. And I advise that the courses at this institution be arranged, first, with special reference to the training of preachers, teachers, lawyers and physicians, because these are most in the public eye, and by precept and example can do most to

uplift mankind, and, second, to instruction in
chemistry, economics and history, especially the
lives of the great of earth, because I believe that
such subjects will most help to develop our resources, increase our wisdom and promote human
happiness.''

I should like, if I may, to dwell somewhat on that statement. It is a formula for our educational problems from
a business man of rare ability and experience and will
repay your earnest consideration. Though brief, it is
most expressive.

He lays down the basis on which to proceed. He says
education, next to religion, is the greatest civilizing influence ''when conducted along sane and practical, as
opposed to dogmatic and theoretical, lines''. This is a
recurrence to fundamentals, a subordination of isms to
the common sense of the job. And it is timely and wise.
There must be provided a broad groundwork of accepted
education, both general and special, totally outside the
controversial fields of thought, for the great body of the
people. Our higher education, so called and all right in
its place, must be nurtured in a soil thus prepared; unless
erected on such a foundation it is the sport of the winds
and a menace. But beyond that, we are the melting pot
of the races, a fact as yet less apparent South than North
and West. Our proclaimed liberty, in whose name so
many crimes are committed, has made us the mecca and
paradise of earth's doctrinaires. While no one would
limit thought or stifle honest expression, a decent regard
for our ideals and institutions demands, at the least and

above all else, a wholesome diet of substantial foods that will produce solid, balanced Americans who can assimilate properly.

He tells us the raw material to get. He says there should be admitted as students only those whose previous record shows "a character, determination and application evincing a wholesome and real ambition for life". Time was when schools went out in search of students. Now, due to growth of population and prolongation of courses, there is an oversupply, despite increase in facilities, and the problem is one of selection. And here Mr. Duke requests that "great care and discrimination be exercised". The subject is too big to discuss now. But among other things I feel sure he meant that the matter should be handled as individually as possible; more so, in my opinion, than by the entrance examination method upon which such great reliance is now being placed. That is too much a rule of thumb for mass production to get the desired results. We should ascertain family facts and antecedents, the record of study and conduct in previous schools and the views of friends and neighbors. Some boys and girls will not take a college education, much to the discouragement of their parents, though there should be none; for no doubt as large a proportion of these will succeed in after life as of attendants at college. And those who take a college education have different types and bents of mind. So our job is to help the young people to find themselves and we can do this only through the care and discrimination which Mr. Duke advocates. This point is really the great cross-roads of life and its method of handling makes or mars more years and lives than all else combined.

He points out the tools to use. They are "men of such outstanding character, ability and vision" for officers, trustees and faculty as will insure the University "attaining and maintaining a place of real leadership in the educational world". No one realized more fully than Mr. Duke that fine buildings do not make a fine school. If possible, the human equation is more vital there than almost any other place. To capability must be added that indefinable thing we call personality. For my own part, I believe the young people get much more from the lives encountered than the books studied. Run back in memory to your own college days and you will find standing out in the perspective some splendid man or woman as the influence that still enthralls you. They meet us at the threshold of life when faith is new and hopes are high and on our open minds for good or bad make impressions that endure. A pebble in the streamlet's flow has changed the course of many a river; a bird upon the tiny bough has warped the giant oak forever.

And may I add, parenthetically, how inadequate seems to me our appreciation of such an important service. I have been really astonished at the little recognition accorded these unsung heroes, not simply in money but in various other ways. How many are in our halls of fame or compendiums of lives worth while? No, look at it as you please, other pursuits are vastly more inviting, other fields far greener. Why, many of those who do take up teaching have to eke out a livelihood by writing, lecturing or otherwise, to the neglect of the students and their own disgust at the inequalities of life. No wonder so many of our boys and girls tire of their studies, get imbued with foolish notions and come home thinking our boasted civilization all wrong.

And he specifies the products he desires, giving the reasons for his preferences. He puts first, the training of preachers, teachers, lawyers and physicians because he considers these are "most in the public eye and by precept and example can do most to uplift mankind". He puts second, instruction in chemistry, economics and history, especially the lives of the great of earth, because he believes such subjects "will most help to develop our resources, increase our wisdom and promote human happiness".

To uplift mankind! To promote human happiness! Such is the true philosophy and the sublime of life. Such, in its essence, is The Duke Endowment I have endeavored to portray to you.

Quite a number of years ago, as Mr. Duke and I sat talking, he fell into one of those reminiscent moods that come to us all now and then. And under the impulse of the fascinating retrospection I asked him what he regarded as the greatest thing he had done. His answer was, assembling in The American Tobacco Company a group of men so capable that each of the large companies into which it was split by the Federal Courts could be amply manned to preserve this great industry and safeguard those interested in it.

The years rolled on. The Endowment became a living fact. And again Mr. Duke and I were talking together. I reminded him of the conversation I have just narrated. And I asked, "What do you say now, Mr. Duke, is the greatest thing you have done?" Without hesitation he replied, "The creation of the Endowment, because through it I make men."

.I often think of those talks, as I do, indeed, of my whole association with Mr. Duke, now, unhappily, but a memory. To me it was an education, a delight, an inspiration. I feel sure there never was a more complete and unreserved relationship between attorney and client. That was his way. He was frankness and simplicity itself. His associates were just members of a big family, laboring to a common end, each putting in his oar according to his talents and training.

Mr. Duke created the fortune he amassed. He did not prosper at any one's expense. On the contrary, he carried his business associates with him to an extent that gained for him the reputation of having made more millionaires than any other American. One of his maxims was never to make any money out of those engaged in an undertaking with him. When I came with him he cautioned me to take pains to draw all papers fairly and plainly, saying no contract was any stronger than the interest of the parties to keep it. He was an early and ardent advocate of the bonus system, whereby a share of the net profits went to both officers and employees in addition to their regular compensation. And this, in various forms, has now been widely adopted and is doing more, perhaps, than any one thing to solve our difficult labor problems by making business a partnership, so to speak, between owners and operators.

Mr. Duke reaped much because he sowed largely and well. His test of a business project was whether or not it would do the job better and cheaper than it was then being done. If careful investigation and consideration showed the proposal to be sound he threw himself into it unsparingly. To realize what I mean you have but to contrast the tobacco industry today and when he entered that field. Then the plant was little more than a weed. Now it forms one of the largest crops, sells in all the markets of earth, gives employment to thousands and returns millions in revenue to the Government and in profits to investors.

Nature endowed Mr. Duke most generously. A truly magnificent mind was supported by a splendid physique and graced with those finer qualities that mark the true gentleman. Common sense, rugged honesty, dynamic energy, tenacity of purpose and courage of conviction were his in abundance. He was most considerate of others, their rights, opinions and pleasures, which made him always a charming host and temperate in his views and expressions. I never heard him use an oath and he rarely spoke disparagingly of any one.

His poise and self-restraint were wonderful. Not many men have been more misrepresented to the public than he. On the hustings and in press and periodicals, by politicians consumed with lust for office or those courting notoriety through cheap sensationalism, Mr. Duke was reviled and held up to scorn and contempt, often in terms so extravagant they overreached themselves and fell upon the other side. This still persists notwithstanding his death. He knew, and I also knew, that these canards were utterly baseless and untrue. Yet he opened not his mouth and held in check the righteous wrath of family and friends.

A striking example of this characteristic occurred in his efforts to obtain an increase in power rates without which I have told you he was unwilling to turn his power properties into the Endowment. To secure this increase an application was made to the proper State Commissions. And to the extent the increase should be allowed it would raise the rates in existing contracts and not simply apply to contracts thereafter made. In order to obviate this effect (though it was a proper effect because the law had made this risk a part of each contract), a good many power users joined in an appeal to the Legislature of the State of North Carolina to pass an act restricting any such increase to future contracts only; and one of their main arguments was that Mr. Duke should not be permitted to use the natural resources of the State to coin more money for his already bulging pockets. I pleaded with Mr. Duke to confound these opponents by making known his plan for the Endowment. But he refused, saying he did not wish to prevail that way, as it was a business proposition with these customers and he was entitled to win out on the merits. And win out he did!

During the world war at the request of the Government Mr. Duke formed and headed a tobacco committee. It was composed of the presidents of various tobacco concerns. Among the members was a splendid citizen of the Old Dominion who for years had been a prominent "so-called" independent tobacconist and so a conspicuous competitor of Mr. Duke. The two met for the first time when the committee assembled in Washington. There were also present representatives of the Army and Navy and they complained bitterly that every little tobacconist in America thought the Government should buy his products. Mr. Duke quietly remarked that he would never advise the Government to ignore the small concerns. On the instant this Virginia gentleman was up and across the room, saying to Mr. Duke, "There's my hand, Sir, I have have been wrong about you all this time." I never saw a more dramatic scene. The two became staunch friends and admirers, and the former adversary is now outspoken in his declaration that Mr. Duke was one of the finest and fairest men that ever lived.

Lastly, I would have you know that Mr. Duke believed devoutly in God and the Future Life. His faith was simple and sincere. During his last illness I remarked to him how I wished that a thousand years hence we might know how the Endowment was faring. He said he had no doubt whatever we would know and understand, that he could not conceive man was but born to die.

No one then realized that the time of his departure was at hand. But soon he passed peacefully into the Great Beyond and became a part of the Ages.

Verily, a workman that needeth not to be ashamed, he rests from his labors, but his deeds abide to bless. And among them shines the Endowment, an enduring lighthouse of humanity which will forever send forth its beams of loving helpfulness across life's storm-tossed sea.

I thank you.

The
Duke Endowment

Annual Report
of
The Hospital Section

1925

427

CHAPTER I

THE DUKE ENDOWMENT

Indenture and Deed of Trust

Mr. James B. Duke, on December 11, 1924, by Indenture and Deed of Trust, established The Duke Endowment and conveyed to the Trustees thereof securities having a value of $40,000,000.

The Deed of Trust provided that the funds should be used as follows:

A. Of the corpus, to establish Duke University as a memorial to his family, $6,000,000.

B. Of the net income from the invested funds, the annual addition to the corpus until a total of not less than $40,000,000 have been so added 20%

C. Of the remainder of the annual net income, that is, 80 per cent of the net income, the apportionment was to be as follows:
   1. To Duke University 32%
   2. To the maintenance and construction of hospitals 32%
   3. To the care of orphans and half orphans 10%
   4. To Davidson College 5%
   5. To Furman University 5%
   6. To Johnson C. Smith University 4%
   7. To superannuated Methodist ministers 2%
   8. To the building of rural Methodist churches . . . 6%
   9. To the maintenance of rural Methodist churches . 4%

Mr. Duke, in the Trust Indenture, states his general purposes in establishing The Duke Endowment as follows:

"For many years I have been engaged in the development of water powers in certain sections of the States of North Carolina and South Carolina. In my study of this subject I have observed how such utilization of a natural resource, which otherwise would run in waste to the sea and not remain and increase as a forest, both gives impetus to industrial life and provides a safe and enduring

428

investment for capital. My ambition is that the revenues of such developments shall administer to the social welfare, as the operation of such developments is administering· to the economic welfare, of the communities which they serve."

He, then, gives his reasons for the several benefactions as follows:

"I have selected Duke University as one of the principal objects of this trust because I recognize that education, when conducted along sane and practical, as opposed to dogmatic and theoretical, lines, is, next to religion, the greatest civilizing influence. I request that this institution secure for its officers, trustees and faculty men of such outstanding character, ability and vision as will insure its attaining and maintaining a place of real leadership in the educational world, and that great care and discrimination be exercised in admitting as students only those whose previous record shows a character, determination and application evincing a wholesome and real ambition for life. And I advise that the courses at this institution be arranged, first, with special reference to the training of preachers, teachers, lawyers and physicians, because these are most in the public eye, and by precept and example can do most to uplift mankind, and second, to instruction in chemistry, economics and history, especially the lives of the great of earth, because I believe that such subjects will most help to develop our resources, increase our wisdom and promote human happiness.

"I have selected hospitals as another of the principal objects of this trust because I recognize that they have become indispensable institutions, not only by way of ministering to the comfort of the sick but in increasing the efficiency of mankind and prolonging human life. The advance in the science of medicine growing out of discoveries, such as in the field of bacteriology, chemistry and physics, and growing out of inventions such as the X-ray apparatus, make hospital facilities essential for obtaining the best results in the practice of medicine and surgery. So worthy do I deem the cause and so great do I deem the need that I very much hope that the people will see to it that adequate and convenient hospitals are assured in their respective communities, with especial reference to those who are unable to defray such expenses of their own.

"I have included orphans in an effort to help those who are most unable to help themselves, a worthy cause, productive of truly beneficial results in which all good citizens should have an abiding interest. While in my opinion nothing can take the place of a home and its influences, every effort should be made to safeguard and develop these wards of society.

"And, lastly, I have made provision for what I consider a very fertile and much neglected field for useful help in religious life, namely, assisting by way of support and maintenance in those cases where the head of the family through devoting his life to the religious service of his fellow men has been unable to accumulate for his declining years and for his widow and children, and assisting in the building and maintenance of churches in rural districts where the people are not able to do this properly for themselves, believing that such a pension system is a just call which will secure a better grade of service and that the men and women of these rural districts will amply respond to such assistance to them, not to mention our own Christian duty regardless of such results. Indeed, my observation and the broad expanse of our territory make me believe it is to these rural districts that we are to look in large measure for the bone and sinew of our country.

"From the foregoing it will be seen that I have endeavored to make provision in some measure for the needs of mankind along physical, mental and spiritual lines, largely confining the benefactions to those sections served by these water power developments. I might have extended this aid to other charitable objects and to other sections, but my opinion is that so doing probably would be productive of less good by reason of attempting too much. I therefore urge the trustees to seek to administer well the trust hereby committed to them within the limits set and to this end that at least at one meeting each year this Indenture be read to the assembled trustees."

CHAPTER II

THE PROBLEM OF DISEASE

The Need of Medical Services

The size of the problem of disease determines the extent of the need of medical services. The problem of disease is measurable in terms of mortality and morbidity rates, that is, death rates and sickness rates. We may, therefore, begin our consideration of the need of medical services with a brief reference to the more important existing death rates, referring those who are interested in greater detail to the very complete analytical consideration of death rates appearing in the official reports, Mortality Statistics of the Bureau of the Census.

Death Rates

The last published general death rate for the United States, that for the year 1923, was 12.3 deaths per thousand population. The average general death rate for the United States for the five years, 1919 to 1923, inclusive, was the same as that for 1923, namely, 12.3.

The general death rates for North Carolina and South Carolina during 1923 were 12.0 and 11.8, respectively.

The colored death rate for the United States during 1923 was 17.1; the white death rate for the same year, 11.8. The racial proportions of population in North Carolina and South Carolina for 1923 were, for North Carolina, white, 70.3 per cent, and colored 29.7 per cent; for South Carolina, white, 49.9, and colored, 50.1. The colored death rate for North Carolina in 1923 was 15.5; the white death rate, 10.5. The colored death rate for South Carolina during 1923 was 14.1; the white death rate, 9.5.

431

Urban and rural death rates for the United States during 1923, the Federal Bureau of the Census classification of urban and rural being based upon places having populations over or under ten thousand, were 13.2 and 11.5, respectively. According to this basis of classifying urban and rural populations, North Carolina, in 1923, was 14 per cent urban and 86 per cent rural; South Carolina, for the same year, was 10.5 per cent urban and 89.5 per cent rural. For North Carolina the urban rate in that year was 16.2 and the rural rate 11.3; for South Carolina, the urban rate was 20.1, the rural rate, 10.9. The higher urban rate for the country generally and especially for the two States is due, in a considerable measure, to the more seriously sick being removed from the country to town, where hospital treatment is available, and to deaths in urban hospitals of rural residents.

The twelve most important causes of death *per hundred thousand population* of the United States for the year 1923, were as follows:

TABLE 1

1. Diseases of the heart 175.3
2. Influenza and pneumonia 106.0
3. Tuberculosis (all forms) 93.5
4. Cerebral hemorrhage (apoplexy) 92.2
5. Acute and chronic nephritis (Bright's disease) 90.1
6. Cancer and other malignant tumors 89.4
7. Congenital malformation and diseases of early infancy 78.0
8. Accidental and non-specific internal causes... 76.4
9. Bronchitis and broncho-pneumonia 56.7
10. Diarrhea and enteritis (under 2 years) 39.9
11. Diabetes 17.9
12. Appendicitis 14.8

The above list of causes of death accounts for three of every four deaths.

Changes in Death Rates

The changes in death rates that have taken place and are taking place in recent times are important to note for the reason that they indicate the more important modifications of the problem of sickness as we face it today. The most important of these changes to be noted in death rates is that of the remarkable decrease in the general death rate since 1880, more especially since 1890, the decade that marks the beginning of modern medicine. The following table, copied from the Mortality Statistics of the Bureau of the Census for 1923, shows the decrease in the general death rate since 1880:

TABLE 2

General Death Rate, 1880 to 1923

Year	Death Rate	Year	Death Rate
1880	19.8	1910	15.0
1890	19.6	1915	13.6
1900	17.6	1920	13.1
1905	16.0	1923	12.3

The decrease in the general death rate above noted is dependent largely upon (1) decreases in certain special death rates, (2) decreases in the infant mortality death rate, and (3) the life-saving influence of modern surgery, the effect of which is distributed throughout a large number of special death rates that enter into and sum up in the general death rate.

Important and interesting decreases in certain special death rates are shown in the following table:

TABLE 3

Disease	1890	1900	1910	1923
Tuberculosis*	245.3	201.9	160.3	93.5
Typhoid fever	46.2	35.9	23.5	6.8
Contagious diseases†	43.0	34.8	35.3	24.0
Diphtheria	97.7	43.3	21.4	12.1
Diarrhea and enteritis‡	‒‒‒‒‒	133.2	117.4	39.9
Deaths per 1,000 population under one year of age	‒‒‒‒‒	162.2	141.5	87.5

A more accurate and significant death rate of infants than the Census estimates of deaths per thousand population under one year of age (the last line of figures in the preceding table), is what is known as the infant mortality rate, by which we mean the number of deaths per year under one year of age per thousand births. As birth registration has developed more slowly than death registration, it is only within recent years that we have been able to obtain reliable infant mortality rates; however, the limited infant mortality rates which are available are worthy of note at this place. In 1900, eight cities in the United States had infant mortality rates ranging from 300 to 419, which is to say that from 300 to 419 of every thousand children born during the year died. In 1923, the average infant mortality rate of all of the large cities of the United States, which includes cities of 50,000 and over, was 78.

The contributions of surgery to improved vitality, as has already been stated, do not express and measure themselves in any particular death rate, but certain it is that surgery has played a great role, perhaps almost as large a part as the reduction in the special death rates, given in the preceding table, has played in reducing the general death rate from 19.6 in 1890 to 12.3 in 1923.

Death rates that have shown a marked decrease during the last 33 years are those, for the most part, of diseases

---

*For 1890: Lungs only; for 1900, 1910 and 1923, all forms.
†Measles, scarlet fever, and whooping cough.
‡Under two years of age.

of infancy and childhood, and, in the case of two diseases, typhoid fever and tuberculosis, those of early adult life. Very little reduction has taken place in the death rate of diseases incident to middle age and later periods of life. On the contrary, the death rates from the more important diseases of middle age and later age periods, especially the death rates of that group of diseases which are referred to as the degenerative diseases, those indicating wear and tear and including heart disease, kidney disease (Bright's disease) and cerebral hemorrhage or apoplexy, have shown a considerable increase. There has also been a considerable increase in the death rate from cancer and malignant tumors. It is true that some part of the increase in the death rate from heart disease, disease of the blood vessels, apoplexy, kidney disease, and cancers or malignant tumors is due to the saving of life in the early years, thereby making it possible for more people to live to the age when cancer and the degenerative diseases come upon the scene. The following table shows the increase that has taken place during the last 23 years in the death rates from the degenerative diseases and cancer:

TABLE 4

Disease	1900	1910	1923
1. Heart disease	132.1	158.8	175.3
2. Cerebral hemorrhage or apoplexy	75.5	79.4	92.2
3. Nephritis or Bright's disease	89.0	99.1	90.1
4. Cancer	63.0	76.2	89.4

There is an interesting difference in the death rates among the higher age groups of the population of the United States and of European countries. In the United States there is an increase in death rates for age groups beyond middle life and an increase in death rates from the degenerative diseases, whereas in European countries there is a decrease in death rates for all age groups. Sir Arthur Newsholme regards the present increase in death rates of the upper age levels as temporary and resulting from the more rapid death of population age groups that in their childhood did not enjoy the sanitary and hygienic advantages of subsequent age groups, the death rates of which, he believes, within a few years, will begin to parallel the death rates of similar age groups in European countries.

Increasing Longevity

Decreased death rates reflect themselves in increased longevity. Longevity within recent times, as compared with the earlier records of longevity, has been and is increasing at an accelerated pace. Professor Irving Fisher of Yale University, in a recent statement, says:

"As I pointed out in 1901, during the Seventeenth and Eighteenth Centuries in Europe human life was lengthening at the rate of about four years per century. During the first three-fourths of the Nineteenth Century, the rate was nine years per century. During the last quarter it was 14 years per century in Massachusetts, 17 years per century in Europe in general, and 27 years per century in Prussia in particular. More recent data show that, in the first quarter of the Twentieth Century, for the United States, England and Germany, life lengthened at the amazing pace of 40 years per century. Raymond Pearl finds that Baltimore, during the last half century, has been lengthening human life at the rate of 30 years per century; while London shows a rate of 45 years per century. But it is Germany which again reaches high water mark with a rate of 60 years per century!"

Dr. Mazyck P. Ravenel, of the University of Missouri, in his recent "Gordon Bell Memorial Address," says:

"In the United States the expectation of life at birth has risen to 58 years, 20 years having been added during a century, and 10 during the past 20 years."

It is necessary in the intelligent planning of ways and means for the conservation of human life that we take note of the fact that the increased longevity of recent times has been effected through the saving of life in the early years. Note, for example, in the following table, which is representative of life tables for the period covered, that is, for the 30 years 1879-1881 to 1909-1911, that the increased expectation of life benefits only those who are under the thirty-fifth year of life, and that for those who have attained half the allotted Biblical span nothing has been accomplished:

TABLE 5

Expectation of Life—New York City

NEW YORK CITY HEALTH DEPARTMENT

Age	Males		Females	
	1879-81	1909-11	1879-81	1909-11
—5	39.7	50.1	42.8	53.8
5	44.9	49.4	47.7	52.9
10	42.4	45.2	45.3	48.7
15	38.2	40.8	41.2	44.2
20	34.4	36.6	37.3	40.0
25	31.2	32.7	34.0	36.0
30	28.2	28.9	31.0	32.1
35	25.3	25.4	28.1	28.4
40	22.5	22.1	25.2	24.7
45	19.8	18.9	22.4	21.1
50	17.2	15.9	19.4	17.7
55	14.5	13.2	16.4	14.6
60	12.2	10.8	13.8	11.8
65	9.9	8.8	11.2	9.4
70	8.5	6.9	9.3	7.5
75	7.1	5.3	7.5	5.7
80	6.2	4.1	6.5	4.5
85	5.4	2.0	5.5	2.4

The practical significance of the distribution of increased longevity, the benefits going largely to those under middle age, is this: Surgery excepted, those who have been concerned with the conservation of life, have interested themselves largely, until very recently, in sanitation, that is, in the improvement of environment, with the consequent cutting off of infection. Water supplies have been purified, milk supplies made safe, contagious disease isolated, carriers of infection at least partially controlled, the susceptible to contagion immunized, in short, the battle of sanitation has been fought—and won. All that remains so far as this first phase of the war on disease is concerned is a mopping-up process. We are now entering upon a new phase of this warfare against man's common enemy, disease, and this new phase has not to do with one's environment but with one's self; it is personal—personal hygiene and personal care—the first to be attained through a more appreciative understanding of the meaning and means of health and the second to be attained by more adequate provisions for the safeguarding of health and the treatment of disease, namely, a more efficient medical service, including both elements, medical personnel and hospitals.

Prevalence of Diseases and Defects

While death rates, trends in death rates and changes in longevity delineate the large outline of disease and its control, a nearer and clearer vision of the immediate problem is obtained through a study of evidence bearing upon the existing prevalence of diseases and defects. This evidence may be assembled under four headings: (1) Evidence furnished through the examination of large numbers of men called up for military service; (2) evidence furnished through the routine examinations of millions of school children from all sections of the country by health departments; (3) evidence furnished by the examination of hundreds of thousands of supposedly well persons by the Life Extension Institute in New York; (4) evidence furnished through many house-to-house sickness surveys by insurance companies, social service agencies, health departments and individuals and agencies engaged in the study of needed provisions, especially hospital provisions, for the care of the sick.

Defects Among Those Examined for Military Service

The evidence furnished through the examination of 2,753,922 selected service men called up for possible enlistment in the World War is the most impressive and perhaps the most convincing with respect to the great prevalence of diseases and defects in the general population. It will be recalled that these examinations were carried out under government supervision. The different defects and defective groups that were listed numbered 269. This list did not include all defects. Only defects of recognizable importance from the military point of view were noted. A large number of defects, including defects of vision, teeth, focal infection, uncured venereal disease, were not noted; moreover, in the examination of the drafted men, when the examiners discovered a defect that disqualified the man for military service, the examination stopped, inasmuch as the purpose of the examination was to ascertain physical fitness for military duty and not to ascertain how many defects the men examined had. The point to be remembered, in this connection, is that the examination conducted by the Draft Boards and the Medical Corps of the Army while listing many defects did not, by any means, list *all* defects. Nevertheless, the following findings in the examination of the selective service men are most impressive in their bearing upon the general prevalence of diseases and defects:

Of the men examined, 21 per cent were disqualified for *any* military service;

28 per cent were disqualified for *active* military service;

33 per cent of those examined in the first draft were disqualified for active service;

46 per cent of the men were found to have defects of military importance;

57 defects per 100 men examined were noted, which is to say that some men had multiple defects;

62 per cent of 113,932 men applying for enlistment in the Navy in 1916, before we entered war and when a greater degree of selection could be exercised, were rejected.

It is regrettable that the defects found in selective service men have not been compiled according to the ages of men examined, in order that the increasing prevalence of disease and defect at the higher age levels, as compared with earlier age groups, might be known. The only facts of this character available with reference to the drafted men is that defects were 30 per cent greater in the combined age group, 21 to 31, than for the age group of 21. In England, where the defects of the men examined for enlistment in the Army of the World War have been tabulated by ages, the following rates are impressive:

Of those of 18 years, 22 per cent were defective;
Of those of 23 years, 48 per cent were defective;
Of those of 40 years, 69 per cent were defective;
Of those of 50 years, 89 per cent were defective.

Defects Found in the Examination of Public School Children

The evidence furnished by the routine physical examinations of school children by health departments is confirmatory of that furnished by the examination of the selective service men. It is and has been the practice of health departments now for a number of years to examine school children, usually the first, third, and fifth grades, for what is known as the common defects of childhood— the term in itself being rather significant. These examinations are rather hasty, economy is necessary, the examination usually requiring from ten to fifteen minutes. Obviously the examination is not a complete one with the object of determining the exact state of the child's health, but to detect defects of such frequent occurrence as to have great importance in their influence on the rate of the child's educational progress. One of the highest authorities in this field of medicine, Dr. Thomas A. Wood, of Columbia University, in a recent publication summarizing the general findings of health departments with reference to defects of school children, furnishes these impressive figures:

School children mentally defective. . . . . 1 to 2%
School children with heart disease. . . . . 1 to 2%
School children with some form of tuberculosis 5 to 10%
School children with defective vision. . . . . 10 to 13%
School children with malnutrition. 20%
School children with diseased tonsils and adenoids. . . 30%
School children with defects of posture. 30%
School children with defects of teeth. . . . . 50 to 75%

Defects Found in the Examination of the Supposedly Well

The evidence of the prevalence of disease and defects accumulated and published by the Life Extension Institute of New York is most illuminating. The Life Extension Institute, since the beginning of its work some fifteen years ago, has been engaged in the examination of large numbers (now approximately 500,000) of supposedly well people, the selection of those examined being by industrial and insured groups and not by individuals. In this way, the Institute has gone into large industrial plants employing hundreds of thousands of workers and has made these group examinations, examining every employee.

The following tabulation, based upon the examination of hundreds of thousands of supposedly healthy people, for the most part of middle age, represents the findings of the Institute:

Individuals with no impairments................. 0%
Individuals with slight physical impairment....... 10%
Individuals with moderate physical impairment..... 41%
Individuals with moderate physical impairment need-
    ing medical supervision...................... 35%
Individuals with advanced physical impairments re-
    quiring systematic medical treatment.......... 9%
Individuals with serious physical impairment demand-
    ing immediate medical attention............. 5%

The Extent of Disabling Illness

In addition to the prevalence of disease and defects that impair vitality and retard efficiency but that do not disable, we have yet to consider the extent of illness of a disabling character, for the most part bedridden illness. Investigations for determining (1) the number of days of disabling illness for the average individual and (2) the number of persons constantly sick for the average thousand population have been made within recent times by many trustworthy agencies.

Professor Irving Fisher, of Yale University, in his report on National Vitality for the National Conservation Commission, appointed by President Roosevelt in 1909, reported that the average individual suffered 13 days of disabling illness each year. Investigating commissions, such as the United States Commission on Industrial Relations and the Social Insurance Commission of California, and the Metropolitan Life Insurance Company, in more recent times, 1913 to 1921, have reported annual disabling illness per individual as ranging from 6 to 9 days. The latter figure is more nearly correct for the reason that most of the studies on which the above conclusions were based concerned themselves with wage-earners and did not include, in all probability, the average proportion of the population that compose the two extremes of life, infancy and old age, where disease of a disabling character is much more prevalent. Assuming that the loss of 9 days per year is a fairly accurate index of the prevalence of disabling illness, the average individual loses one-fortieth of his time from incapacitating disease. Ernst C. Meyer, of the Rockefeller Foundation, in summing up a study of the results of a number of recent sickness surveys, states that ordinarily 25 persons for every thousand of the population are at all times sick and in bed. This statement is in line with the 9 days of sickness per individual, or the loss of one-fortieth of the individual's time from sickness, as 25 cases of sickness per thousand population is equivalent to saying that ordinarily one-fortieth of the population is at all times in bed from disabling illness.

The aforestated general findings are in harmony with what hospital authorities, in their surveys of communities to determine hospital needs, usually find, namely, this number—about 25 people per thousand population incapacitated from disabling illness. Of the incapacitated, 10 per cent, or 2½ cases per thousand population, are so seriously ill as to need hospital care. This does not mean, of course, that there are not additional cases of *ambulatory* illness that require hospital treatment—cases of malignant tumors or cancers, of tuberculosis, of heart disease, of arterial disease, of kidney disease, of gallstones and kidney stones, of unrepaired injuries following childbirth, of hernias, etc. The hospital cases, including both disabling and ambulatory illness, approximate 3.75 cases per thousand population. With the ordinary allowance in hospital planning of a surplus or reserve of 25 per cent of hospital beds over the needs of ordinary times, such a number of hospital cases, 3.75 per thousand, would call for five beds per thousand population.

CHAPTER III

MEDICAL SERVICES

Conditions at the Time The Duke Endowment Was Established

As a matter of record and as a point of departure from which bearings may be taken from time to time for the purpose of measuring the influence and effect of the Hospital Section of The Duke Endowment, it is most important that the present condition of medical services be noted carefully and recorded accurately. Furthermore, the record should include the present condition of medical services both for the country generally and for the more restricted field—the two Carolinas—in which The Duke Endowment is at work. With an available record of medical services both for the country in general and for the Carolinas in particular, it will be possible at future times to distinguish between improvements which may be a part of general changes and, therefore, not directly related to the work of The Duke Endowment, and improvements which are localized in the field to which The Duke Endowment is more closely related.

What Constitutes Medical Services

Much misunderstanding and controversy comes out of discussions that fail in their outset to establish a corner, a mutually acceptable starting point, a definition.

The term medical services, as here used, includes considerably more today than it included fifty years ago. Then, it included little more than medical personnel, the doctor and his paraphernalia, limited portable equipment, saddlebags and drugs. Since that time the modern hospital and professional nursing have developed. Take away the 7,000 hospitals with their 800,000 beds, the 55,000 nurses in training and the 150,000 graduate nurses, and the medical services of the United States would be paralyzed. Medical personnel with the right proportion of nurses and technical assistants and with adequate hospital facilities means medical personnel with potential service doubled, quadrupled, multiplied many times.

Nurses save the time of physicians which would otherwise have to be given to such essential services in the care of the sick as the taking and recording of temperature, pulse and respiration, the bathing of the patient, catheterizing patients, giving enemas, poulticing, bandaging, etc. Technicians save the time of physicians that would be given or should be given in large measure to simple laboratory tests, such as ordinary urinary analyses, examinations of expectorations for tubercle bacilli, examinations of swabs from the throat for diphtheria bacilli, examinations of pus for cocci, examinations of excreta for worms or their eggs, examinations of blood for malaria, blood counting, the Widal test, examinations of gastric juice, etc. Hospital facilities eliminate distances between patients and time consumed in travel and make one visit to patients grouped in a hospital do where many would be required with patients in scattered homes. In connection with this last statement it is evident that nursing and hospital facilities will multiply to a much larger extent the potential services of rural medical personnel than of urban personnel, because under rural conditions, long travel and poorer roads, the saving in travel time is so much greater. It is, therefore, safe to say that while a physician whose services are valued by his community and who practices under ordinary urban conditions is enabled with hospital facilities and with the assistance of nurses and technicians to do from two to three times the work that he could do without such supplementary services (not to mention the enhanced quality of his work), a physician in a rural section with his practice scattered over a large territory, given the assistance of hospital facilities, nurses and technicians, may accomplish from three to six times the work that would be possible in the absence of such facilities and assistance.

Medical service rests on a tripod of services, medical personnel, nursing and technical personnel, and hospital facilities and the weakness or absence of any one of the supports results in a service breakdown. The three, doctors, nurses, and hospitals, are interdependently related, and any complete and satisfactory consideration of the care of the sick must think of these three services not fractionally but as a whole. Unintentional failure to do this, by some who have engaged in recent discussions of this subject, has resulted in misunderstandings and controversy which might otherwise have been avoided. With this general consideration of what is included under the term medical services, we may now formulate a definition.

Medical services are such services as are rendered or made possible by a personnel especially trained and facilities especially designed for the purposes of saving human life, restoring health, and preventing disease.

With the above stated content of medical services, and for the sake of an easier grasp of the subject, we may now proceed to a consideration of this triad of services: (1) medical personnel, (2) nursing service, and (3) hospitals.

Medical Personnel

With the professed purpose of medicine in mind, and with the general welfare uppermost in thought, it is safe to say that the public interest requires that two conditions with respect to medical personnel be supplied: (1) a normal supply of doctors and (2) a normal distribution of doctors.

Significance of Either Excess or Deficiency

If the supply of doctors be either excessive or deficient, an abnormal social condition exists.

Too many doctors in a country or community is harmful to both the profession and the public. For the profession, an excessive medical personnel brings about a competition that inhibits professional understandings, sympathetic purposes and coöperative enterprises; that encourages and results in high fees, split fees, unnecessary specialists and excessive references; that, in short, tends toward selfishness with the loss of the professional spirit and outlook. For the public, an excessive medical personnel means just one thing, supernumeraries and waste. For example, if a county may be served by twenty physicians and it is served by thirty, there are ten unnecessary physicians and physicians' families which that community supports.

Too few doctors in a country or community means inadequate medical care for the sick, unnecessary suffering and premature deaths, vital losses, to be sure, but economic losses, too, because human efficiency, dependent to a very large per cent on vitality, is the basic and most valuable asset of society.

The great basic law of supply and demand, which regulates the quantity of commodities and services alike, appears to have left during a seventy-five year period little discernible effect upon the proportion of doctors to population. On the one hand, the supply has remained fairly constant except as influenced by the effect of (1) war and (2) the elevation of medical standards on the output of medical colleges; and, on the other hand, the general demand for the services of medical personnel has likewise remained fairly constant. This apparent balancing of the forces of supply and demand, with respect to medical personnel, is due, in all probability, to an equipoise of those forces or factors which, on the one hand, tend to decrease, and, on the other hand, tend to increase the demand for medical service.

Factors Tending to Decrease the Demand for Medical Personnel

Decrease in the prevalence of certain diseases: Many diseases have been found to be largely preventable and to a considerable extent have been prevented, thereby obviating the need for a large amount of medical service. Table 3, on page 16 of this Report, showing the downward trend of certain important death rates, measures, to some extent, this factor in decreasing the demand for medical service.

The automobile: Improved transportation, made possible through the automobile and better roads, enables, especially, the rural practitioners, where the demand exists, to do at least twice the work that was possible under conditions antedating the coming of the automobile.

Rural telephones: The telephone, and especially the rural telephone, not only saves the time of the family in reaching the doctor, but it is a great conservator of the doctor's time. In the first place, the doctor may obtain information and give advice over the telephone that would otherwise require a visit; and in the second place, the doctor may be reached not only at his office, but at the homes of patients in the vicinity of the family which makes the call, thus saving the time of the physician in returning to his office, finding the new call and having to drive over much of the same territory over which he has just driven.

Hospitals: The hospital, by bringing the patients to the doctor and segregating them under conditions where the physician has the assistance of nurses and technicians, has a tremendous influence in decreasing the demand which otherwise would be made on medical personnel; moreover, it is precisely those patients, the more seriously ill, who would require frequent visits that are brought to the hospital. Under rural conditions, it is possible with the assistance of hospital facilities for a physician to give from two to five times the service, and much better service, too, than he could give without such facilities. The development of hospitals is comparatively of recent times, as indicated in the following table:

TABLE 8

Year	No. of Hospitals	Year	No. of Hospitals
1873	149	1914	5,057
1900	2,000*	1918	5,323
1906	2,411	1923	6,830
1909	4,359	1925	7,370

Professional nursing: Much of the work which the physician was called upon to do before the development of professional nursing is now cared for by the nurse. It may be said here that the more resourceful the physician and the greater demand upon his time, the larger the sphere of service which he will find for his assistant nurse. There are practicing physicians in rural communities whose time is highly valued and heavily drawn upon that use nurses to keep their records, to take much of the history of their patients, to do much of their surgical dressings, to assist them in their obstetrical work, to perform most of their simple laboratory tests, to do their vaccinations and immunizations, to give salvarsan and neo-salvarsan, etc. There are busy practitioners who without the aid of their assistant nurses would not be able to do more than 40 or 50 per cent of the work which they accomplish with such help. Professional nursing, like hospitals, is of rather recent development. In 1879, according to United States

*Estimate based on graph, Journal American Medical Association, January 12, 1924, page 118.

Government reports, there were 11 schools for training nurses, 298 pupils, and that year 141 graduates; now there are nearly 2,000 schools for nurses with 55,000 pupils and a little more than 15,000 graduates each year.

Having considered the more important factors which lessen the demand on medical personnel, we now turn to the other side of the picture to note those factors which increase this demand.

Factors Tending to Increase the Demand for Medical Personnel

Increase in incidence of certain diseases: While the infectious diseases, largely diseases of infancy, youth, and young adults, have been decreased, the degenerative diseases, diseases of late middle age and old age, have increased, claiming as victims many who under former conditions would have lost their lives in infancy and childhood.

The prevalent belief that the medical profession in the prevention of certain diseases stands in its own way from a business standpoint rests upon superficial and fallacious reasoning. To illustrate: The death rate of babies under two years of age from diarrhea and enteritis has been decreased in the last 20 years from 133.2 to 39.9 per 100,000 population, but the infant whose life is saved and who lives his three score years and ten requires and uses the medical profession some fifty to one hundred times more than the baby that dies in its early months or years. So it is that while some diseases have been greatly reduced in incidence and fatality, more people are living and living longer and sending for doctors oftener than would be the case if conditions of vitality were as formerly. It is almost certainly true that an improved vitality plus a more intelligent and larger appreciation of health has increased, more than the elimination of certain diseases has decreased, the demand on medical personnel.

The enlarged field of medicine: It has been said on high authority that medical science has advanced further in the last 50 years than in the 2,000 years preceding that time. The medical profession, through the discoveries of medical science and the improved methods of treating diseases, is in a position to render a far larger service in both the maintenance and restoration of health than ever before. Moreover, the public is better informed through popular education, as carried on by the press and the school, as to the value of medical service than at any previous time in history. There is, therefore, on the one hand, a greater appreciation and demand on the part of the public for medical service and, on the other hand, a larger content of service which the profession may render.

The recent and great expansion of the sphere of medical service is realized to some extent, at least, when we recall that forty years ago one could so completely master the science and art of medicine as to be able to practice after one year of training; that thirty-five years ago two years of training were all that was necessary to master the science and art to the extent of being permitted to practice; about 1903, three years of special training were required in order to qualify to practice; and that within the last few years most of the licentiates of medicine have had two years of academic work in a college or university, four years in a medical school and from one and a half to two years in a hospital, a total of from seven to nine years' training. Such has been the growth of the science and art of medicine as indicated by the longer time required to so master its science and art as to be qualified to attend the sick. Consider the recent development of medicine from another point of view: Twenty-five years ago one might obtain a complete examination and diagnosis in the course of an hour or an hour and a half and at the hands of a single physician, whereas, this same service today, including all the laboratory and X-ray examinations and special examinations, will require from six to ten hours and the coöperation of from four to six or eight physicians.

The public appreciation of medical service has grown step by step with the increasing ability of the profession to render service. For example, in many of the more enlightened centers of the country, specialists in the diseases of children are not only treating the sick babies but are supervising the raising of the well babies—in short, the pediatrician, instead of restricting his services to the 4 to 8 per cent of sick babies, is rendering service to 100 per cent of the babies, to the sick and the well. We are all familiar with this practice in dentistry. A generation ago the dentist saw only the badly decayed teeth, but today the dentist is not occupied so much with the treatment of bad teeth as in the preservation of good teeth, and the more enlightened people come to the dentist regularly every six months just as they take their automobiles at periodic intervals to the garage for a general inspection. And so, too, we see the rapid development of periodic health examinations, frequently referred to as the birthday examination, that is a complete physical invoicing of the individual once a year. It will not be long until a very large part of the population comes to physicians, as they take their automobile to the garage, before a break occurs. And so, the time approaches when, with the better services which the medical profession can render and with a more intelligent appreciation of the public for such services, the doctors will concern themselves not only with the 2 or 3 per cent who are obviously sick but with 100 per cent of the population.

In concluding this consideration of factors that have, on the one hand, tended to decrease and, on the other hand, tended to increase the demand for medical service, we may say that there seems to have been such a balancing of the opposing forces of supply and demand as to have maintained a fairly uniform proportion of physicians to population over the 75-year period from 1850 to 1925.

The Distribution of Physicians

In considering the distribution of physicians, it will be well to note both the number and the type of physicians affected by the several factors which influence distribution —in short, to study the distribution of physicians from both a quantitative and qualitative viewpoint.

Quantitative Distribution of Physicians

The report by Mayers and Harrison, "The Distribution of Physicians in the United States," gives the proportion of physicians to population, for the year 1923, in places of variable sizes as shown in the following table:

TABLE 9

Places having a population of:	Population Per Physician*
Less than 1,000	1,238
Between 1,000 and 2,500	910
" 2,500 and 5,000	749
" 5,000 and 10,000	688
" 10,000 and 25,000	721
" 25,000 and 50,000	647
" 50,000 and 100,000	628
More than 100,000	536

In order to appreciate what part of the general population of the country is affected by the distribution of physicians as stated in the preceding table, we may now glance at a second table, also from the report of Mayers and Harrison, which gives (1) the *number* of *places* falling within the population classification used in the preceding table and (2) the *percentage of the total population of the country* that lives *in* and *about* such places. The table follows:

---

*Population both *in* and *about* places.

TABLE 10

All Places	Number Places Having Physicians	Percentage Pop. In and About
Less than 1,000	15,724	32.5
Between 1,000 and 2,500	3,167	11.3
Between 2,500 and 5,000	1,227	6.7
Total	20,118	50.5
Between 5,000 and 10,000	636	5.6
Over 10,000	632	43.9
Total	1,268	49.5

If we accept the town of 1,000 population as the dividing line between urban and rural conditions, as used by Mayers and Harrison in their Report, then we find 32.5 per cent of the population of the country living under rural conditions, and of this population, 3.4 per cent live *in* 15,724 places of 1,000 people, and 29.1 per cent live *about* these settlements.

If we accept the practice followed by the Bureau of the Census of the United States Government, which classifies as rural those who reside in places of 2,500 people and less, and as urban those who reside in larger places, then we have 43.8 per cent of the total population living under rural conditions. Of these, 8.8 per cent live *in* 18,891 towns of less than 2,500 and 35 per cent live *about* such places.

It would seem from the conditions which ordinarily obtain in medical practice that a more logical basis of classification would be to regard places of 5,000 people as the dividing line between rural and urban populations. The reason for this is that there is very little difference in the conditions of practice and medical care in places of less than 5,000 population. In places of larger population, 5,000 and over, hospitals become more frequent, and occasionally specialists are found. If we use the 5,000 population basis as the dividing line between rural and urban conditions in the practice of medicine, then we have 50.5 per cent of the population living *in* and *about* 20,118 towns of 5,000 people and less, and of the 50.5 per cent, 13.3 per cent live *in* the towns and 37.2 per cent *about* the towns.

Qualitative Distribution of Physicians

In 1906, 51 per cent of the graduates of the preceding four-year medical college course located in places of 5,000 population and less, and 49 per cent of these graduates located in places of population in excess of 5,000. By 1923, that is, in 17 years, only 22.9 per cent of the graduates of the preceding four-year course located in places of 5,000 and less, and 77.1 per cent located in places of 5,000 or more. These statistics show that there has developed a well marked tendency on the part of the more recent graduates of medicine to seek urban locations.

Now, we turn from the younger graduates to the older graduates. Mayers and Harrison point out that between 1906 and 1923 there was an 18 per cent decrease in the number of physicians practicing *in* and *about* places of not more than 1,000 population, that is, in clearly rural practices. Of greater significance is that of the 18 per cent decrease, 6 per cent occurred in the *ten-year* period between 1906 and 1916, and 12 per cent in the *seven-year* period between 1916 and 1923.

There are two types of physicians who leave the small rural practice and move to the city. The first type has been successful as a physician or in business and, usually, has a family of children to be educated. This type moves to the larger center of population for educational and social reasons rather than to build up a new practice. The second type is the progressive, industrious, wide-awake physician who has kept abreast of the advances in medicine, who has accumulated enough property to afford him financial assurance for the time between moving to a larger city and the time when he can reëstablish himself professionally under more advantageous conditions of practice. These two types, the successful physician who has retired, and the well-abreast-of-the-times doctor who has no fears in challenging the keener competition of a city profession, leave the country for the city.

Dr. William Allen Pusey, in a recent study of rural medical service which covered 283 representative rural counties, counties in which there were no towns with populations in excess of 5,000 and counties distributed over 41 states, found that the average age of physicians in these counties was 52 years, and that an average of only 1.4 recent graduates of medicine had located in these counties in the last ten years.

From the foregoing, we are to note a movement of growing strength which operates to locate not only the larger number of physicians among urban people, but that operates to locate the best physicians, the more recent graduates of medicine and the older men who have kept abreast with the advances in medical science, in city practices. In short, we have both a *quantitative* and a *qualitative* dislocation of medical personnel, and of the two dislocations the qualitative one is by far the more important.

Factors Influencing the Distribution of Physicians

We have already noted two important facts with reference to the distribution of physicians. First, that in proportion to population the number of physicians in cities is and has always been greater than in rural sections. Second, that within recent years, the disproportion in the number of urban and rural physicians has become greater. These facts call forth two questions: (1) Why has the city always claimed more doctors in proportion to population than the country? (2) Why, within recent years, has the disproportion between the number of urban and rural physicians increased?

The answer to the first question is that the greater advantages which the city offers in the way of personal comforts, social attractions, and business opportunities have always appealed to physicians, as they have to all others, members of the various professions and trades, and has resulted in the choice of urban conditions of life by the larger number.

The answer to the second question, namely, why the recent accentuation of the tendency of physicians to seek city practices, is more involved. It will be recalled that this accentuated movement of physicians to cities within recent years has influenced the choice of location for two types of physicians in particular, namely, (1) the more recent graduates in medicine, and (2) the older physicians who have kept abreast of the advances of medical science. Two explanations of this recent tendency of these better qualified physicians to choose urban locations are offered. These explanations are: (1) the marked industrial development of cities within the last two decades; (2) the presence in cities, as will later appear, of facilities, hospitals, for the practice of modern medicine and the absence of such facilities from rural communities. We will turn, now, to a brief consideration of each of these two influences in the choice of locations on the part of the more up-to-date physicians.

Recent urban industrial development: In their report on "The Distribution of Physicians in the United States," Mayers and Harrison state: "During the two decades, 1900 to 1920, the population of the United States increased by nearly 30,000,000—an increase of nearly 40 per cent. Of this vast increase only about 4,000,000 occurred in the territory outside of incorporated towns and villages." This great increase in population of city over country was obviously not due to differences in the birthrate of the urban and rural communities; nor was it due to foreign immigration. It could, therefore, have come about in but one way, namely, by the movement of people from country to city. Herein lies the explanation of the concurrent loss of population of large rural sections. Again, to quote Mayers and Harrison: "The counties that show a decrease of population from 1910 to 1920 comprised over 30 per cent of the area of the country. In the east north central section (Ohio, Indiana, Illinois, Michigan and Wisconsin) counties showing a decrease in population comprise over 45 per cent of the area." This rapid growth of the urban population at the expense of the rural population became especially marked with the rapid, industrial development incident to the Great War, that is to say, its effect was more noticeable after 1916 than before that year. In this general movement of population cityward the medical personnel of rural sections was caught. This is one explanation, although perhaps not the most important one, in the recent movement of physicians from rural to urban locations.

Facilities for the practice of modern medicine: Comment has already been directed to the great developments in medical science within recent years, but it may be permissible to recur to that thought for the purpose of pointing out, briefly, some of the more important changes in the art of medicine. Forty years ago, where one surgical operation was performed, fifty are performed today. Then the surgical risk was great; now, it is slight. There was no such thing as the X-ray at that time. The X-ray was discovered in 1895. As late as 1905 its use was restricted very largely to the big hospitals of the country. Forty years ago, the diagnostic laboratory was in its very beginnings. For every ten square feet of space set apart for laboratories then there are a thousand square feet used for laboratory work today. When Sir William Osler went in 1884 to the University of Pennsylvania he owned and used the only microscope in the hospital.

The practice of modern medicine requires such a breadth of knowledge, such extensive technical procedure, and such an expensive outlay for equipment, laboratory apparatus, X-ray equipment, operating room and sterilizers, that the average physician, who forty years ago carried all of his needs in a pair of saddlebags, can neither *purchase* nor *use* the absolute necessities for the practice of medicine. Such equipment is needed and such coöperative participation in its use is required that the pooling of resources of both bank and brain in the institutionalization of medicine, that is, in hospitals, has come as nothing less than a necessity.

The physician with ideals of thoroughness and efficient service breaks through the limitations of circumstance and finds a way and a place where he can practice his profession in the light of scientific knowledge and in accordance with his ideals. So it is that the recent graduate of medicine and the older doctor who has continued a student of medicine leaves the rural section, where he has no access to the facilities necessary for the practice of modern medicine, and moves to the urban community where he may have the advantages of a hospital.

Hospitals

The Background of Scientific Discovery Out of Which Hospitals Developed

Improvements in the microscope, its more general use during the last half of the last century in the study of disease, and the discovery of the causative factors in disease caused medical science to shift its chief interest from the study of the phenomena or symptoms of disease to the study of the causes of disease. It was this change in the dominant interest of medicine from symptoms to causes, resulting from the microscopic study of disease, that marks the point of departure of modern medicine from ancient medicine—the medicine of the great Hippocrates and all of his disciples down to the middle of the nineteenth century.

Pasteur, following the new interest in medicine, established, during the seventies and eighties of the last century, the infectious nature of many diseases, overthrowing the old idea of spontaneous generation. Koch confirmed the findings of Pasteur and simplified his methods and made them of general application. Lister made practical application of the work of Pasteur and Koch and brought forth antiseptic or modern surgery. So it is that these three, Pasteur, a great Frenchman; Koch, a great German; and Lister, a great Englishman, constitute the high tribune of modern medicine.

Antiseptic surgery, born at the hands of Lister, brought with it certain conditions for its performance. First of all, it required a room or place that could be made exceptionally clean, that was free from dust, that could be well-heated and ventilated without draughts, that could be well-lighted, with the lights so arranged as to prevent shadows. Second, it required certain equipment, equipment rather elaborate and expensive, equipment for sterilizing water, for sterilizing utensils, for sterilizing instruments and dressings, and all of this equipment conveniently related to the room or place where the surgery was to be done. Third, modern surgery required the assistance of specially trained personnel. We have here, then, as conditions for the performance of modern surgery, requirements that the individual physician cannot supply and requirements that cannot be met in domestic establishments; in short, we have conditions required for the performance of modern surgery that make absolutely necessary a place, an equipment, a personnel that represents a pooling of professional and public interests and that only a hospital can supply.

The microscope that made possible the work of Pasteur, and Koch, and Lister, and that brought in its train the operating room with its accessories in equipment and personnel, brought also the diagnostic laboratory. The microscope, as a means of demonstrating the causative relation existing between certain microscopic forms or germs and certain diseases, made it possible, through the discovery of the causative agent, to diagnose disease. To illustrate: The finding of the tubercle bacillus in the expectoration of a person with a cough and loss of flesh and strength not only serves as (1) an explanation of the cause of the disease but as (2) an incontrovertible diagnostic evidence of tuberculosis. The finding of the malarial germ in the blood of a person serves not only as an explanation of the cause of the disease but also as a diagnostic clincher for the recognition of the disease. Again, when men began to peer into the discharges and structure of the body with the magnified vision of the microscope, they noted not only the presence of germs that might be used as above stated for the purpose of diagnosis, but they began to note microscopic changes in the tissues or the flesh which were found subsequently to be constantly present in certain diseases, and, therefore, to be of diagnostic value. To illustrate: The microscopic changes in a lump or growth are as characteristic of inflammatory processes and tumors of various kinds as is the presence of the tubercle bacillus in the expectoration of a consumptive. So it was that the microscope began to be used, to be found necessary and important, in the diagnosis of diseases through the findings of either (1) characteristic germs or (2) characteristic tissue changes. And, again, having entered into the minute recesses of the body for diagnostic evidences of disease in the form of physical changes (addition of germs or alteration of tissue), it was but a step to note slight chemical changes in the juices, liquids, secretions and excretions of the body, which also had diagnostic value, as albumen or sugar in the urine or an excess of acid in the secretions of the stomach. So through the influence and use of the microscope the diagnostic laboratory came into existence. Now the diagnostic laboratory, as in the case of surgery, calls for equipment and special training which prohibits its satisfactory use by the individual physician and necessitates a pooling of resources that only the hospital can supply.

In 1895, another discovery, the X-ray, accentuated the movement, already well under way, in the direction of the pooling of professional resources. X-ray equipment costs anywhere from $3,000 to $10,000, and for its satisfactory use requires one with special training. Here, again, we have a condition for the modern practice of medicine which lies beyond the individual physician and which can be made available only through the organized practice of medicine as it is found in hospitals.

In more recent years the electrocardiograph, metabolism outfits for the study of nutrition, and other appliances, both too expensive and too highly technical for the average practitioner to purchase and to use, have come into existence. These appliances are not refinements but necessities in the practice of modern medicine. As in the equipment for surgery, for the diagnostic laboratory, for the X-ray, so here again these facilities for the modern diagnosis and treatment of disease can be made available only through a pooling of professional and public resources, and this means just one thing—hospitals.

As one would naturally expect, along with and keeping pace with the aforementioned developments in medi-

cine, developments leading inevitably to the pooling and
organization of professional resources, hospitals came into
use.   The chronology of the growth of. hospitals is the
chronology of the development of modern medicine.   Keeping in mind the fact that the interest, studies and discoveries out of which modern medicine has evolved have
spanned the last half century, note the parallel growth of
hospitals from 1873 to the present time, as shown in the
following table:

TABLE 11

Hospital Growth in the United States

Year	Number of Hospitals	Year	Number of Hospitals
1873	149	1914	5,057
1900	2,000*	1918	5,323
1906	2,411	1923	6,830
1909	4,359	1925	7,370

The following table shows the increase in the number
of hospitals and in the number of hospital beds along with
the increase in the population of the United States in the
fifty-year period between 1873 and 1923:

TABLE 12

Hospitals in the United States and Its Possessions·

	1873	1923	Per Cent of Increase
Number of hospitals. . .	149	7,095†	4,661
Number of hospital beds	35,453	792,069	2,162
Population	38,558,371	105,710,620	174

· The following graph, which we reproduce by courtesy
of the Modern Hospital Publishing Company, shows the
growth of hospital facilities in the United States for the
fifty-year period, 1873 to 1923.

---

*Estimate based on graph, Journal of the American Medical Association,
·January 12, 1924, page 118.
†Hospitals of less than 10 beds excluded from this figure.

****

Distribution of Hospitals by Urban and Rural Conditions

The distribution of hospitals in the United States according to the size of cities is shown in the following table:

TABLE 15

UNITED STATES

Size of Cities	Number of Cities	Number of Hospitals	Average No. of Hospitals
100,000 population and over...	68	1,546	22.7
50,000 to 100,000.........	76	446	5.8
25,000 to 50,000.........	143	532	3.7
10,000 to 25,000.........	459	1,001	2.1
10,000 and under.........14,946		3,366	.22

The important lesson from the above table is this: *In* places of 10,000 population and under, 17.8 per cent of the population of the United States lives; *about* such places, in the surrounding rural area, 38.3 per cent of the population of the United States lives. The hospitals in

465

these smaller places serve 17.8 plus 38.3 or 56.1 per cent of the population. In only a little more than one out of every five such places is there a hospital.

Distribution of Hospitals by Ownership

According to the survey of hospitals for the year 1926, as made by the Modern Hospital Publishing Company, the ownership of hospitals in the United States was as follows:

Government 31%
Associations, Communities, and Orders......... 36%
Individuals 33%

Total 100%

Government-owned hospitals were divided as follows:

Federal Government 8.0%
State Government 10.5%
County Government 7.0%
City Government 5.5%

Total 31.0%

The Federal Government hospitals consist largely of Army Hospitals, Naval Hospitals, U. S. Marine Hospitals, Veterans' Hospitals, and National Homes for disabled soldiers.

The State Government hospitals consist largely of hospitals for the insane and tuberculosis.

The 36 per cent of hospitals that are owned and operated by religious orders, fraternal orders, industrial and community organizations, are divided as to ownership as follows:

Denominational 17%
Independent Associations 14%
Industrial 3%
Fraternal 2%
                                         _____
Total 36%

What Constitutes Adequate Hospital Provisions

Hospital authorities consider provisions of five general hospital beds per 1,000 population for cities as adequate. In the cities of 100,000 population and over, the number of hospital beds per 1,000 population ranges from 1.9 beds per 1,000 in Akron, Ohio, to 8.8 beds per 1,000 in St. Paul, Minnesota. The general average for these larger cities is approximately five beds per 1,000 population.

In addition to the above provisions of five general hospital beds per 1,000 population, hospital authorities consider that cities should provide hospital facilities for special conditions as follows:

Contagious diseases per 1,000 population...... .5 beds
Diseases of Children per 1,000 population..... .5 "
Maternity per 1,000 population............. .45 "
Tuberculosis, as many beds as annual deaths.

Cities, on account of their living conditions—hotels, boarding houses, tenements, and a large non-resident population—and on account of the attraction of their comparatively highly specialized medical profession for medical cases within the sphere of the city's commercial influence, need a larger number of hospital beds in proportion to population than do rural communities.

For North Carolina and South Carolina counties with towns not exceeding 10,000 population and where the people are not accustomed to the use of a local hospital, the Director of the Hospital Section of The Duke Endowment is suggesting that the initial hospital provision should be not five, nor two, but one bed per 1,000 population. For example, in a county of 30,000 population, a 30-bed hospital; in a county of 40,000 population, a 40-bed hospital.

Professional Nursing

Development of Professional Nursing

We cannot conceive intelligently of medical services and leave out of consideration the enormously important, essential and supplemental role of professional nursing.

When the sick person was carried from the home to the hospital, there had to be some one to take the place of the gentle hands and loving hearts hitherto drawn from the family, near relatives and sympathetic neighbors. So professional nursing came into existence—came with the development of the institutional care for the sick. Hospitals not only called for the services of the nurse but supplied the means—a training center—for providing such services. So it is that the development of professional nursing runs a parallel course with the development of hospitals. If one will note Table 11, on page 48, of this Report, which shows the development of hospitals, beginning in the 70's of the last century, and then examine Table 16, on page 59, showing the development of professional nursing, the interesting and close parallelism between the growth of hospitals and professional nursing will be at once apparent.

TABLE 16

United States

SHOWING THE DEVELOPMENT OF PROFESSIONAL NURSING

Years	Schools	Nurse pupils	Yearly Graduates	Capacity of hospitals (beds)	Average* daily number of patients
1	2	3	4	5	6
1879	11	298	141		
1880	15	323	157		
1881	17	414	133		
1882–83	22	475	124		
1883–84	33	579	221		
1884–85	34	793	218		
1885–86	29	837	349		
1886–87	31	989	335		
1887–88	33	1,093	421		
1888–89	33	1,248	431		
1889–90	35	1,552	471		
1890–91	34	1,613	527		
1891–92	36	1,862	582		
1892–93	47	2,338	786		
1893–94	68	2,710	970		
1894–95	131	3,985	1,498		
1895–96	177	5,094	1,773		
1896–97	208	7,263	2,498		
1897–98	377	8,805	3,027		
1898–99	303	10,018	3,132		
1899–1900	432	11,164	3,456	84,227	
1900–1901	448	11,599	3,710	95,180	
1901–2	545	13,252	4,015	108,435	
1902–3	552	13,779	4,206	112,467	
1903–4	724	17,713	5,333	130,930	
1904–5	862	19,824	5,795	145,506	
1905–6	974	21,052	6,400	166,063	
1906–7	1,023	21,119	6,759	176,026	
1907–8	1,026	26,457	6,759	185,932	
1908–9	1,096	29,320	7,017	199,012	
1909–10	1,129	32,636	8,140	214,597	
1910–11	1,121	29,906	7,720	194,236	
1911–12	1,057	32,389	8,062	199,172	158,606
1912–13	1,094	34,417	9,937	202,887	158,389
1913–14	1,327	39,597	10,234	233,748	173,640
1914–15	1,509	46,141	11,118	256,325	185,408
1915–16	1,520	47,611	11,520	265,332	198,174
1916–17					
1917–18	1,770	55,251	13,751	303,193	225,890
1919–20	1,755	54,953	14,980	321,619	252,823

*See Bulletins Nos. 73 and 51 — — Trades Schools Dept. of the Interior

CHAPTER VII

PROVISIONS, PURPOSES AND PLANS OF THE HOSPITAL SECTION

Provisions

The provisions which determine the *income* of the Hospital Section of The Duke Endowment are fully set forth in Chapter I of this Report. The provisions which determine the *expenditure* of the funds available to the Hospital Section will now be considered.

Under the provisions of the Trust, the Trustees may give a sum not exceeding one dollar for every day a patient who is unable to pay is treated free of charge in a hospital not operated for private gain. It is provided further that the Trustees of the Endowment may expend any surplus of funds over the expenditure needed for the maintenance of charity patients, for the construction and equipment of hospitals. These two provisions, the one for the *maintenance* and the other for the *construction and equipment* of hospitals, are restricted in their application to the two States, North Carolina and South Carolina, until the hospital needs of the two States are adequately supplied, and then, when there is a surplus of funds over those needed for hospital work in the two States or when there is no longer a need of assistance from the Endowment, the Trustees may use the funds available to the Hospital Section in the hospital work of other States, the states contiguous to the Carolinas being given the position of preferred beneficiaries.

Explanatory Consideration of Provisions

In the provision for the maintenance of hospitals there are three conditions that are deserving of comment. The *first* condition is one that, by excluding hospitals operated

470

for private gain, limits the financial assistance which the
Trustees may give to community hospitals. The *second*
condition is one that limits financial assistance on the basis
of the charity work which a hospital is called upon to
carry. The *third* condition is one that limits financial assistance for charity work to one dollar a day for each
free patient.

The Limitation of Assistance to Community Hospitals

The explanation of this limitation does not lie in any
lack of appreciation, on the part of either the Founder or
the Trustees of the Endowment, of the work of private
hospitals. The private hospital, like the private school,
has been a necessary forerunner of the community hospital.
As private schools antedated public schools, so private
hospitals have prepared the way for public hospitals.
Those who have developed private hospitals have assumed,
not infrequently, in addition to their heavy professional
responsibilities, serious financial risks. Evidence in support of this statement is abundant. The Trustees of the
Endowment, in a study of hospitals early in 1925, found
for forty-nine of fifty-eight private hospitals from which
information was available and which were located in North
and South Carolina a total annual deficit of $87,000.
Moreover, instances are numerous where a progressive
physician, in order that he might be able to practice modern
medicine and his community have the advantage of a
hospital, has seriously involved his estate in an investment
which at his death is worth about thirty cents on the dollar. This is true for the reason that the value of a hospital
is about seventy per cent professional skill and thirty per
cent plant. From these considerations it is clear that society is deeply obligated to those who have given it the
private hospital; and especially is this true for the people
of North Carolina and South Carolina whose hospital
facilities, until within very recent years, have been sup-

plied to a very large extent by private resources. The Trustees of the Endowment, recognizing the paternal relation of the private hospital to the public hospital, share in the feeling of appreciation which society should have for those who have assumed unassisted the heavy burden of providing modern institutional care for the sick.

With this genuine appreciation of the private hospital, we turn now to consider the reasons which restrict the assistance of The Duke Endowment to those hospitals which incorporate a community interest.

The first and chief reason is that sickness is too big a problem for private resources and too socially important a problem to be neglected, avoided or shirked by the community.

The size of the problem of sickness is at once apparent when we consider the sick in the aggregate. In a type county, for example, a county of 30,000 population, there are present constantly 750 cases of bedridden sickness (25 cases per 1,000 population) and at least three times that number (75 cases per 1,000 population), 2,250, with serious physical impairments, people not in bed but on their feet, anywhere from twenty to fifty per cent inefficient. In this latter group of the impaired, including at one extreme those who are "just able to be up and about" and at the other extreme those who are "not quite up to the scratch," we find the great majority of those afflicted with heart disease, high and low blood pressures, tuberculosis, cancers, diseases of the gall bladder, gallstones, kidney stones, Bright's disease and other diseases of the kidneys, intestinal kinks and adhesions, constipation, hemorrhoids, hernias, displacements of organs, especially the female generative organs, unrepaired injuries following childbirth, chronic poisonings from the various forms of focal infection, etc. Among the 3,000 incapacitated and impaired there are 112 so seriously ill as to need hospital care. Of the 112 seriously ill who need hospital care, one-third, or 37, are not financially able to obtain it. They are charity cases. There is the problem of sickness in the aggregate. Who can look upon it and not see in it a community problem of the first magnitude—a problem too big to be left to the unassisted interest of from twenty to twenty-five men, the physicians of the county?

Sickness is a community problem not only by reason of the size of the problem, but by reason of its social significance. Any condition that involves one-tenth of the units of society in incapacity and serious impairment is of exceptionally large social importance.

The important relation which health and disease bears to civilization and history is just beginning to be understood and appreciated. The most fertile part of the globe has been closed to civilization because of climatic conditions and tropical diseases, against both of which protection is now available. Epidemics and endemic disease, the bringing of malaria to Greece by returning soldiers, venereal diseases, falling birth rates and mounting death rates have played no minor role in the history of nations. The strength of contending armies, until within very recent times, has been far more affected by disease than by battles. In this connection a quotation from the chapter on military hygiene in "Preventive Medicine and Hygiene," by Rosenau will be illuminating:

"In 1809, during the Walcheren expedition the mortality in the British army from disease was 346.9 per 1,000 effectives, while only 16.7 per 1,000 were killed by the enemy. In the Russian campaign against Turkey, in 1828, it was estimated that 80,000 men died of disease and 20,000 in consequence of wounds. During General Scott's campaign in Mexico the losses from disease alone exceeded 33 per cent of the effective strength of the forces under his command; and of a single regiment of Indiana volunteers, which entered the service 1,000 strong, only 400 returned to the State for muster out. Laveran states that in the Crimean War the allies lost 52,000 men in six months, of which number 50,000 men were unharmed by the Russians. During the entire war, according to Viry, the French lost no less than 95,000, of whom 75,000 died of disease.

"The mortality among the United States forces in the Civil War was divided as follows:

Mortality	White	Colored	Total
Killed in battle	42,724	1,514	44,238
Died of wounds	47,914	1,817	49,731
Died of disease	157,004	29,212	186,216
Died, cause unknown	23,347	837	24,184
Total	270,989	33,380	304,369

"From the most reliable data available, the deaths in the armies of the Confederate States during this struggle did not fall short of 200,000, three-fourths of which number were due to disease and one-fourth to the casualties of battle."

Industrial competition, not only as between competing plants, competing industries, competing sections of the country, but as between the great industrially competing countries of the world, is going to be determined more and more by the factor of vitality, group and national vigor.

The foregoing considerations with respect to the social significance of disease lead, as do considerations of the size of the problem of sickness, to the unavoidable conclusion that sickness is a community problem and has been ever since Cain raised the question: "Am I my brother's keeper?"

In passing, it may be well to consider, briefly, what happens when a community either thoughtlessly or deliberately, by omission or commission, neglects or shirks its responsibility to the sick. In the first place, there is much needless suffering and many unnecessary deaths. In the second place, the community pays a great deal more, both in blood and in money, than the more humane and intelligent course would have cost. When a community avoids the initiative in providing hospital care for its sick, one of the more progressive physicians or several such physicians are forced into building a private hospital. As these physicians cannot provide hospital facilities for the entire profession, and as other physicians or small groups cannot compete without hospitals with those who have them, a second private hospital goes up and so on as the community grows. Such a community may save a little tax money which would otherwise go into the one overhead cost of a single well-organized and efficient hospital, where it loses many times the taxes saved in the payment of fees which are necessary to maintain multiple hospital overhead costs. The community pays either in taxes or fees—but pays in both instances.

The limitation of the assistance of The Duke Endowment to community hospitals is a limitation dictated by wisdom. Sickness is a community problem. For an outside agency to assume the normal obligation which a community has to its sick is not helpful, in the larger sense, but harmful. To help those who help themselves, and not the converse, is the part of The Duke Endowment.

The Limitation of Assistance in Proportion to the Charity Burden of a Hospital

The Bureau of the Census of the United States Government, in its studies of the population of hospitals, has found that about one-third of the patients who are treated in hospitals are charity cases, those who are economically unable to pay for their treatment. In some communities this proportion is larger; in others, smaller. In proportion to the size of the burden of charity which a hospital is called upon to carry, the Trustees of The Duke Endowment are permitted to render financial assistance. If a community has no poverty, if there is no need to provide for the treatment of charity cases in hospitals, such a community does not need any assistance from The Duke Endowment. If a community has a large number of sick and suffering who are in need of hospital care that they themselves cannot supply, and if the community will not recognize its obligation to these, such a community does not deserve the assistance of The Duke Endowment. If, on the other hand, a community has a charity problem for its hospital, if it assumes it and in proportion as it assumes it, The Duke Endowment will help.

The fact that the Trustees of The Duke Endowment measure their financial assistance to hospitals by the amount of charity which these institutions are called upon to carry does not mean that The Duke Endowment is of no material assistance to patients who can pay. Ordinarily, the two-thirds of the patients in the hospitals of the United States who pay for themselves pay also for that part of the treatment of the one-third charity cases that is not assumed by the community or some philanthropic interest. When, therefore, a community or philanthropic agency provides the cost for the charity cases in a hospital, it becomes unnecessary for the hospital to collect from the pay cases enough to cover the cost of service to *both* pay and charity cases. The Duke Endowment, in contributing to the charity burden of a hospital and to the extent that it contributes, lifts the cost of charity from those who can pay and who would ordinarily have to pay for the limited amount of charity which the hospital would undertake. The financial contribution of The Duke Endowment to a hospital is, therefore, of direct material assistance not only to the poor but to those who are able to pay for their hospital care.

The Limitation of a Dollar a Day to the Charity Patient

The wisdom of this limitation appears when we consider the necessary part which distress, sickness and suffering plays in the development of character. If no one suffered, if no one was in distress, there would be no one with whom to sympathize. The source of sympathy in character is suffering, experienced and understood, and without suffering that quality of character, sympathy, would be lacking. Sympathy, born in the travail of suffering, is perhaps the finest quality in human character. It gives the individual the capacity to feel with and feeling with to become identified with others and, in this way and to the extent of this identification of the individual interest with the interest of others, to develop greatness of character. This identification of the one self with the other selves, this reflection of the interest of the individual in others, the work of sympathy, brings about the development of another constituent of the character close akin to sympathy, namely, love. Love, in its turn, generates service. Service, in its turn, results in sacrifice, not symbolically but literally, since all work, manual and mental, is accomplished through cellular activity and cellular activity is effected through the actual consumption and wearing out, in short, the sacrifice of the cells of the body, of parts of the body, and ordinarily, in a period of 70 years of service of the body in toto. And so it is of suffering that sympathy is born; of sympathy, love is born; of love, service is born; and of service sacrifice is born, and thus it is that out of trial and tribulation the finer elements of human character develop.

If it is true that distress, need and suffering are great and necessary forces in the process of character-building— the larger purpose and end in human life—then it follows that any agency that *completely* relieves the individual or the community of the necessity of responding to human need and relieving distress inhibits and renders inoperative one of the great and beneficent forces of life. If the Founder of the Endowment had provided that communities might be completely relieved of all obligations to their unfortunate neighbors, of all opportunities to render fine human service, great harm would have been done; if, on the other hand, the Founder of the Endowment makes it possible to extend the helping hand and to speak the word of encouragement to those who are just beginning to stand alone and walk uprightly; in short, if he has made possible assistance that encourages and does not substitute community effort, he has done great good, both to those who receive needed relief and to those who have been assisted in the more blessed role of giving. Two and a half or three dollars a day for each charity patient would relieve and tend to paralyze community interest and effort, would splint and waste the arm that needs exercise; one dollar a day for the charity case encourages, assists, develops. Hence the wisdom of the limitation of a dollar a day for each charity case.

Purposes

The major purpose of the Trustees of The Duke Endowment in the administration of the Hospital Section is not to be confused, as it is likely to be, with the maintenance and building of hospitals.

The assistance provided by The Duke Endowment for the development of adequate hospital facilities is not regarded by the Trustees as an end in itself, but as a necessary means to a much larger objective, namely, an improved medical service that reaches not only the ten per cent of the more seriously sick who constitute the hospital cases of a community but also the other ninety per cent who are cared for outside of the hospital, in the community at large. The explanation of the foregoing statement lies in the fact that, generally speaking, the more capable physicians, that is to say, the older graduates of medicine who have kept abreast of the advances of medical science and the younger graduates, and especially those with hospital experience, either leave or refuse to enter practices where hospital advantages are absent. Hospitals hold and attract the better type of physicians. A few able physicians in a community set the pace and fix the standards for the entire local profession. So it is that a local hospital builds up a profession, raises professional standards and serves to improve the practice of medicine not only for patients in the hospital but for patients in the whole county.

A concrete illustration will serve to make clear the influence of the hospital on the practice of medicine, both *in* and *about* the local institution. A county of 36,000, with a county town of 4,000, opened a hospital in 1923. Since the hospital was opened and because of the hospital, there have located in that county within the last few years, a graduate of the Johns Hopkins Medical School, with from two to three years hospital surgical experience, and two graduates of the Medical Department of the University of Pennsylvania, both well-trained hospital men. Only one other graduate of the last ten years has located in the county. These three doctors serve as a court of diagnostic appeal for the seriously sick and for the cases of difficult diagnosis of the entire county. The existence of such a court of appeal in the county has a most wholesome and stimulating influence on all the doctors of the community. This example is by no means an exception.

In conclusion, we repeat that *the purpose of the Trustees of The Duke Endowment in the administration of the Hospital Section is an improved local medical service;* their means for bringing about this desirable end is a local hospital.

Plan

The plan of the Trustees of The Duke Endowment for the administration of the Hospital Section is, in principle, simple; in execution, rather detailed.

In principle, the plan is to submit a form or application blank to a hospital that wishes to apply for assistance. When the application blank is filled out and returned, it supplies such information about the hospital as enables the Trustees to do two things: (1) to ascertain (a) whether the hospital comes within the terms of the Trust, and, if it does, (b) to what extent it is entitled to assistance; (2) to establish a clearing house of information through which each hospital may take advantage of the experience of the entire group of hospitals that apply to the Endowment for assistance.

Through the information collected from all beneficiary hospitals, censored, corrected, set up in comparative tables and returned to the hospitals, the superintendent and trustees of any particular hospital may (1) compare their income, both as to sources and extent, with that of all other beneficiary hospitals; (2) may compare their expenditures, their per capita per diem cost, and how much of the per capita per diem cost was for food and cooking, for nursing services, for surgical supplies and medicines, for laundry, etc., etc., with that of all other beneficiary hospitals and also with that of the group of hospitals of similar size, work, and race admissions as their own; (3) may compare the results of their professional work, the percentage of admissions which terminated fatally, the percentage of the more important surgical conditions which terminated fatally, the percentage of obstetrical conditions and complications which terminated fatally, the percentage of children under treatment which terminated fatally, etc., with similar information from all other beneficiary hospitals and also with that of the group of hospitals of similar size, work, and race admissions as their own.

Such comparative information enables the management of any hospital to know in what respects its work compares, satisfactorily, unsatisfactorily or questionably with that of similar institutions. The management of a hospital, having had its attention brought to bear upon work which appears unsatisfactory or questionable, is in a position, through the clearing house of information available to it through its connection with The Duke Endowment, to be placed in touch with those hospitals whose work in the particular item under consideration appears to be of an exceptionally high order. For example, a hospital finds that its laundry cost per patient per day is 30 per cent above the average. The hospital asks The Duke Endowment to give it the advantage of the experience of well-managed hospitals known to have a lower than the average patient day cost on laundry. The Hospital Section, referring to its list, picks out some 5, 6, 7, or 8 well-managed hospitals with laundry costs less than the average, addresses a letter of inquiry to these hospitals and receives their replies explaining their method of handling laundry. These replies are copied and the copies mailed to the hospital making the inquiry. So the individual hospital is given the advantage of the group experience.

In summary, it may be said that the plan of the Trustees in the administration of the Hospital Section contemplates a two-fold service: (1) a financial service and (2) an information service, and of the two, it is probable that in time the latter may prove to be the more valuable.

THE

Duke Endowment

FOURTH ANNUAL REPORT

OF

The Hospital Section

1928

OFFICERS AND TRUSTEES

THE CONSTRUCTION AND EQUIPMENT PROGRAM*

Provisions

Under that section of the Trust Indenture that makes financial provision (to the extent of one dollar a day for every day patients who are unable to pay have been treated free of charge), for operating hospitals that are not used for purposes of private gain and that are located in North Carolina and South Carolina, the Trustees of The Duke Endowment are permitted to use any *surplus* funds accruing to the Hospital Section for assisting communities in constructing or otherwise securing additional hospital facilities. Under this provision of the Trust, the Trustees may contribute (1) to the purchase of new equipment, (2) to the construction of additions to hospital buildings, (3) to the construction of entirely new hospital plants, and (4) to the purchase of privately owned hospitals for community use.

Policies

Financial Assistance: The Trustees are permitted to exercise greater discretion in assisting communities in the construction and equipment of hospitals than they are permitted to exercise in contributing to the maintenance or operation of hospitals.

In the operation of hospitals, the proportion of operating cost that the Trustees may provide is definitely fixed by the Trust Indenture at not more than one dollar a day

---

*We are repeating here what was said in last year's annual report under the subdivisions "Provisions" and "Policies." This repetition seems to be called for for the reason that the work of The Duke Endowment has not extended over a sufficient period of time for those who may be interested in applying for assistance in the building and equipment of hospitals to have become reasonably informed as to the scope and the limitations of the Trustees of The Duke Endowment in assisting in the building and equipment of additional hospital facilities.

for all patients who are unable to pay, whereas, in contributing to the construction of hospitals, no fixed sum or proportion of the cost is named. However, where the Trust Indenture is silent, circumstances are audible and binding. Two conditions, namely, (1) the amount of the surplus (which is dependent upon the earnings of the invested funds), and (2) the number and the character of applications for assistance determine how much the Trustees may appropriate for any given proposal.

The number of applications directly influences the size of the appropriations that the Trustees may make to different communities. To illustrate: With earnings that produce a surplus of $400,000, the Trustees can be more generous with ten applications for building than with twice that number.

The character of an application for assistance, as well as the number of pending applications, influence the response of the Trustees. Some applications are more meritorious and urgent than others. To illustrate: Two communities apply for assistance in building a hospital; in one community there is no hospital of any kind, public or private; in the other community there is a private hospital with eight-tenths of a hospital bed per thousand population. The first community is in greater need, and, other things being equal, deserves first consideration. However, other things may not be equal, and the community with eight-tenths hospital bed per thousand people may be more deserving of assistance than the other community with not a single hospital bed per thousand population. If, for example, the community with eight-tenths hospital bed per thousand population is willing to contribute 60 per cent of the funds that are needed for additional hospital facilities and the other community will contribute but 35 per cent of the funds needed for a hospital, and if both communities are of like per capita wealth, then the second community with some hospital beds, but with an inadequate number of beds, would make the stronger appeal.

Again, two communities apply for financial assistance in the building of hospitals: In one community the funds are subscribed—volunteer dollars; in the other the funds are obtained by voting bonds—drafted dollars. Other things again being equal, the first community should, perhaps, receive first consideration.

And, again, two communities apply for financial help for building hospitals: In one community there is an alert, well-organized medical profession in which there is an unusual number of graduates of medicine of the last ten-year period; in the other community there is an unprogressive, divided, indifferent group of doctors, with a high average age and few graduates of the last ten-year period. Other things being equal, the first of these communities should receive first consideration.

These illustrations serve to indicate rather clearly that there are a number of varying local conditions that are necessary factors in arriving at a sound judgment as to the relative merits of applications from different communities for assistance in the building of hospitals. These varying local conditions should and do influence the Trustees in both (1) the order in which applications are taken up and (2) in the measure of assistance that is extended to the applicants. In order that these local conditions should have their proper weight in passing upon the hospital needs of any given community, the Trustees ordered prepared and adopted at their November meeting in 1927 an application for the general use of those communities which are interested in applying for assistance in the building of local hospitals. * * *

Advisory Assistance: The Trustees anticipated that most communities which might be interested in the building of local hospitals would need and desire, in addition to any financial assistance that they might receive, certain preliminary advice with respect to the planning of their hospital—advice as to how to choose a proper location, advice for estimating the size or number of beds necessary for local requirements, and advice concerning the general arrangement of the various services included in a well-conceived hospital. To meet this anticipated need, a study of the rather limited literature on the subject of the small general hospital was made and a firm of architects of large experience and approved reputation was employed to assist in the preparation of a publication, designed to assist both the general and professional groups in the planning and building of small local hospitals.

"The Small General Hospital" or "Bulletin No. 3," was published in December, 1927. This publication consists of seventy-five large size pages suitable for architectural drawings. The bulletin is divided into three parts. Part I deals with such general considerations as (1) the larger social purposes of a hospital, (2) problems of location, (3) adaptability of hospitals to different communities, (4) the various types of buildings to be considered, (5) material and structural considerations, and (6) the relations of the more important services, such as that of (a) the out-patient service to the in-patient service, (b) the dietetic service to patients, (c) the diagnostic and operating services to each other and the other services, and (d) the proportion of beds that should be in wards, semi-private rooms, and private rooms, etc. Part II is more detailed and is intended largely for those directly concerned with the building of the hospital, architects, contractors, and building committees. Part III consists of thirty full-page drawings showing floor plans and details of every wall of every room, as well as structural details and, in addition, the location of all furniture and equipment.

The relation of the ideal to the attainable is taken care of in the following way: The hospital, as it should be constructed and equipped, provided sufficient resources are available, is described fully, and then a chapter on possible economies follows, so that those communities that may wish and can afford to have the very best have the ideal set before them, and those communities that are more limited in resources are given practical suggestions as to where economies are possible and may be effected with least departure from the model.

Bulletin No. 3 will be revised from time to time, possibly every three or four years, so as to incorporate the best lessons of accumulating experience. In the revisions there will be included photographs, floor plans, and structural descriptions of actual hospitals that seem to represent the best thought in hospital planning combined with high investment values. Along with such descriptive matter, the names of the architects and contractors and the cost of construction and equipment of each hospital will be given.

Participation in New Construction and Equipment During 1928

During 1928 the Trustees of The Duke Endowment participated with local communities in providing additional hospital facilities as shown in Table 32 on page 165.

New Hospitals Completed in 1928

Three new hospitals opened in 1928, to the construction and equipment of which The Duke Endowment contributed, the Haywood County Hospital, the Marion General Hospital, and the Garrett Memorial Hospital.

****

Haywood County Hospital

The Haywood County Hospital, Waynesville, North Carolina, was constructed and equipped with funds raised by a county bond issue voted by the people and contributions from The Duke Endowment and individuals and organizations in the county. The county bond issue of $100,000 and other gifts by the county governing authorities totaled $106,516.08, The Duke Endowment gave $10,000, and individuals and organizations in the county contributed $2,209.96.

The hospital is well located on a five-acre lot, approximately 300 feet by 800 feet, overlooking State Highway No. 10, and about one mile from the center of the town. The hospital was opened to receive patients January 1, 1928.

The hospital is of fireproof construction.

The hospital, including the basement, is four stories in height and has a cubic content of 213,700 cubic feet.

The hospital has a capacity of 45 beds, including eight bassinets in the nursery, divided as follows: Wards, 16; two-bed rooms, 8; private rooms, 21.

The walls are of brick and are trimmed with Indiana limestone.

The partitions are of four-inch hollow tile.

The floors have a total area of 21,810 square feet. The floors are constructed of hollow tile and reënforced concrete.

The floor covering is as follows:

Area covered with tile .... 11 per cent
Area covered with terrazzo.............. 14 per cent
Area covered with cement............... 23 per cent
Area with composition covering (marbeloid) 52 per cent

The roof of the hospital consists of reënforced concrete covered with gravel and tar.

The stairs consist of steel frame with slate treads.

The cost of the hospital was as follows:

(a) Lot and improvements $10,284.61
(b) Structural branches 73,869.48
(c) Plumbing 2,700.00
(d) Heating 8,370.50
(e) Electric work 4,473.50
(f) Elevator 2,908.80
                                    _____
(g) Total cost, without equipment......$102,606.89

Cost per cubic foot without equipment, 48.01 cents.
Cost per bed without equipment, $2,280.15.
Cost of equipment, $16,119.15.
Cost of equipment per bed, $358.20.
Cost per bed equipped, $2,638.35.

****

Marion General Hospital

The Marion General Hospital, Marion, McDowell County, North Carolina, was constructed and equipped with funds raised by public subscription and contributions from The Duke Endowment and the city. Public subscriptions from individuals and organizations amounted to $34,675.33, The Duke Endowment gave $29,000, and the city gave $1,756.85.

The hospital is located on a lot of seven-eighths of an acre, about four blocks from the center of town, and is easily seen from State Highway No. 10, being about half a block away from Highway No. 10 on James Street. This hospital was opened to receive patients November 1, 1928.

The hospital is of semi-fireproof construction.

The hospital, including the basement, is three stories in height, and has a cubic content of 160,000 cubic feet.

The hospital has a capacity of 40 beds, including 10 bassinets in the nursery, divided as follows: Wards, 26; two-bed rooms, 8; private rooms, 6.

The walls consist of concrete blocks, veneered with variegated brown and red face brick. The ground floor walls are 17 inches thick and the other walls 13 inches thick. The boiler-room walls and ceiling are of fireproof masonry construction.

The partitions are of wood frame construction.

The three floors have a total area of 12,326 square feet. The floors are of wood frame construction. The floor covering is as follows:

Area covered with tile . . . . 3.2 per cent
Area covered with cement. . . . . 36.2 per cent
Area covered with linoleum. . . . . 18.2 per cent
Area covered with wood . . . . 42.4 per cent

The roof of the hospital consists of slate-coated shingles on the steep roofs and composition and tin on the deck roofs.

The stairs are of wood frame construction.

The cost of the hospital was as follows:

(a) Lot and improvements...............$ 7,975.52
(b) Structural branches 39,685.76
(c) Plumbing 5,700.00
(d) Heating 4,500.00
(e) Electric work 2,646.08
(f) Elevator 1,599.82
                                    _____
(g) Total cost, without equipment........$62,107.18

Cost per cubic foot without equipment, 38.19 cents.
Cost per bed without equipment, $1,552.68.
Cost of equipment, $8,325.00.
Cost of equipment per bed, $208.13.
Cost per bed equipped, $1,760.81.

****

Garrett Memorial Hospital

The Garrett Memorial' Hospital, Crossnore, Avery County, North Carolina, was constructed and equipped with funds raised by public subscription and a contribution by The Duke Endowment. Public subscriptions amounted to $9,149.37 and The Duke Endowment gave $8,250.

The hospital is well located on a two-acre lot, approximately 300 by 300 feet, about half a block from State Highway No. 194. The hospital was opened to receive patients on August 6, 1928.

The hospital is not of fireproof construction.

The hospital, including the basement, is two stories in height, and has a cubic content of 56,000 cubic feet.

The hospital has a capacity of 18 beds, divided as follows: Wards, 12; two-bed rooms, 6.

The walls consist of native stone.

The partitions are of wood frame construction.

The basement and first floor have a total area of 4,150 square feet. The floors are of wood frame construction. The floor covering is as follows:

Area covered with cement............... 36 per cent
Area covered with wood................ 64 per cent

The roof of the hospital consists of cement tile shingles.

The stairs are of wood frame construction.

The cost of the hospital was as follows:

(a) Lot and improvements...............$ 939.55
(b) Structural branches 9,206.84
(c) Plumbing 454.46
(d) Heating 786.50
(e) Electric work 270.93

(f) Total, without equipment...........$11,658.28

Cost per cubic foot without equipment, 20.8 cents.
Cost per bed without equipment, $647,68.
Cost of equipment, $5,741.09.
Cost of equipment per bed, $318.95.
Cost per bed equipped, $966.63.

THE
DUKE ENDOWMENT

HOSPITAL SECTION

■

A SIX-YEAR REVIEW
OF THE ACTIVITIES OF
ASSISTED TUBERCULOSIS SANATORIA
IN THE CAROLINAS

*(Reprinted from the Annual Report of the Hospital
Section for the Year 1930)*

THE DUKE ENDOWMENT
POWER BUILDING, CHARLOTTE, N. C.

CHAPTER IV
TUBERCULOSIS SANATORIA

Introduction

In *North Carolina the* Winyah Sanatorium in Asheville, a private institution, opened in 1888 and closed in May, 1930, appears to have been the first tuberculosis sanatorium. The Violet Hill Sanatorium in Asheville, also a private institution, was opened in 1895. The best obtainable information indicates that these two were the only institutions of this type in existence at the beginning of the century. St. Joseph's Sanatorium in Asheville was opened by the Sisters of Mercy in 1900 and was apparently the first non-profit tuberculosis sanatorium in North Carolina. The state sanatorium, opened in 1907, was the next and the Red Cross Sanatorium in Wilmington, opened in 1912, largely through the efforts of the local tuberculosis association, was the first non-profit sanatorium exclusively for local or community use. There were seven non-profit sanatoria, including the state institution, at the time The Duke Endowment was established and at that time there were twenty-four private tuberculosis sanatoria located, with one exception, in the mountains around Asheville.

In *South Carolina* Aiken Cottages, opened in 1897 largely through the efforts of winter residents of Aiken, appears to have been the first tuberculosis sanatorium. It was not intended primarily for residents of the county. Eighteen years later the next tuberculosis sanatorium came into existence. Hopewell Sanatorium in Greenville, opened in 1915 through the efforts of the local tuberculosis association, and merged with the Greenville County Tuberculosis Sanatorium in 1930, was the second institution of this type in the state and the first intended primarily for residents of the community in which it was located. The state sanatorium came into existence the same year. At the time The Duke Endowment was established there were six sanatoria in South Carolina, including the state institution. So far as the records show, there has never been a tuberculosis sanatorium operated for profit in South Carolina.

Growth During the Past Six Years

When The Duke Endowment was established there were 37 tuberculosis sanatoria in the Carolinas, exclusive of the sanatorium operated by the United States Veterans Bureau at Oteen, North Carolina. Six years later the number was 40. The private group had decreased in number from 24 to 21 and the non-profit group, exclusive of the two state institutions, had increased from 11 to 17. Sixteen of these institutions applied to The Duke Endowment for assistance as such at the end of 1930 and Table 27 on page 3 is a record of their names, location, auspices, number of beds for patients at the end of 1930, total days of care of patients, the number and per cent that were free, and the contribution by The Duke Endowment during 1930 for the free days of care during 1929 at one dollar a day. The new tuberculosis sanatorium in Spartanburg, South Carolina, which opened on October 6, 1930, and cared for a comparatively small number of patients to the end of the year, is not included in this table for the reason that it is under the same management as the Spartanburg General Hospital and applied for assistance as a department of this hospital.

TABLE 27

LOCATION, AUSPICES, BEDS, DAYS OF CARE, AND THE DUKE ENDOWMENT CONTRIBUTION FOR 1929

Sanatorium	Location	County	Auspices	Patient Beds	Days of Care Total	*Free Days Number	*Free Days Per Cent	Contribution For 1929
16 TUBERCULOSIS SANATORIA	16 Towns	15 Counties		904	252,889	208,124	82.3	168,538
10 NORTH CAROLINA SANATORIA	10 Towns	9 Counties		673	192,152	158,914	82.7	122,815
Forsyth County Sanatorium	Winston-Salem	Forsyth	County	178	34,593	34,496	99.7	13,134
Mecklenburg Sanatorium	Huntersville	Mecklenburg	County	162	54,254	53,725	99.0	45,404
Guilford County Sanatorium	Jamestown	Guilford	County	106	36,473	34,450	94.5	32,888
St. Joseph's Sanatorium	Asheville	Buncombe	Religious	94	31,444	5,415	17.2	7,981
Red Cross Sanatorium	Wilmington	New Hanover	Community	36	9,356	7,434	79.5	7,309
Catawba County Sanatorium	Newton	Catawba	County	25	7,436	7,368	99.1	972
Halifax County Sanatorium	Halifax	Halifax	County	24	6,829	6,829	100.0	6,134
Edgecombe County Sanatorium	Tarboro	Edgecombe	County	22	5,141	5,141	100.0	4,733
Scott Parker Sanatorium	Henderson	Vance	County	14	3,707	3,458	93.3	3,726
Bethel Home	Weaverville	Buncombe	Religious	12	2,919	598	20.5	534
6 SOUTH CAROLINA SANATORIA	6 Towns	6 Counties		231	60,737	49,210	81.0	45,723
Ridgewood Camp	Columbia	Richland	Community	67	19,158	13,411	70.0	12,985
†Greenville County Sanatorium	Greenville	Greenville	County	55	10,897	10,514	96.5	8,657
Pinehaven Sanatorium	Charleston	Charleston	Community	50	16,727	13,233	79.1	12,793
Camp Alice	Sumter	Sumter	Community	26	8,467	7,508	88.7	6,365
‡Aiken Cottages	Aiken	Aiken	Community	20	3,273	2,329	71.2	2,012
Marion County Tuberculosis Camp	Mullins	Marion	County	13	2,215	2,215	100.0	2,911

*Includes days of care that part pay patients did not pay for.   †Formerly Hopewell Sanatorium.   ‡Open only part of the year.

Beds for Patients

A comparison of the gains or losses in beds available for patients at the end of the years 1924 and 1930 is of interest:

	Beds for Patients		
	1930	1924	Gain or —Loss
BOTH STATES	2,329	1,549	780
Private Sanatoria	716	827	—111
Non-Profit Sanatoria	939	409	530
State Sanatoria	674	313	361
NORTH CAROLINA	1,789	1,282	507
Private Sanatoria	716	827	—111
Non-Profit Sanatoria	673	250	423
State Sanatorium	400	205	195
SOUTH CAROLINA	540	267	273
Non-Profit Sanatoria	266	159	107
State Sanatorium	274	108	166

While beds in all of these tuberculosis sanatoria increased 50 per cent in number, 40 per cent in North Carolina and 100 per cent in South Carolina, the group of local non-profit sanatoria which were assisted by The Duke Endowment shows an increase of 130 per cent, 169 per cent in North Carolina and 67 per cent in South Carolina. It is not probable that The Duke Endowment has had any influence on the decrease in number and beds in the private sanatoria or on the increase in beds in the state sanatoria, but the gain in the local non-profit sanatoria, both in number and in beds used, can be attributed in no small degree to the contribution of one dollar a day for free days of care.

Several of the tuberculosis sanatoria increased their bed capacity during 1930 by additions or by new building projects and the number of beds shown in Table 28 on page 5 is the average number in use during the year by the institutions applying for assistance. The bed occupancy was 56 per cent in 1924, as compared with 79 per cent in 1930. In North Carolina the gain was from 61 per cent

TABLE 28
BEDS FOR PATIENTS
BY RACE AND UTILIZATION

	Total Beds	Beds by Race		Beds Occupied	
		White	Negro	Number	Per Cent
16 TUBERCULOSIS SANATORIA____	872	693	179	692.8	79.4
5 Community_____	189	126	63	156.1	82.6
2 Religious_____	106	106		94.1	88.8
9 County_____	577	461	116	442.6	76.7
10 IN NORTH CAROLINA_____	673	558	115	526.4	78.2
1 Community_____	36	21	15	25.6	71.1
2 Religious_____	106	106		94.1	88.8
7 County_____	531	431	100	406.7	76.6
6 IN SOUTH CAROLINA_____	199	135	64	166.4	83.6
4 Community_____	153	105	48	130.5	85.3
2 County_____	46	30	16	35.9	78.0

to 78 per cent and in South Carolina from 49 per cent to 84 per cent.

The ratio of beds to population was one for every 2,940 people six years ago and one for every 2,130 people at the end of 1930. In the two states taken separately the ratios at the end of 1924 were one to 2,220 in North Carolina and one to 6,400 in South Carolina, but elimination of the private sanatoria, which draw the great majority of their patients from other states, and which for the most part are located in western North Carolina, gives a ratio in the two states of one bed for every 6,300 people and in North Carolina of one bed for every 6,260 people. At the end of 1930 the corrected ratios would be, for both states one to 3,070, for North Carolina, one for 3,000, and for South Carolina one for 3,230. The Carolinas still have a long way to go to reach the national average, as evidenced by the fact that there is one sanatorium bed for every 1,880 people in the United States, and one out of every 2,200 persons in the United States was occupying a bed in a tuberculosis sanatorium at the average time during 1930, as compared with one bed occupied, the private sanatoria excluded, for every 3,800 people in the Carolinas.

While the number of beds for patients in these local non-profit sanatoria at the end of 1930 was 2.3 times the number six years ago, the average number of patients per day in 1930 was three times the number in 1924, as indicated by the following tabulation:

	Average Number of Patients Per Day		
	1930	1924	Gain or —Loss
BOTH STATES	696	229	467
Community	156	88	68
Religious	94	97	—3
County	446	44	402
NORTH CAROLINA	526	152	374
Community	25	11	14
Religious	94	97	—3
County	407	44	363
SOUTH CAROLINA	170	77	93
Community	131	77	54
County	39		39

The large increase in the number of patients receiving treatment has come about in the group operated by counties. The number of these institutions has increased from three to ten, one of the community group having become a county institution in 1930.

The average number of patients per day in the two state sanatoria increased from 293 in 1924 to 606 in 1930, a gain of 313. The group of private sanatoria shows a loss of 238 patients, from 630 to 392. This makes a net gain in the average number of patients per day of 542 in all tuberculosis sanatoria, from 1,152 in 1924 to 1,694 in 1930.

Days of Care

If the days of care that part pay patients did not pay for are added to the free days of care of patients who were not able to pay anything for their care, including the Spartanburg County institution, the total free days for these

TABLE 29
DAYS OF CARE
BY ECONOMIC STATUS OF PATIENTS

	Total Days	Full Pay		Part Pay		Free	
		Number	Per Cent	Number	Per Cent	Number	Per Cent
16 TUBERCULOSIS SANATORIA	252,889	27,181	10.7	36,039	14.3	189,669	75.0
5 Community	56,981	2,592	4.5	17,560	30.8	36,829	64.7
2 Religious	34,363	24,315	70.8	5,622	16.3	4,426	12.9
9 County	161,545	274	.2	12,857	8.0	148,414	91.8
10 IN NORTH CAROLINA	192,152	24,444	12.7	20,866	10.9	146,842	76.4
1 Community	9,356			2,778	29.7	6,578	70.3
2 Religious	34,363	24,315	70.5	5,622	16.3	4,426	12.9
7 County	148,433	129	.1	12,466	8.4	135,838	91.5
6 IN SOUTH CAROLINA	60,737	2,737	4.5	15,173	25.0	42,827	70.5
4 Community	47,625	2,592	5.4	14,782	31.1	30,251	63.5
2 County	13,112	145	1.1	391	3.0	12,576	95.9

institutions in 1930 would be approximately 209,000. Even more striking than the increase in the number of beds for patients and the average number of patients per day in these sanatoria assisted by The Duke Endowment, is the fact that the number of free days of care in 1930 was five and one-half times the number in 1924. The following tabulation brings out this fact:

	Free Days of Care		
	1930	1924	Gain or —Loss
BOTH STATES	209,000	37,300	171,700
Community	44,791	21,689	23,102
Religious	6,013	2,745	3,268
County	158,196	12,866	145,330
NORTH CAROLINA	158,914	19,434	139,480
Community	7,434	3,823	3,611
Religious	6,013	2,745	3,268
County	145,467	12,866	132,601
SOUTH CAROLINA	50,086	17,866	32,220
Community	37,357	17,866	19,491
County	12,729		12,729

The free days of care made up 45 per cent of the total in 1924, 35 per cent in North Carolina and 63 per cent in South Carolina. In 1930 these percentages were 82, 83, and 81 respectively. The county sanatoria reported 20 per cent of their days of care paid for by the patients in 1924 and two per cent in 1930.

A division of days of care as between races was first made in 1927. This division for the past four years is as follows:

| | Days of Care by Races | | | |
| | Total | White | Negro | |
			Number	Per Cent
BOTH STATES	810,565	649,530	161,035	20
1927	166,755	138,401	28,354	17
1928	181,796	148,263	33,583	18
1929	209,125	165,430	43,695	21
1930	252,889	197,436	55,453	22
NORTH CAROLINA	596,050	492,399	103,651	17
1927	118,598	100,912	17,686	15
1928	131,271	109,094	22,177	17
1929	154,029	128,209	25,820	17
1930	192,152	154,184	37,968	20
SOUTH CAROLINA	214,515	157,131	57,384	27
1927	48,157	37,489	10,668	22
1928	50,525	39,169	11,356	23
1929	55,096	37,221	17,875	32
1930	60,737	43,252	17,485	29

The population of the two states is 35 per cent Negro, 29 per cent in North Carolina and 45 per cent in South Carolina. The days of care of Negroes in these sanatoria made up approximately 22 per cent of the total in 1930, 20 per cent in North Carolina and 29 per cent in South Carolina. The Negro death rate from tuberculosis is approximately twice the death rate for white people, which would appear to indicate that the incidence of the disease in its active stages among Negroes is about double the incidence among white people.

Four of the ten sanatoria in North Carolina do not admit Negroes, the two institutions operated by religious organizations, one county institution that admits only white children, and one small county sanatorium open only to white adults. One of the institutions in South Carolina is open only to white adults. This makes twelve institutions in the two states in as many counties open to Negroes. These institutions limit their admissions almost entirely to patients from the counties in which they are located. The other 134 counties are dependent upon the 76 beds in the state sanatoria for what institutional care the Negroes get. The Negro population of the two states is 1,718,500 and there are 281 beds in the local non-profit and state institutions to care for tuberculosis in this group, or one bed for every 6,100 Negroes, as compared with one bed for every 2,400 white people. In other words, there are approximately two and one-half times as many beds for white people in proportion to population as there are beds for Negroes.

TABLE 30
PATIENTS DISCHARGED
BY ECONOMIC STATUS

	Total Patients	Full Pay		Part Pay		Free	
		Number	Per Cent	Number	Per Cent	Number	Per Cent
16 TUBERCULOSIS SANATORIA	996	123	12.3	196	19.7	677	68.0
5 Community	259	17	6.6	110	42.5	132	50.9
2 Religious	129	102	79.1	18	14.0	9	6.9
9 County	608	4	.7	68	11.2	536	88.1
10 IN NORTH CAROLINA	706	106	15.0	90	12.7	510	72.3
1 Community	37			10	27.0	27	73.0
2 Religious	129	102	79.1	18	14.0	9	6.9
7 County	540	4	.7	62	11.5	474	87.8
6 IN SOUTH CAROLINA	290	17	5.9	106	36.6	167	57.5
4 Community	222	17	7.7	100	45.0	105	47.3
2 County	68			6	8.8	62	91.2

Patients Discharged

The free patients are a comparatively small proportion of the patients discharged from the two sanatoria operated by religious organizations. They are located in the mountains and draw most of their patients from other states.

The 11 institutions in this group that were operating during 1924 discharged 588 patients, as compared with 996 discharged by the 16 institutions in 1930, an increase of 408. The state sanatoria discharged 644 patients in 1924 and 944 in 1930, a gain of 300.

Patients were first divided by race in 1927 and this division of patients discharged during the past four years follows:

	Patients Discharged by Races			
			Negro	
	Total	White	Number	Per Cent
BOTH STATES_____	3,650	2,695	955	26
North Carolina_____	2,584	1,954	630	24
South Carolina_____	1,066	741	325	30

The fact will be brought out later in this discussion that the ratio of Negro patients to white patients discharged is greater than the ratio of days of care of Negroes to days of care of white patients. This is due to the fact that many Negro patients are brought into the institutions in the far advanced stage of the disease and die within a short time.

Average Stay of Patients

One method of arriving at an average stay of patients according to their economic status that is of some value is by dividing days of care of all patients during the past six years, 1,048,000, by the number of patients discharged, 4,940. This gives an average stay of 212 days, or approximately seven months. The 187,000 full pay patient days, divided by 925 full pay patients discharged, gives an average of 202 days for this group, about six and one-half months. The 1,050 part pay patients stayed 201,000 days, or an average of 191 days, a fraction over six months. About two-thirds of the days of care, 660,000, were of free patients, 2,965 in number, and they stayed an average of 222 days, almost seven and one-half months.

Total days of care in the North Carolina sanatoria numbered 763,200 and 3,523 patients were discharged. The average stay arrived at on this basis would be 217 days, as compared with 200 days for South Carolina, where there were 1,417 patients discharged and 284,800 days of care.

The two sanatoria operated by religious organizations, with an average stay of 235 days, account for the longer average stay in North Carolina. The community group, located in South Carolina with one exception, shows an average stay of 202 days, as compared with 211 days for the county sanatoria as a group.

The community and county groups combined, which cared for 80 per cent of the patients during these six years, show an average stay for full pay patients of 163 days, 177 days for part pay patients, and 220 days for free patients. The only value of these averages is to show that the free patient, as a general rule, stays about two months longer than the full pay patient and about 40 days longer than the part pay patient in these local tuberculosis sanatoria. These averages, while not absolutely accurate because total days of care of all patients cared for during this period are divided by the number of patients discharged and the days of care prior to 1925 did not include days of care for some 250 patients in these institutions at the beginning of that year, may be considered accurate, for all practical purposes, certainly with an error of not over ten per cent.

Beginning with the year 1926 these sanatoria have reported their days of care of patients discharged, divided as between those who stayed over ninety days and those who stayed less than ninety days. The average stay of patients discharged over the five-year period has been 181 days, or approximately six months. The variation in the average stay from year to year has been as follows: 1926, 134 days; 1927, 181 days; 1928, 217 days; 1929, 174 days; 1930, 191 days. The community group shows an average of 206 days, the religious group 216 days, and the county group 155 days. The high average for the community group, as compared with the county group, practically all of the community sanatoria being in South Carolina and the county sanatoria in North Carolina, gives North Carolina an average of 172 days for the five years as compared with 204 days in South Carolina.

The average patient who stayed over ninety days was in the sanatorium 300 days, or approximately ten months, 285 days in North Carolina and 337 in South Carolina. The community group again shows a long average stay of 340 days, as compared with 260 days in the county group. The religious group average was 345 days.

The average patient who stayed less than ninety days was in these institutions 42 days and there is not much variation in these figures from year to year or as between states and the different groups. Of the patients discharged, 46 per cent either died or were discharged in less than ninety days after they were admitted.

Deaths and Death Rates

Almost 1,000 patients were discharged from the 16 tuberculosis sanatoria during 1930, of which 227, or 22.8 per cent were dead. These facts are brought out in Table 31 on page 13. The North Carolina institutions discharged 70 per cent of the total and the South Carolina institutions 30 per cent. The patients suffering from pul-

TABLE 31

DEATHS AND DEATH RATES

Stage on Admission	Both States Patients Number	Both States Patients *Per Cent	Both States Deaths Number	Both States Deaths Per Cent	North Carolina Patients Number	North Carolina Patients Per Cent	North Carolina Deaths Number	North Carolina Deaths Per Cent	South Carolina Patients Number	South Carolina Patients *Per Cent	South Carolina Deaths Number	South Carolina Deaths Per Cent
PATIENTS DISCHARGED	996	100.0	227	22.8	706	70.0	168	23.8	290	30.0	59	20.3
Minimal	154	18.8			103	18.1			51	20.3		
Moderately Advanced	282	34.4	20	7.1	207	36.4	17	8.2	75	29.9	3	4.0
Far Advanced	384	46.8	202	52.6	259	45.5	150	57.9	125	49.8	52	41.6
Total Pulmonary	820	82.4	222	27.1	569	80.6	167	29.3	251	86.6	55	21.9
Non-Pulmonary	122	12.2	1	.8	115	16.3			7	2.4	1	14.3
Non-Tuberculous	41	4.1	3	7.3	16	2.3	1	6.3	25	8.6	2	8.0
Not Diagnosed	13	1.3	1	7.7	6	.8			7	2.4	1	14.3
WHITE PATIENTS	730	73.3	94	12.9	533	75.5	76	14.3	197	67.9	18	9.1
Minimal	127	22.3			93	23.3			34	19.9		
Moderately Advanced	236	41.4	9	3.8	169	42.4	6	3.6	67	39.2	3	4.5
Far Advanced	207	36.3	84	40.6	137	34.3	69	50.4	70	40.9	15	21.4
Total Pulmonary	570	78.1	93	16.3	399	74.9	75	18.8	171	86.8	18	10.5
Non-Pulmonary	118	16.2			115	21.6			3	1.5		
Non-Tuberculous	34	4.7	1	2.9	13	2.4	1	7.7	21	10.7		
Not Diagnosed	8	1.0			6	1.1			2	1.0		
NEGRO PATIENTS	266	26.7	133	50.0	173	24.5	92	53.2	93	32.1	41	44.1
Minimal	27	10.8			10	5.9			17	21.3		
Moderately Advanced	46	18.4	11	23.9	38	22.4	11	28.9	8	10.0		
Far Advanced	177	70.8	118	66.7	122	71.7	81	66.4	55	68.7	37	67.3
Total Pulmonary	250	94.0	129	51.6	170	96.3	92	54.1	80	86.0	37	46.2
Non-Pulmonary	4	1.5	1	25.0					4	4.3	1	25.0
Non-Tuberculous	7	2.6	2	28.6	3	1.7			4	4.3	2	50.0
Not Diagnosed	5	1.9	1	20.0					5	5.4	1	20.0

*Of the total admitted in the various stages and by race.

monary tuberculosis numbered 820. Slightly more than one-half, 53 per cent to be exact, were admitted to the institutions in the minimal and moderately advanced stages of the disease.

Almost one-half of the patients suffering with pulmonary tuberculosis were admitted in the far advanced stage of the disease and over one-half of these died in the institutions. The report of far advanced patients who stayed more than ninety days indicates that the disease was arrested when four of the far advanced cases were discharged, 11 cases were apparently arrested, and 11 others were quiescent, or a total of 24 far advanced patients that the stay in the institutions definitely helped. Of the remaining 360 far advanced patients, 48 showed some improvement. A great many of these far advanced cases who did not die in the sanatoria probably died a short time after leaving. It is the policy of some institutions to send patients about to die to their homes, because of the depressing effect a death in a sanatorium has upon other patients.

Practically all of the 122 patients discharged who were suffering from other forms of tuberculosis than pulmonary were children with tracheo-bronchial tuberculosis cared for in three North Carolina sanatoria, the Mecklenburg Sanatorium, the Guilford County Sanatorium, and the Catawba County Sanatorium. The last named institution is for children only. The group of 41 patients found not to have tuberculosis stayed a comparatively short time. No diagnosis was made of 13 cases. These patients also stayed a comparatively short time.

The white patients make up 73 per cent of the total, 76 per cent in North Carolina and 68 per cent in South Carolina. The population is 65 per cent white in the two states, 71 per cent in North Carolina and 55 per cent in South Carolina.

In the minimal and moderately advanced stages the proportion of white patients is slightly more than twice the ratio for Negroes, while in the far advanced stage the proportion of Negroes is almost twice the ratio for white people. Two out of every three Negroes suffering from pulmonary tuberculosis in the far advanced stage died in the institutions, as compared with two out of every five whites, but that is not a good index of end results. It is probable that a great many of the white patients died soon after they were discharged.

Approximately 600 patients were discharged during 1925 from the 12 sanatoria in existence at the end of that year, 440 white patients and 160 Negroes. Practically all of them were suffering from pulmonary tuberculosis and 142 of the 600 patients, 23 per cent, were dead when discharged, the same proportion that died in 1930. The North Carolina institutions discharged 432 of the 600 patients, of which 317 were white and 115 were Negro, and 23 per cent of these patients were dead when discharged. In South Carolina 123 white patients were discharged and 45 Negroes and 23 per cent were dead when discharged.

Additional facts as to the stage of the disease on admission and the condition of the patients on discharge are not available until 1926. In that year 20 per cent of the white patients discharged from the 14 sanatoria assisted were in a minimal stage of the disease on admission, 49 per cent were moderately advanced, and 31 per cent far advanced. The Negro patients were divided 6 per cent minimal, 32 per cent moderately advanced, and 62 per cent far advanced. A comparison with the same figures for 1930 indicates that there is a tendency to admit a somewhat larger proportion in the minimal stage, a much smaller proportion in the moderately advanced stage, and a much larger proportion in the far advanced stage, particularly among Negroes. This condition is brought about to a certain extent by the fact that the sanatoria that have been built and enlarged during the past three or four years have at first admitted a large proportion of far advanced cases. One encouraging factor is the larger proportion of cases which are being admitted in the minimal stage.

Patients Staying Over 90 Days: In addition to the patients suffering with pulmonary tuberculosis who stayed 90 days or over, there were 87 white patients in North Carolina and one white and three Negro patients in South Carolina with non-pulmonary tuberculosis. None of these patients died and practically all of them were children suffering with tracheo-bronchial tuberculosis.

There were five non-tuberculous white patients, three in North Carolina and two in South Carolina, and one of the South Carolina patients died. The one non-tuberculous

TABLE 32

CONDITION OF PATIENTS ON DISCHARGE
WHO REMAINED 90 DAYS OR OVER

Condition on Discharge	Total Patients		Minimal		Moderately Advanced		Far Advanced	
	Number	Per Cent	Number	Per Cent	Number	Per Cent	Number	Cent Cent
PATIENTS DISCHARGED	484	100.0	90	18.6	198	40.9	196	40.5
Arrested	85	17.6	55	61.1	26	13.1	4	2.0
Apparently Arrested	64	13.2	19	21.1	34	17.2	11	5.6
Quiescent	56	11.6	5	5.6	40	20.2	11	5.6
Improved	127	26.2	11	12.2	68	34.3	48	24.5
Unimproved	36	7.4			10	5.1	26	13.3
Dead	116	24.0			20	10.1	96	49.0
WHITE PATIENTS	361	74.6	73	20.2	167	46.3	121	33.5
Arrested	70	19.4	46	63.0	22	13.2	2	1.7
Apparently Arrested	49	13.6	15	20.5	28	16.8	6	4.9
Quiescent	53	14.7	5	6.9	40	23.9	8	6.6
Improved	106	29.4	7	9.6	58	34.7	41	33.9
Unimproved	28	7.7			10	6.0	18	14.9
Dead	55	15.2			9	5.4	46	38.0
NEGRO PATIENTS	123	25.4	17	13.8	31	25.2	75	61.0
Arrested	15	12.2	9	53.0	4	12.9	2	2.7
Apparently Arrested	15	12.2	4	23.5	6	19.4	5	6.7
Quiescent	3	2.4					3	4.0
Improved	21	17.1	4	23.5	10	32.2	7	9.3
Unimproved	8	6.5					8	10.6
Dead	61	49.6			11	35.5	50	66.7

Negro patient in a South Carolina sanatorium did not die.

It appears from this table that 484, or 59 per cent of the 820 patients discharged in 1930 who were suffering from pulmonary tuberculosis, stayed longer than ninety days. In 1926, the first year for which these figures are available, 48 per cent of the patients discharged stayed over ninety days. In 1927 it was 51 per cent, in 1928, 59 per cent, and in 1929, 53 per cent.

Of the white patients discharged in 1926, 54 per cent stayed more than ninety days and 31 per cent of the Negroes. In 1930, 63 per cent of the white patients stayed over ninety days and 49 per cent of the Negroes. This increase in the proportion of patients staying longer is reflected in the longer average stay of patients.

Stage on Admission: Of the white patients discharged in 1926, 20 per cent were admitted in the minimal stage of the disease, 50 per cent in the moderately advanced stage, and 30 per cent in the far advanced stage. A comparison with 1930 indicates that the ratio admitted in the minimal stage of the disease is the same, the moderately advanced group ratio is slightly less, 46 per cent, and the far advanced group correspondingly greater, 33 per cent.

In 1926 the ratio of Negro patients admitted in the minimal stage was 10 per cent of the total, the moderately advanced group was slightly more than one-third of the total, and 54 per cent were in the far advanced stage. In 1930 there had been an increase in the proportion of Negro patients admitted in the minimal stage from 10 per cent to 14 per cent, the moderately advanced ratio had decreased from one-third to one-fourth of the total, and the far advanced group had increased from 54 per cent to 61 per cent. The medical directors of these sanatoria say that it is very difficult to get Negroes into the institutions before they reach the far advanced stage. One factor is the fear of hospitals that is inherent in the race. Another factor is the economic status of the race. The bread winner has to work or the family will suffer, because there are no accumulated savings, as a rule, or family wealth.

A comparison of the white and Negro ratios in 1926 of patients discharged who were admitted in the minimal stage of the disease indicates that the proportion of white patients was twice the ratio for Negroes, two to ten as compared with one to ten, but in 1930 the difference had been lessened considerably. Of the Negro patients discharged, 14 per cent were admitted in the minimal stage and the white ratio was the same as in 1926.

One-half of the white patients in 1926 were moderately advanced and slightly more than one-third of the Negro patients. Both races show a decrease in 1930 to 46 per cent for the white patients and to 25 per cent for the Negroes.

In 1926, 30 per cent of the white patients discharged were admitted in the far advanced stage of the disease, as compared with 54 per cent of the Negro patients. In 1930 these ratios had increased to one-third of the white patients and 61 per cent of the Negroes.

It appears from Table 32 on page 16 that, of all the patients discharged in 1930, one out of every five was admitted in the minimal stage of the disease, two in the moderately advanced stage, and two in the far advanced stage. In 1926 the ratio of patients discharged who were admitted in the minimal stage was the same, but the ratio for the moderately advanced group was much greater and the far advanced group correspondingly less. The moderately advanced group made up almost one-half of the patients discharged in 1926.

Condition on Discharge: In 1926, of all patients discharged, the unimproved and dead made up 28 per cent of the total and 31 per cent in 1930. Of all white patients discharged in 1926, 21 per cent were in this group and 23 per cent in 1930. The Negro group shows 56 per cent in 1926 and the same ratio in 1930. There is not much variation in these ratios as between the two states.

A further comparison on this basis, according to the stage of the disease on admission of the patients, shows that the ratio of white patients discharged unimproved or dead in the moderately advanced and far advanced cases was slightly less in 1930 than in 1926, and the same holds true of the moderately advanced Negro patients discharged, but 81 per cent of the far advanced Negro patients were dead or unimproved in 1926 as compared with 77 per cent in 1930.

A comparison of the other groups discharged in 1926 and 1930 is not possible, because in 1926 patients discharged were classified only as arrested, improved, unimproved, and dead. A comparison of the 1930 ratios with 1927 shows not a great deal of variation.

None of the patients admitted in the minimal stage of the disease went out without some improvement being indicated in their condition and 61 out of every 100 had the disease definitely arrested, as contrasted with 13 in the moderately advanced stage and two out of every 100 in the far advanced stage. About 20 per cent of the patients in the minimal stage had the disease apparently arrested, as compared with 17 per cent in the moderately advanced stage and with six per cent of those in the far advanced stage. Twenty per cent of the moderately advanced cases were quiescent when they left and six per cent of both the minimal and far advanced cases were quiescent on discharge. The chances of the white patient showing some improvement in the far advanced stage is about three and one-half times greater than for the Negro. This may be accounted for by a greater natural resistance to the disease on the part of white patients, or it may be due to the Negro patients being in a more serious condition, that is even more far advanced than the far advanced white patient when admitted. The chances that a patient will go out unimproved or dead are about four times as great in the far advanced group as in the moderately advanced stage.

Patients Staying Less Than 90 Days: In addition to the patients suffering from pulmonary tuberculosis, as indicated in Table 33 on page 21, there were 30 white patients suffering from non-pulmonary tuberculosis, 28 in North Carolina and two in South Carolina, and practically all of them were children with tracheo-bronchial tuberculosis. None of these 30 patients died, but the one Negro patient in a South Carolina sanatorium with non-pulmonary tuberculosis did die.

There were 29 white patients found to be non-tuberculous, 19 in South Carolina and 10 in North Carolina, and none of them died. Two of the three non-tuberculous Negro patients in the South Carolina sanatoria died. The three discharged from the North Carolina sanatoria did not die in the institutions.

No diagnosis was made on eight white patients, six in North Carolina and two in South Carolina, and none of them died. No diagnosis was made on five Negro patients, all in South Carolina, and one of them died.

The proportion of Negro patients admitted in the far advanced stage of the disease was about twice the proportion of white patients. The ratio is two to five for the white patients and four to five for the Negroes.

An institutional stay of less than ninety days cannot do a far advanced case much good and it is doubtful whether the 82 patients discharged alive lived very long after they left these sanatoria. The stay in the institutions probably helped a few of the 64 minimal cases and some of the 84 moderately advanced cases. Much was accomplished by taking these patients out of their homes, particularly the far advanced cases, where they were a constant source of infection to other members of their families, and from a standpoint of disease prevention the expense involved was justified. There are three or four small county sanatoria in North Carolina that restrict their work almost entirely to the care of these hopeless cases, their major purpose being to prevent rather than to cure.

TABLE 33
DEATHS AND DEATH RATES OF PATIENTS WITH PULMONARY TUBERCULOSIS
WHO STAYED LESS THAN 90 DAYS

	Total Patients	Minimal	Moderately Advanced	Far Advanced
16 SANATORIA	336	64	84	188
Deaths	106			106
Per Cent	31.5			56.4
WHITE PATIENTS	209	54	69	86
Deaths	38			38
Per Cent	18.2			44.2
NEGRO PATIENTS	127	10	15	102
Deaths	68			68
Per Cent	53.5			66.7
10 NORTH CAROLINA SANATORIA	224	43	58	123
Deaths	78			78
Per Cent	34.8			63.4
WHITE PATIENTS	136	39	46	51
Deaths	29			29
Per Cent	21.3			56.9
NEGRO PATIENTS	88	4	12	72
Deaths	49			49
Per Cent	55.7			68.1
6 SOUTH CAROLINA SANATORIA	112	21	26	65
Deaths	28			28
Per Cent	25.0			43.1
WHITE PATIENTS	73	15	23	35
Deaths	9			9
Per Cent	12.3			25.7
NEGRO PATIENTS	39	6	3	30
Deaths	19			19
Per Cent	48.7			63.3

Age of Patients on Admission

A comparison with 1927, the first year the sanatoria reported patients discharged by age groups, indicates that the greatest variation has taken place in the group under fourteen years of age. In 1927 there were 58 children discharged, seven per cent of the total, and 154 in 1930, almost 16 per cent of the total. This is explained largely by the erection of the Catawba County Sanatorium for children only and by the addition of special buildings for children at the Mecklenburg Sanatorium and Guilford County Sanatorium. In North Carolina the gain has been from 22 to 129 in this group, from less than four per cent

TABLE 34

AGES ON ADMISSION OF PATIENTS DISCHARGED

	Total		Over 90 Days		Under 90 Days	
	Num-ber	Per Cent	Num-ber	Per Cent	Num-ber	Per Cent
16 SANATORIA	996	100.0	581	58.3	415	41.7
Under 14 years	154	15.5	113	19.4	41	9.9
14 to 19 years	105	10.5	57	9.8	48	11.5
20 to 24 years	171	17.2	99	17.0	72	17.4
25 to 29 years	156	15.7	88	15.2	68	16.3
30 to 34 years	115	11.5	67	11.5	48	11.5
35 to 39 years	87	8.7	49	8.5	38	9.2
40 to 44 years	65	6.5	31	5.4	34	8.3
45 years and over	143	14.4	77	13.2	66	15.9
10 NORTH CAROLINA SANATORIA	706	70.9	435	61.6	271	38.4
Under 14 years	129	18.3	99	22.8	30	11.1
14 to 19 years	69	9.8	41	9.4	28	10.3
20 to 24 years	123	17.4	71	16.3	52	19.2
25 to 29 years	100	14.2	58	13.3	42	15.5
30 to 34 years	80	11.3	50	11.5	30	11.1
35 to 39 years	60	8.5	37	8.5	23	8.5
40 to 44 years	46	6.5	21	4.8	25	9.2
45 years and over	99	14.0	58	13.4	41	15.1
6 SOUTH CAROLINA SANATORIA	290	29.1	146	50.3	144	49.7
Under 14 years	25	8.6	14	9.5	11	7.6
14 to 19 years	36	12.4	16	11.0	20	13.9
20 to 24 years	48	16.5	28	19.3	20	13.9
25 to 29 years	56	19.3	30	20.5	26	18.1
30 to 34 years	35	12.1	17	11.6	18	12.5
35 to 39 years	27	9.3	12	8.2	15	10.4
40 to 44 years	19	6.5	10	6.9	9	6.2
45 years and over	44	15.3	19	13.0	25	17.4

of the total to over 18 per cent; in South Carolina 36 children were discharged in 1927, as compared with 25 in 1930, a reduction in proportion of patients discharged from 15 per cent to less than nine per cent.

A division of patients discharged into three age groups, under twenty years, twenty to forty years, and over forty years, and a comparison with the year 1927, indicates that the proportion of patients over forty years has remained practically the same, one out of every five discharged, the proportion of patients discharged in the age group between twenty and forty years has decreased, and a corresponding increase is noted in the proportion discharged who were admitted when less than twenty years of age.

Out-Patients

Of the 16 sanatoria applying for assistance, 11 reported out-patient work. Only two sanatoria reported out-patients in 1924, one in North Carolina and one in South Carolina.

In North Carolina the non-profit tuberculosis sanatoria, with the exception of the two institutions operated by religious organizations and the state sanatorium, are operated as a part of and largely under the supervision of the health departments in the counties where they are located. The three largest county sanatoria developed within the last seven years in the wealthiest and most populous counties, have full-time resident physicians and these physicians conduct the out-patient clinics, either at the sanatorium or at the county health department. When this activity is a part of the larger program of tuberculosis prevention and control, it is difficult to define what patients should be considered out-patients. The two sanatoria operated by religious organizations do not have any out-patients and two of the county sanatoria did not report any out-patients, because this activity is conducted by the county health departments away from the institutions. As the number and bed capacity of these institutions have increased, the out-patient work has also increased.

In South Carolina the tuberculosis sanatoria, other than the state institution, have developed largely as part of the activities of the local tuberculosis associations, but in the last two or three years sanatoria have opened in Marion, Spartanburg, and Greenville Counties as county owned and operated institutions. In Greenville County the sanatorium operated by the tuberculosis association merged with the county sanatorium when it was opened the latter part of 1930. This indicates a tendency on the part of counties to take over tuberculosis control and prevention as part of the public health activities, but these local tuberculosis associations have done and are continuing to do very effective work, assisted to a considerable extent by county and municipal tax funds. For example, the sana-

TABLE 35
OUT-PATIENT SERVICE

	Out-Patients			Total Visits
	White	Negro	Total	
11 SANATORIA	3,066	1,955	5,021	7,567
Minimal	225	112	337	630
Moderately Advanced	220	61	281	1,051
Far Advanced	174	117	291	985
Total Pulmonary	619	290	909	2,666
Non-Pulmonary	123	29	152	236
Non-Tuberculous	1,584	1,105	2,689	3,050
Not Diagnosed	740	531	1,271	1,615
6 NORTH CAROLINA SANATORIA	1,301	183	1,484	1,615
Minimal	109	25	134	150
Moderately Advanced	150	29	179	227
Far Advanced	87	41	128	155
Total Pulmonary	346	95	441	532
Non-Pulmonary	119	16	135	151
Non-Tuberculous	701	56	757	770
Not Diagnosed	135	16	151	162
5 SOUTH CAROLINA SANATORIA	1,765	1,772	3,537	5,952
Minimal	116	87	203	480
Moderately Advanced	70	32	102	824
Far Advanced	87	76	163	830
Total Pulmonary	273	195	468	2,134
Non-Pulmonary	4	13	17	85
Non-Tuberculous	883	1,049	1,932	2,280
Not Diagnosed	605	515	1,120	1,453

torium in Charleston is owned by the county and operated by the tuberculosis association, a somewhat unusual arrangement but one which appears to work very satisfactorily.

The same difficulty is found in defining the out-patient activities of the sanatoria in South Carolina as in North Carolina. The South Carolina sanatoria report a much larger volume of out-patient work and it appears probable, from what is known about the activities of the organizations operating these sanatoria, that they are more active in the prevention and control of tuberculosis, particularly among Negroes, than the North Carolina institutions. They appear to have a more effective follow-up service through the media of clinics and visiting nurses.

Diagnostic Services

Laboratory: In North Carolina the three largest county sanatoria and the county sanatorium exclusively for children report well-equipped laboratories with technicians in

TABLE 36
LABORATORY SERVICE

	In-Patients			Out-Patients		
	13 Sanatoria	*7 North Carolina Sanatoria*	*6 South Carolina Sanatoria*	*9 Sanatoria*	*5 North Carolina anatoria*	*4 South Carolina Sanatoria*
ALL EXAMINATIONS	8,456	6,268	2,188	2,128	666	1,462
Routine Urinalysis	1,095	700	395	47	29	18
Blood Examinations:						
Red Blood Count	707	593	114	24	16	8
White Blood Count	820	599	221	36	25	11
Differential	801	583	218	34	25	9
Hemoglobin	817	600	217	31	18	13
Wassermann	625	399	226	181	63	118
Widals	3	1	2	1		1
Cultures	46	23	23	9	7	2
Tissues Microscopic	136		136	7		7
Gastric Analysis	11	6	5	1	1	
Stool Examination	369	369		151	151	
Sputum Examinations	2,924	2,326	598	481	324	157
Throat Cultures	1	1				
Miscellaneous	101	68	33	1,125	7	1,118

charge, three of the smaller sanatoria report their laboratory work done in local hospitals or health departments, while the two sanatoria operated by religious organizations and one small county sanatorium report no laboratory work at all, except what is done for the patients before they are admitted or by the attending physicians at their offices.

The three largest sanatoria in South Carolina apparently are doing very effective diagnostic work with well-equipped laboratories, while in the three smaller institutions it is done by doctors or technicians in other hospitals.'

The sanatoria in existence six years ago reported a very small amount of laboratory work.

X-ray: All except one of the ten sanatoria in North Carolina report X-ray work for their patients and six of them have their own equipment. Only one sanatorium had its own equipment six years ago and a very small amount of X-ray work for patients was reported.

In South Carolina two of the sanatoria report ownership of their own X-ray equipment and the others have access to these departments in local general hospitals. One sanatorium owned its equipment six years ago and a very small amount of work was reported by any of them.

TABLE 37
X-RAY SERVICE

	15 Sanatoria	9 North Carolina Sanatoria	6 South Carolina Sanatoria
ALL PATIENTS EXAMINED	2,184	1,606	578
Per Cent Examined	36.3	73.3	15.1
Films Made	2,602	1,891	711
Fluoroscopic	2,650	2,159	491
IN-PATIENTS EXAMINED	1,039	833	206
Per Cent Examined	104.3	118.0	71.0
Films Made	1,502	1,160	342
Fluoroscopic	1,464	1,018	446
OUT-PATIENTS EXAMINED	1,145	773	372
Per Cent Examined	22.8	52.1	10.5
Films Made	1,100	731	369
Fluoroscopic	1,186	1,141	45

TABLE 38

PLANT VALUES, INVESTMENTS, AND CAPITAL DEBTS

	Plant Values	Investments, Endowment	Capital Debts
16 TUBERCULOSIS SANATORIA	1,765,299.54	108,310.03	164,000.00
5 Community	204,322.27	108,310.03	
2 Religious	419,686.83		164,000.00
9 County	1,141,290.44		
10 IN NORTH CAROLINA	1,389,367.43	2,200.00	164,000.00
1 Community	18,380.40	2,200.00	
2 Religious	419,686.83		164,000.00
7 County	951,300.20		
6 IN SOUTH CAROLINA	375,932.11	106,110.03	
4 Community	185,941.87	106,110.03	
2 County	189,990.24		

Property Valuation

Plant Value: The 11 non-profit sanatoria, exclusive of state institutions, in existence six years ago, reported plant values at $809,647. If to the total in the above table is added the cost of the new sanatorium in Spartanburg County, approximately $175,000, the total value of the 17 institutions would be only $60,000 short of $2,000,-000 at the end of 1930. In other words, plant values have increased almost two and one-half times in six years.

The six institutions in North Carolina six years ago reported plants valued at $676,367 and $400,000 of this amount was reported by one of the institutions operated by religious organizations. Most of the balance was reported by the recently constructed Guilford County Sanatorium. Plant values have more than doubled in the six-year period.

The five community sanatoria in South Carolina six years ago had a plant value of $133,280 and a considerable part of this amount was invested in the recently constructed sanatorium in Charleston County. At the end of 1930 the seven sanatoria had a plant value of over $550,000.

The 409 beds in the 11 sanatoria in existence at the end of 1924 represented an investment per bed of $1,720, $789 for the community group, $4,100 for the religious group, and $1,958 for the county group. The 1,000-bed capacity of the 17 sanatoria six years later represented an investment per bed of $1,940, an increase of $220 per bed. The community group shows an increase of $238 per bed, the religious group, which has only two more beds than six years ago, decreased $141 per bed, and the county group also shows a decrease per bed of $64. This is caused by the fact that the county sanatoria in a number of instances have been able to enlarge their bed capacity considerably at a comparatively small expense.

Leaving out the religious group entirely, the investment per bed in the community and county groups was $1,256 six years ago and $1,700 now, $1,710 in North Carolina and $1,684 in South Carolina. Six years ago in North Carolina these two groups showed an investment per bed of $1,712 and $838 in South Carolina. In other words, the investment per bed is more than twice what it was six years ago in South Carolina and almost the same in North Carolina.

Investments: Only four sanatoria, all in the community group, three in South Carolina and one in North Carolina, have any income-producing investments, and two institutions have most of it, over $72,000 for Aiken Cottages and almost $32,000 for Camp Alice. Invested funds have increased only $10,000 during the six-year period and the number with invested funds has increased only one. It is hoped now that The Duke Endowment has withdrawn support from these tuberculosis sanatoria they will make an effort to build up endowment funds.

Capital Debts: The two institutions in the religious group were the only sanatoria with capital debts six years ago, amounting to $270,800. Only one institution (in the religious group) had a capital debt of $164,000 six years later. County and municipal bond issues for the purpose of building or maintaining tuberculosis sanatoria are not counted as capital debts for the reason that they are not direct obligations of the institutions concerned.

Operating Indebtedness: At the end of 1930, only one of the sanatoria had a capital debt and only three owed any money on account of operating expenses. The total operating debt amounted to $27,826.32.

Receipts

By Main Purposes: The 11 sanatoria in existence at the end of 1924 reported receipts that year of $227,058 and very little of this amount was for capital purposes. If to the $800,000 received by the 16 sanatoria in 1930, is added approximately $175,000 received and spent for the Spartanburg County Sanatorium, the total for the year would be some $25,000 less than $1,000,000. Receipts in the operating account alone are almost three times the total receipts in 1924. These receipts do not include borrowed money.

TABLE 39
RECEIPTS BY MAIN PURPOSES

	Total Receipts	Operating Account	Capital Account
16 TUBERCULOSIS SANATORIA	800,209.56	649,920.09	150,289.47
5 Community	139,103.67	135,003.67	4,100.00
2 Religious	129,327.91	129,327.91	
9 County	531,777.98	385,588.51	146,189.47
10 IN NORTH CAROLINA	516,257.38	489,229.39	27,027.99
1 Community	23,813.23	23,813.23	
2 Religious	129,327.91	129,327.91	
7 County	363,116.24	336,088.25	27,027.99
6 IN SOUTH CAROLINA	283,952.18	160,690.70	123,261.48
4 Community	115,290.44	111,190.44	4,100.00
2 County	168,661.74	49,500.26	119,161.48

Operating Account: Receipts from patients for services rendered were only $10,000 more in 1930 than in 1924. In both years most of this money was received by the two sanatoria operated by religious organizations. Contributions in 1924 amounted to $73,270, $34,938 in North Carolina and $38,332 in South Carolina. Contributions in 1924 to the community group amounted to $45,054, to the religious group to $11,495, and to the county group to $16,721. Contributions in 1930 were more than six times what they were in 1924, the largest increases being in the community and county groups, the religious group showing an increase of about $1,000.

Income from invested funds amounted to $5,908 in 1924 and all of this was received by two community sanatoria in South Carolina with endowment. The number of institutions showing receipts from this source had increased to four in 1930, but there is not much change in the amount.

TABLE 40

OPERATING RECEIPTS
BY PRINCIPAL SOURCES

	In-Patients	Contributions	Investments, Endowment	Out-Patients	Miscellaneous
16 TUBERCULOSIS SANATORIA	151,619.16	487,308.42	6,617.90	3,344.29	1,030.32
5 Community	27,295.62	100,162.44	6,308.16	484.80	752.65
2 Religious	116,790.83	12,477.72			59.36
9 County	7,532.71	374,668.26	309.74	2,859.49	218.31
10 IN NORTH CAROLINA	127,527.39	358,693.65	204.86	2,473.49	330.00
1 Community	4,020.50	19,738.20			54.53
2 Religious	116,790.83	12,477.72			59.36
7 County	6,716.06	326,477.73	204.86	2,473.49	216.11
6 IN SOUTH CAROLINA	24,091.77	128,614.77	6,413.04	870.80	700.32
4 Community	23,275.12	80,424.24	6,308.16	484.80	698.12
2 County	816.65	48,190.53	104.88	386.00	2.20

TABLE 41

OPERATING ACCOUNT CONTRIBUTIONS
BY PRINCIPAL SOURCES

	County	Municipal	Religious	The Duke Endowment	Other
16 TUBERCULOSIS SANATORIA	291,386.81	11,224.96	5,003.27	168,533.00	11,155.38
5 Community	36,912.00	10,999.96	4,181.45	41,464.00	6,605.03
2 Religious			821.82	8,515.00	3,140.90
9 County	254,474.81	225.00		118,559.00	1,409.45
10 IN NORTH CAROLINA	223,902.18	4,000.00	4,451.02	122,815.00	3,525.45
1 Community	4,800.00	4,000.00	3,629.20	7,309.00	
2 Religious			821.82	8,515.00	3,140.90
7 County	219,102.18			106,991.00	384.55
6 IN SOUTH CAROLINA	67,484.63	7,224.96	552.25	45,723.00	7,629.93
4 Community	32,112.00	6,999.96	552.25	34,155.00	6,605.03
2 County	35,372.63	225.00		11,568.00	1,024.90

Contributions

Operating Account: Contributions from county tax funds amounted to $38,988 in 1924, municipalities gave $10,-686, religious organizations $9,877, and contributions from other sources amounted to $13,719. The Duke Endowment did not make a contribution until 1926 for the free days of care in 1925. A comparison with 1930 indicates that there has not been a great deal of change in the amounts received from municipalities, religious organizations, and other sources. The increase has come about largely in county contributions and the addition of The Duke Endowment contribution. For example, the contribution by counties to county institutions in North Carolina amounted to $16,721 in 1924 and to $219,102 in 1930.

Capital Account: Contributions for capital purposes in 1924 amounted to very little, if anything. Counties made contributions in 1930 to seven county sanatoria that applied for assistance as such amounting to $143,453.41. Addition of the Spartanburg County Sanatorium contribution, which appears in the Spartanburg General Hospital report as part of that institution, would make the total from this source about $318,000 to county sanatoria. The contributions to six county sanatoria in North Carolina were in comparatively small amounts and totaled $25,-174.18. The contribution for the building of the new Greenville County Sanatorium in South Carolina amounted to $118,279.23.

Municipalities, religious organizations, and The Duke Endowment made no contribution for capital purposes to these institutions and contributions from interested individuals and organizations to four institutions amounted to $6,836.06. One community institution in South Carolina reported a gift amounting to $4,100 and one county institution in the same state had $882.25 given to it. Two of the county institutions in North Carolina reported gifts amounting to $1,853.81 for capital purposes.

Capital Expenditure

Only one institution (in the religious group) reported no capital outlay during 1930. The increase in plant values, counting the Spartanburg County Sanatorium, amounted to approximately $273,000 and practically all

TABLE 42
CAPITAL EXPENDITURE

	Grand Total	Capital Outlay	Corporation Expense	Funds Invested
16 TUBERCULOSIS SANATORIA	170,755.27	158,645.31	4,959.04	7,150.92
5 Community	13,685.44	6,204.52	330.00	7,150.92
2 Religious	1,578.50	940.73	637.77	
9 County	155,491.33	151,500.06	3,991.27	
10 IN NORTH CAROLINA	33,986.21	32,958.44	1,027.77	
1 Community	1,034.00	1,034.00		
2 Religious	1,578.50	940.73	637.77	
7 County	31,373.71	30,983.71	390.00	
6 IN SOUTH CAROLINA	136,769.06	125,686.87	3,931.27	7,150.92
4 Community	12,651.44	5,170.52	330.00	7,150.92
2 County	124,117.62	120,516.35	3,601.27	

of it was in the county group. This group also spent over $350,000 in 1929. Capital outlay, if anything, amounted to very little in 1924.

Corporation expense, most of which includes the organization expenses in connection with the new Greenville County Sanatorium, includes small amounts paid for rent, travel expenses of trustees, contributions to charity and the like. Five of the 16 institutions report such expense.

The three community sanatoria in South Carolina with invested funds reported additions during the year amounting to $7,150.92.

The one institution (in the religious group) with a capital debt reported $12,000 paid on the principal and $4,207.50 interest.

Cost of Operation

The operating cost of these institutions in 1924 amounted to $197,044, $144,556 in North Carolina and $52,488 in South Carolina. The cost of operating the community group was $59,991, the religious group $108,-918, and the county group $28,135. The cost of operation in 1930 was $577,136, $437,308 in North Carolina and $139,828 in South Carolina. The community group cost was $123,961, the religious group $98,225, and the county group $354,950.

In-Patients: The average cost per in-patient per day in 1924 was $2.36, $2.61 in North Carolina and $1.86 in South Carolina. The group costs were as follows: Community, $1.86; religious, $3.09; county, $1.74. The average costs for 1930 and by states appear in Table 43 on the opposite page. The group costs in 1930 were as follows: Community, $2.09; religious, $2.86; county, $2.14. The religious group cost shows very little change over the six-year period, but the community and county groups have had a decided increase. A comparison with 1925 cost

529

figures indicates that a considerable part of this increase has come about in the food cost. Apparently the patients are getting more and better food than they were getting five or six years ago, an important consideration in the treatment of tuberculosis. Improved diagnostic facilities have also added to the cost, as well as the additional cost incident to the employment of full-time resident physicians. Only one institution had a full-time resident in 1924. At the end of 1930 there were six institutions with full-time residents.

The amount actually spent for ordinary replacement and repair of buildings and equipment is included in the cost figures, but the buildings become obsolete over a period of years or deteriorate to such an extent, particularly the frame structures, that it is more satisfactory to abandon or tear them down than it is to attempt to make repairs.

TABLE 43

IN-PATIENT COST PER DAY

	16 Sanatoria	10 North Carolina	6 South Carolina
1. Administrative, Housekeeping, Plant Operation, and Dietary Salaries and Wages (A1, C1, D1, E1)	.3694	.3737	.3557
2. Nursing Salaries and Expense (B1-7)	.3215	.3309	.2920
Sub-Totals, Items 1 and 2	.6909	.7046	.6477
3. Food (E2-6)	.8769	.9242	.7273
4. Fuel, Light, Power, Ice, and Water (D2-5, E8)	.1422	.1414	.1447
5. Medical and Surgical Supplies (B10-13)	.0651	.0586	.0858
6. Laundry (C5-6)	.1099	.1064	.1209
7. Household and Dietary Supplies (C2-4, E7, E9)	.0738	.0685	.0904
8. Administrative Supplies and Expense (A2-8)	.0589	.0572	.0641
Sub-Totals, Items 3 to 8 inclusive	1.3268	1.3563	1.2332
Totals, Items 1 to 8 inclusive	2.0177	2.0609	1.8809
9. Laboratory Salaries and Expense (B18-20)	.0062	.0063	.0056
10. X-ray Salaries and Expense (B14-17)	.0199	.0234	.0091
Totals, including Laboratory and X-ray	2.0438	2.0906	1.8956
11. Medical and Surgical Salaries (B8-9)	.0643	.0501	.1093
12. Motor Service (C7-10)	.0128	.0125	.0138
Totals, except Replacement and Repair	2.1209	2.1532	2.0187
13. Replacement and Repair (D6-13)	.1087	.1011	.1325
In-Patient Cost Per Day	2.2296	2.2543	2.1512

This is a real cost that is not included. Estimated depreciation, figured on the basis of the average life of these buildings, from two to four per cent per annum according to the type of construction, would add 13 cents to the average cost and $33,026 to the total cost. This would bring the total cost of in-patient service up to almost $597,000, or an average of $2.36 per patient per day, $2.20 for the community sanatoria, $3.05 for the religious group, and $2.29 for the county sanatoria. The average cost in North Carolina would be $2.38, as compared with $2.29 for South Carolina.

Interest on investment is not included in these cost figures. As a matter of fact, only one institution had a capital debt on which it was paying interest and that is not included in these cost figures, but the money spent for new construction in recent years came largely from county bond issues on which interest is being paid by the taxpayers. Interest on investment at six per cent, amounting to $100,622, added to the cost of operation in 1930 would bring the total up to $697,481, or an average cost of $2.76 per day, which would be the basic cost figure with a reasonable return on investment, if these institutions operated as business enterprises for profit.

Out-Patients: The 16 sanatoria reported $13,303.12 as the cost of treating out-patients. The North Carolina sanatoria spent $4,134.95 and the South Carolina sanatoria $9,168.17. The average cost per visit for both states was $1.76, for North Carolina it was $2.56 and for South Carolina it was $1.54. If to the amount spent for the treatment of out-patients is added an allowance for depreciation, amounting to $1,738.20, and interest on investment, amounting to $5,295.90, the total cost would be $20,337.22, or an average cost per visit of $2.95.

Income and Expense

Table 44 on page 38 balances the sources of operating income against the cost of caring for in-patients (exclusive of allowance for depreciation and interest on investment) and in this way indicates what part of the cost is paid by the in-patients, what part The Duke Endowment contributes, and what part comes from other sources, such as income from investments or endowment, donations and subsidies from counties, cities, churches and other religious organizations, community chests and civic organizations, and gifts by individuals.

An interesting fact brought out is that the in-patients, The Duke Endowment, and other contributors each paid almost exactly one-third of the cost of caring for all in-patients as reported by these institutions during the past six years. In-patients paid slightly more than one-third of the cost. The Duke Endowment contributed exactly one-third, and the other contributors made up slightly less than one-third. In other words, The Duke Endowment paid one-half of the operating deficit, but these ratios change radically when the religious group is eliminated and only community and county sanatoria are considered. In these two groups patients paid only ten per cent of the cost, The Duke Endowment contributed 41 per cent and the balance, 49 per cent, came from other sources. The North Carolina in-patients paid only seven per cent of the cost, The Duke Endowment gave 42 per cent and 51 per cent came from other sources, while in South Carolina almost 17 per cent came from patients, The Duke Endowment gave 38 per cent, and 45 per cent came from other sources. As a matter of fact, the religious group collected approximately $108,000 more from in-patients than it cost to care for them and the contribution by The Duke Endowment boosted their surplus for the six years to almost $136,000.

The first year The Duke Endowment contributed 31 per cent of the cost, the next year when the large sanatorium operated by a religious organization applied for the first time this was reduced to 26 per cent, the third year it was 32 per cent, in 1928 one-third of the cost, in 1929 36 per cent, and 37 per cent in 1930. When the religious group is eliminated and only the county and community sanatoria considered, there is a steady gain in the proportion of the cost contributed by The Duke Endowment from 31 per cent in 1925 to 43 per cent in 1930. The increase in the proportion of free days of care accounts to a large extent for this gain.

As stated in the previous discussion, two sanatoria did not apply for assistance in 1925, and, in addition, there was one small county institution which was not assisted for 1927 and one new sanatorium, opened late in 1930, which applied as part of a general hospital. If to the cost of caring for in-patients during these six years shown in the table is added the cost of the missing institutions for the years indicated, the total would be about $2,500,000, or an average cost of approximately $2.40 per patient per day for the six-year period.

Summary

To summarize briefly the facts brought out in this discussion, the number of sanatoria in the group to which The Duke Endowment has extended assistance during the past six years has increased from 11 to 17, the bed capacity from 409 to 1,000, the average number of patients per day from 229 to 696, free days of care from 37,300 to 209,000, in-patients discharged from 588 to 996, the death rate remains the same, a larger proportion of patients are being admitted in the minimal and the far advanced stages of the disease, more children are being cared for, the volume of out-patient service shows a decided increase, and diagnostic facilities have improved considerably. From a finan-

TABLE 44

IN-PATIENT COST, IN-PATIENT RECEIPTS, THE DUKE ENDOWMENT CONTRIBUTION

		1925	1926	1927	1928	1929	1930	6 Years
	SANATORIA ASSISTED	10	14	14	14	16	16	17
ALL SANATORIA	In-Patient Cost	147,780.77	316,832.12	363,437.91	419,149.59	471,327.27	563,833.18	2,282,360.75
	In-Patient Receipts { Amount	23,369.52	155,021.89	164,024.39	151,524.92	142,612.03	151,619.16	788,171.91
	{ Per Cent	15.8	48.9	45.1	36.2	30.3	26.9	34.5
	The Duke Endowment { Amount	45,710.20	81,146.00	116,015.00	139,333.00	168,538.00	208,124.00	758,866.20
	{ Per Cent	30.9	25.6	31.9	33.2	35.8	36.9	33.3
	*Other Sources { Amount	78,701.05	80,664.23	83,398.52	128,291.58	160,177.24	204,090.02	735,322.64
	{ Per Cent	53.3	25.5	23.0	30.6	33.9	36.2	32.2
COMMUNITY AND COUNTY SANATORIA	In-Patient Cost	145,847.63	207,591.78	270,290.67	324,246.60	374,388.80	455,607.85	1,787,883.33
	In-Patient Receipts { Amount	21,141.25	29,747.51	34,573.61	30,858.96	34,458.91	34,828.33	185,608.57
	{ Per Cent	14.5	14.3	12.8	9.5	9.2	7.5	10.4
	The Duke Endowment { Amount	45,284.60	76,639.00	112,430.00	134,499.00	160,023.00	222,111.00	730,986.60
	{ Per Cent	31.0	36.9	41.6	41.5	42.7	43.4	40.9
	*Other Sources { Amount	79,421.78	101,205.27	123,197.06	158,888.64	179,906.89	223,668.52	871,288.16
	{ Per Cent	54.5	48.8	45.6	49.0	48.1	49.1	48.7
RELIGIOUS SANATORIA	In-Patient Cost	1,933.14	109,240.34	93,237.24	94,902.90	96,938.47	98,225.33	494,477.42
	In-Patient Receipts { Amount	2,228.27	125,274.38	129,450.78	120,665.96	108,153.12	116,790.83	602,563.34
	{ Per Cent	115.3	114.7	138.8	127.1	111.6	118.9	121.9
	The Duke Endowment { Amount	425.60	4,507.00	3,585.00	4,834.00	8,515.00	6,013.00	27,879.60
	{ Per Cent	22.0	4.1	3.9	5.1	8.8	6.1	5.6
	Surplus { Amount	720.73	20,541.04	39,798.54	30,597.06	19,729.65	24,578.50	135,965.52
	{ Per Cent	37.3	18.8	42.7	32.2	20.4	25.0	27.5

NORTH CAROLINA SANATORIA

Sanatoria Assisted	11	10	10	9	9	9	6
In-Patient Cost	1,683,497.96	433,172.86	355,831.08	312,758.35	269,928.46	226,322.99	85,484.22
In-Patient Receipts — Amount	687,773.07	127,527.39	122,880.39	136,633.57	149,012.61	139,378.67	12,340.44
Per Cent	40.9	29.4	34.5	43.7	55.2	61.6	14.4
The Duke Endowment — Amount	528,676.05	155,914.00	122,815.00	96,095.00	75,888.00	49,562.00	25,402.05
Per Cent	31.4	36.7	34.5	30.7	28.1	21.9	29.7
*Other Sources — Amount	467,048.84	145,731.47	110,135.69	80,029.78	45,027.85	37,382.32	47,741.73
Per Cent	27.7	33.9	31.0	25.6	16.7	16.5	55.9

COMMUNITY AND COUNTY SANATORIA

In-Patient Cost	1,189,020.54	334,947.53	258,892.61	217,855.45	176,691.22	117,082.65	83,551.08
In-Patient Receipts — Amount	85,209.73	10,736.56	14,727.27	15,967.61	19,561.83	14,104.29	10,112.17
Per Cent	7.2	3.2	5.7	7.3	11.1	12.0	12.1
The Duke Endowment — Amount	500,796.45	153,901.00	114,300.00	91,261.00	72,303.00	45,055.00	24,976.45
Per Cent	42.1	45.7	44.1	41.9	40.9	38.5	29.9
*Other Sources — Amount	603,014.36	171,309.97	129,865.34	110,626.84	84,826.39	57,923.36	48,462.46
Per Cent	50.7	51.1	50.2	50.8	48.0	49.5	58.0

RELIGIOUS SANATORIA

In-Patient Cost	494,477.42	98,225.33	96,938.47	94,902.99	93,237.24	109,240.34	1,933.14
In-Patient Receipts — Amount	602,563.34	116,790.83	108,153.12	120,665.96	129,450.78	125,274.38	2,228.27
Per Cent	121.9	118.9	111.6	127.1	138.8	114.7	115.3
The Duke Endowment — Amount	27,879.60	6,013.00	8,515.00	4,834.00	3,585.00	4,507.00	425.60
Per Cent	5.6	3.1	8.8	5.1	3.9	4.1	22.0
Surplus — Amount	135,965.52	24,578.50	19,729.65	30,597.06	39,798.54	20,541.04	720.73
Per Cent	27.5	25.0	20.4	32.2	42.7	18.8	37.3

SOUTH CAROLINA COMMUNITY AND COUNTY SANATORIA

Sanatoria Assisted	6	6	6	5	5	5	4
In-Patient Cost	598,862.79	139,660.32	115,496.19	106,391.15	93,509.45	90,509.13	62,296.55
In-Patient Receipts — Amount	100,398.84	24,091.77	19,731.64	14,891.35	15,011.78	15,643.22	11,029.08
Per Cent	16.8	18.4	17.1	14.0	16.1	17.3	17.7
The Duke Endowment — Amount	230,190.15	49,210.00	45,723.00	43,238.00	40,127.00	31,584.00	20,308.15
Per Cent	38.4	37.7	39.6	40.6	42.9	34.9	32.6
*Other Sources — Amount	268,273.30	57,358.35	50,041.55	48,261.80	38,370.67	43,281.91	30,059.32
Per Cent	44.8	43.9	43.3	45.4	41.0	47.8	49.7

*Income from investments, donations and subsidies from counties, municipalities, religious organizations, community chests, civic organizations, and individuals, and miscellaneous items.

cial standpoint plant values have increased during the six years from $809,647 to $1,940,000, receipts per annum from $227,058 to almost $1,000,000, contributions from $72,271 to $812,000, and the cost of operation from $197,044 to $577,136. The Duke Endowment contributed one-third of the cost of caring for in-patients in the assisted sanatoria during the six years, 41 per cent of the cost in the community and county groups and six per cent of the cost in the religious group.

The W. K. Kellogg Foundation

Report of a Survey of the W. K. Kellogg Foundation Made in 1937

by Drs. William S. and Lena K. Sadler

Part I. THE FOUNDATION PLAN AND PURPOSE

Section I. The Foundation Progam as a Whole.   While the
Foundation's purpose as defined in the charter is child   welfare, the
revised articles of incorporation provide a very broad scope for the
execution of this purpose. A careful examination of the charter, together
with the bylaws as amended on August 31, 1936, has served to convince us that
the present set-up is entirely adequate to provide for proper authorization,
as well as efficient execution of all the present activities of the
Foundation. Nothing we have observed during this very complete and thorough-
going survey has disclosed any plan of work or project of activity which is
not adequately provided for in the charter under which the Foundation is at
present working.

This survey was carried out during a succession of three-day periods
throughout the spring and summer of 1937, and included not only an
examination of the methods and procedures of the home office in Battle Creek,
but numerous visits to the seven County Health Units for the detailed
observation of their work, and are suggestions relative to these various
activities will be incorporated in the succeeding sections of this report.

Each of the officers of the Foundation discussed with us fully, and
disclosed to us in detail, the plans, policies, techniques, and methods of
administration, including accounting, and most freely answered all of our
inquires respecting every phase of the Foundation's work. This included a

1

full opportunity to learn all of the plans for the ensuing fiscal year which were being formulated during the time of our later survey trips.

We were permitted to attend a regular board meeting to observe the workings of a general session of the County Directors and heads of departments functioning as coordinated by the Records Committee and under the supervision of the Foundation officers as they presented their recommendations for the more complete coordination and unification of the work of various units constituting the Michigan Community Health Project.

This report will not only embody the findings of fact as related to the nature, character, and efficiency of the Foundation's plan of work and the character and competency of its personnel, but will frankly embody all of our personal reactions of approval, on the one hand, and such suggestions as we have been led to make looking toward the possible improvement and extension of the work, on the other hand, which suggestions, if they seem to be in the nature of criticisms, we sincerely trust will be regarded as an attempt on our part to offer constructive criticism.

We have taken time to "season" our observations and to mature our suggestions regarding the Foundation's work; having prepared our field notes soon after the completion of the survey, this matter has been allowed to rest almost six months before the preparation of this final draft of observations and recommendations. We have been thus deliberate in the making of this report because we early discovered in our trips to Battle Creek that we were in contact with a new thing as Foundations go. It was disclosed to us that the Foundation was working in a somewhat new field; as regards many phases of its activities there was little or no precedent to guide its directors in the making of plans and execution of objectives. We are strongly impressed that

2

the Foundation is carrying on a great social experiment, the purposes and importance of which can only be disclosed in later years.

We early learned that while this combined "social experiment" and "university without bricks" was firmly predicated on well-established principles of public health administration, its ramifications extended out into a far-flung field in a direct and indirect attempt at child betterment which included manifold phases of both preventive and curative medicine and dentistry, and went on to include within its embrace the whole domain of sanitary science as well as many aspects of the educational and school systems of these seven counties, and we later discovered that it went on into other avenues of social welfare. In fact it was so comprehensive as to recognize that child welfare includes the whole domain of health, education, and prosperity of the rural community, for we observed that the larger part of the Foundation's activities pertain to work among these rather typical seven rural counties since only one county contains a large city (Battle Creek) and that municipality was exempt from the Foundation's immediate activities, but we would emphasize that we found none of the work of the Foundation in these seven counties, but what was relevant to the health, welfare, and happiness of children.

We were thoroughly impressed with the fact of the unique combination between hard-headed, scientific public health administration and a very high philanthropic but practical idealism. At first we felt that such a complex and unusual combination of motivation would not work out when it came to its actual application in the field, but we are glad to record that our fears were without justification, for we actually saw such a unique program being effectively executed in a very practical manner in the Health Unit and staffs

3

of these seven counties.

We wish to record our believe that the Foundation's officers have been very wise in the type of counties they have selected for this socio-health experiment. These seven counties afford sufficient diversification, on the one hand, and uniformity of rural life problems, on the other, to constitute a very typical proving ground for this far-flung experiment in child welfare. On careful analysis of the population of these counties, we were convinced still more of the wisdom of their choice, since their aggregate population is near 300,000 people, presenting a child welfare problem of ministering to around 50,000 school children, not to mention the pre-school group.

Since the work of the Michigan Community Health Project is limited to these seven counties situated so near Battle Creek where the home office is located, it is apparent that such an arrangement contributes to efficiency and economy of administration, but before we had finished our study of the work we wondered if such proximity of activities did not in some way prevent those who were charged with the responsibilities of administration, from clearly appraising the actual results of these multiform activities. When we are too close to our work it does sometimes interfere with detecting mistakes, on the one hand, and of fully appreciating the results accomplished, on the other.

We found in these seven counties that the work was organized about what appeared to be a standard full-time county health officer. As we studied the work and methods of this county unit plan it appeared to us to be on the whole effectively organized, and we had opportunity to check our opinions as they were being formed, by numerous conferences with experienced health officers, such as Dr. Grant Fleming, of McGill University, and Dr. Wilson

4

Smiley, of Cornell.

We have heard the Foundation's work criticized as consisting of a somewhat faddish and sentimental over-developed county health service, but we did
not find this to be the case on careful examination. We found the seven
health departments being administered, as regards their public health
service, at little or no more cost per capita than that of other standard
public health services throughout the country, and for the educational
expenditures we found in operation a wide-spread health and educational
program which, in our opinion will prove to be of inestimable worth to the
children growing up in these rural communities.

We discovered that the expenditure of the Foundation in these counties
consisted of two distinct phases: First, that which pertains to public
health administration, which we believe to be along accepted and well-
standardized lines, albeit, it is progressive and up-to-date, and second,
expenses embraced in the definitely experimental, new, and somewhat
idealistic attempts to improve community life and enhance child welfare by
extending public health administration to fields additional to and beyond the
ordinary work of preventing communicable diseases and the commonly accepted
activities of sanitary science.

5

Confidential Report

W. C. Smillie to the Director of the Kellogg Foundation

May 10, 1937

COMMUNITY HEALTH CENTERS

The most important and far-reaching innovation in the Foundation's program during the past two years is the conception of the community health center. Although I did not indicate the fact to anyone, I was greatly disappointed when I went over the plans and visited the hospital buildings under construction at Coldwater and Hillsdale. After discussing the whole matter with Dr. Morrison, I found that your ideas coincide almost exactly with mine, but you did not think that the time had come to develop the program in its entirety. It seemed at first that the Foundation had planned little more than a presentation of a nice hospital to each of these communities. The buildings are well planned and well constructed, and meet adequately the purpose for which they are obviously intended. The physicians, and the people of these communities as well are delighted with this handsome gift, and thoroughly appreciative of the generosity of the donor.

But it is a hospital, not a community health center, and furnishes only one major community health service. It is my conception that a hospital -- a place for the care of the very sick -- is an essential community service and an important one, but the hospital should be but a part of the Community Health Center. As constructed, it would appear that the various essential community health center activities are intended to be simply a small and

6

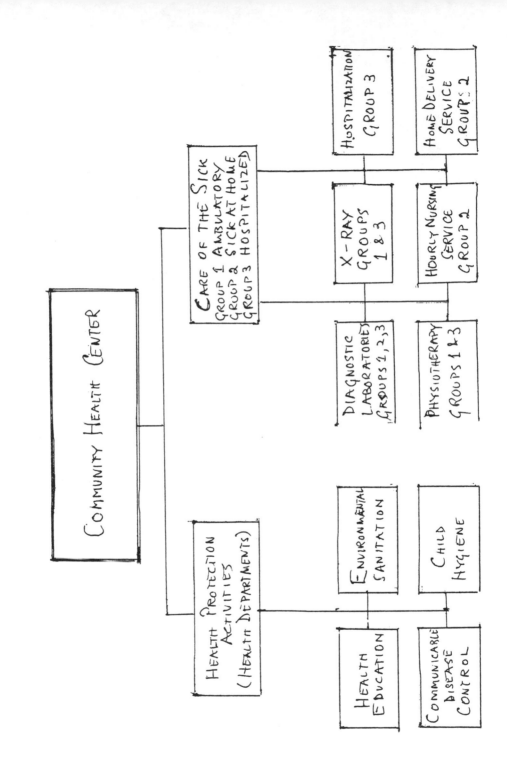

secondary part of the hospitalization program.

We have three major types of sick people:

1. The ambulatory patient.

2. The patient who may be adequately cared for at home.

3. The patient requiring hospitalization.

A county health center must have, as its objective, the prevention of illness in all; and, in case of illness, it must make provision for medical and nursing care of all of the above three groups, and not for group three only. (See diagram).

The two diverse functions of a Community Health Service -- namely, health protection, and care of the sick - should be uld be conducted as a unit enterprise. It seems most reasonable that the personnel should work under the same roof, and in close cooperation. There should be a meeting place in the building for the local medical society, and all matters pertaining to the health promotion of the community should be centered here.

Certain of the above community functions, such as the activities of the health department, are obviously the responsibility of the whole community, and should be paid for from the tax funds. The medical and nursing care of the indigent sick is in this same category. But the great proportion of the services rendered may well be considered as individual personal services for which each individual should pay.

I am frank to say that I sincerely believe that payment for these various services can best be met by a system of voluntary hospital insurance. The Brattleboro plan has also developed a separate insurance scheme for home nursing care and other limited benefits. These are administrative details; suffice it to say that this whole program is doomed to financial stress and

7

possible failure unless some satisfactory plan of limited benefit voluntary

hospital insurance is worked out for the community.

I shall watch the development of this plan with great interest, and

extend to you my best wishes for success and carrying out your significant

activities in this important field.

A Report Upon the Organization and Activities of the

W. K. Kellogg Foundation

To the President and Board of Trustees of the W. K. Kellogg Foundation,

Battle Creek, Michigan

Sirs:

This brief report has been prepared after a month's residence in Battle

Creek, Michigan. During this time I had an opportunity to visit the seven

rural counties in which the Foundation has engaged in work. The Foundation

activities were discussed with the field staff in each county and trips were

made with various members of the staff in order to understand the nature of

the work.

Each of the officers of the central staff in Battle Creek discussed with

me the whole program of the Foundation and presented in detail that part of

the activities for which he was directly responsible.

The plans for the work of the next fiscal year were being formulated

during my stay in Battle Creek. The last week was almost wholly occupied in

general staff conferences concerning the details of proposed work for next

year. This gave me an unusual opportunity to become acquainted with the

8

whole Kellogg Foundation plan of work in the seven counties in southern Michigan.

At the request of the President, [I] am pleased to submit certain observations concerning past activities and future plans of the Foundation. It is quite obvious that these observations must be taken for what they are worth, namely, the personal opinion of a disinterested, but unavoidably biased, individual. I find it impossible to view any piece of work objectively, but always relate whatever I may observe to past experience and formed prejudices.

The Foundation is working in an uncharted field. It has chosen to develop a great social experiment. The experiment is not limited to the field of public health administration, but invades the more intangible social science fields of social welfare, public education and rural economics. An attempt, courageous almost to the point of the impossible, is being made to mold the whole pattern of life of a large rural population.

The primary purpose of the Foundation as set forth in its charter is to provide the means and develop methods whereby the health, welfare, and happiness of children may be promoted. No finer philanthropic ideal could be conceived, nor one fraught with greater difficulties. To achieve these ends, it is necessary to mold the thought, break down the prejudices, change governmental procedures and improve the mode of life of a whole people.

The officers of the Foundation have been intelligent in the selection of the field of work in the limitations they have placed upon themselves. The area selected is relatively small consisting of seven typically rural counties in southern Michigan, adjacent to Battle Creek, where the central administrative offices are located. The population includes approximately

9

200,000 people, with about 40,000 children of school age.

The officers have found a great advantage in having all the Foundation activities close at hand. This is, however, a disadvantage as well. They are so close to the work that they find it difficult to make an appraisal of its effectiveness. Administrative details sometimes assume undue proportions. It is no easy matter to separate the fortuitous from the essentials when one is disturbed by the sound of the wheels of the machinery in motion all around.

Furthermore, the field of work is new. Basically the Foundation's work in the seven counties is organized along the general lines of standard, full-time county health unit procedure. This is advantageous since experience has shown that a well-balanced, full-time personal with a medical health officer in charge is an effective administrative unit. The plan has its distinct disadvantages, however, since most public health authorities consider the Foundation's work as a glorified and expensive county health unit service, when, as a matter of fact, the fundamental purpose of the work reache[s] much deeper into community life than does the standard full-time public health services.

An analysis of any of the county budgets reveals the fact that the number of personnel and money expended does not exceed the standards commonly recommended for adequate rural health services. The supplementary budget, which provides for the new and experimental phases of the work, represents the excess cost, but can be justified on the basis that this part of the work is frankly experimental.

Another difficulty encountered in the work of the Foundation is that since most of the activities are in a new field, it becomes almost impossible

10

550

to develop any criteria as to success or failure of a given project. It will
not be possible to determine for many years to come whether or not the
efforts will have been worth the expenditures in thought and effort. Thus
the officers must develop an unlimited patience, and a thorough immunity to
the withering blasts of rigorous criticism. One should always be alert to
stop a piece of experimental work when it becomes certain that it is not
worthwhile. A given project should not be stopped, however, solely because
of the fact that it is receiving severe criticism.

I am not at all sure that I can be of any real help to the officers of
the Foundation in presenting my opinion of the Foundation's plan of work, but
I am willing to give this opinion for what it is worth. I shall take up in
some detail those different activities that were observed, and shall then
present a brief discussion of the plan as a whole.

Respectfully submitted,

Wilson G. Smillie, M.D.

May 14, 1937

The Kellogg Foundation Plan as a Whole

In the previous paragraphs we have discussed the various elements of the
work of the Foundation. This analysis does not give a true picture of the
Foundation's activities as a structural unit. The policies and aims can be
understood only if seen in their entirety.

The officers are conducting a unique social experiment. The work as it
has gradually developed is a splendid and altruistic conception. The plans
carry out on a large scale the universal human desire to do good to others.
It must be recognized, of course, that the best intentioned and most

11

philanthropic purposes can do more harm than good. We have learned that the real achievement of philanthropy is not the help that is given to others. Rather it should teach and aid the recipients to help themselves.

Thus the primary aid of a great social foundation must be, not direct aid, but development of methods which can be assimilated by the family and the community as a means of self-improvement.

The easiest and most delightful course to follow in philanthropic work is to be "Lady Bountiful" and dispense charity with open hands. The hardest thing to do is to weigh every new activity, measure every new policy by the single yardstick, which may be stated as follows:

Is there a reasonable expectation that this policy can become, in the near future, an integral part of the machinery of normal community life - supported by taxation or voluntary contributions and carried on under the direction of official agencies?

The Foundation has set as its goal the improvement of the methods of society and the promotion of the health, welfare and happiness of children. The experiments have been limited to seven rural counties in southern Michigan, all quite similar in area and type of population. It is clear, of course, that the efforts in money expended would not be justified, if the principles that are developed have but a limited geographic application. A project of this type has greatest value if the newer methods that are developed on a small scale can eventually be adapted to meet community needs in areas far removed from that where the demonstration was made. It is quite wise, during the early stages of development, to limit the experiments to limited areas.

The Foundation's plan is based on the principles of established official

12

rural health service. Each county director is a full-time county health officer appointed on the same basis and responsible for the same official activities as any other full-time county officer in the state. Thus it is quite essential that there should be close cooperation between each of the health units and the state health department. The state is the sovereign power and the state health commissioner is responsible, directly or indirectly, for all the health promotion activities that are carried out in every section of the state. Thus he should be quite familiar with the policies and activities of each local health organization, whether official or voluntary.

The County Board of Supervisors are the responsible governing body in each county. They appoint the county health officer and advise him in matters relating to policy. They are the elected representatives of the people, and in the end, they are the ones that are most directly responsible for the health and welfare of the people of the county. Thus it is quite obvious that the County Board of Supervisors must be thoroughly familiar with the work of the county health unit. They must be familiar also with the special supplementary activities of the Foundation in their respective counties, and the Foundation must work in close harmony with them.

The basic organization of the health units to which the Foundation contributes in each county is similar in principle to that of currently accepted rural public health practice. The classification of personnel, division of responsibility and form of budget are like those adopted throughout the United States. The cost of this work in the southern Michigan area is approximately 77 cents per capita. This is in the upper quartile of current county health unit cost, but is not out of line with accepted

13

standards. But the greater proportion -- 65 cents per capita -- of this expenditure is furnished by the Foundation, with only 12 cents per capita from official agencies. Most of the official funds come from the State Health Department and only small amounts from local official sources.

As a general rule, people appreciate services in direct proportion to their participation. I believe that the local officials, such as Board of County Supervisors should not only assume definite responsibilities in the planning of the program, but should also contribute from county funds toward standard activities at least as large a percent per capita appropriation as the average county of like population and wealth in the state now contributes to existing county health unit services.

This official appropriation should be made to standard items and should be applied toward commonly accepted activities and not to the supplementary budget. It may not be feasible at the present time to secure this local official support, but this goal should be achieved as rapidly as possible.

The items in the supplementary budget represent the expenditures of the Foundation toward the social experiment. As such, they are a legitimate charge against the Foundation. Many of the items are temporary in nature and not continuous. For example, one may be quite certain that the expenditures for medical and dental post graduate training will be terminated within a few years.

Some of the activities that are at present supported by the supplementary budget, may, in time, prove of such continuing worth that they should be incorporated into the standard budget and paid for by local tax funds. Most of the expenditures for the supplementary budget relate to education of professional personnel, -- physicians, dentists and particularly

14

school teachers. It is reasonable to expect that, in the near future, the professional personnel of the whole state of Michigan will receive adequate training. It does not seem probable, therefore, that this part of the Foundation program need be adopted by other communities and supported from local tax funds. Educational standards are essentially a state-wide responsibility. It is not improbable that nation-wide unification of educational standards of professional personnel is a real possibility in the future.

The most novel and interesting part of the Foundation's program to me are:

    1.   The medical participation experiment.

    2.   The winter camp program.

    3.   The utilization of the county public health nurses in a much broader social field, and wider scope of activity than has been attempted elsewhere.

Each of these activities has been developed to meet an obvious community need. I am not at all sure that the plans, as carried out at present, will prove in the end to be the most effective and workable methods of accomplishing their purposes. But each of these activities of the Foundation is exploring a new field and the only manner in which one can find out whether or not a plan will work is to try it out and see.

The Foundation plans must remain flexible. No policy should be considered a permanent one but each project should be considered on its own merits, the results reviewed at proper intervals, and if one method is not satisfactory, then the Foundation is under no obligation to continue it for a longer period. In the end, the Foundation will have served a very useful and

15

important purpose -- the development of the experimental method in promotion
of child health. Each of the activities is carefully worked out to achieve a
definite goal. As in all experimental work, some of the results will be
unsuccessful; others will work out in so satisfactory a manner that they will
not only be of great permanent benefit to the children of the area, but they
will also be of such simple and practical value that they will become a
definite part of community life of the demonstration area. It is quite
probable that some of the methods that are developed may be utilized for far
and wide in all parts of the rural areas of the nation.

16